Current Topics in Zoonoses

Edited by Alfonso J. Rodriguez-Morales

Published in London, United Kingdom

Current Topics in Zoonoses
http://dx.doi.org/10.5772/intechopen.110908
Edited by Alfonso J. Rodriguez-Morales

Contributors
Abdelrahman Abdel Hai Moukhtar, AbdulRahman A. A Saied, Adedotun Ayodeji Bayegun, Adil M. Allahverdiyev, Ahmet Berkay Civan, Albany Reséndiz Mora, Anahi Sotelo-Rodríguez, Andrew W Taylor-Robinson, Anil Sukumaran, Archana Mootha, Asli Pinar Zorba Yildiz, Asmaa A. Metwally, Benjamin Obukowho Emikpe, Benjamín Nogueda, Betsy Joseph, Burcak Yavuz, Carlos Wong-Baeza, Deepali Kalambhe, Emrah Sefik Abamor, Faten F. Mohammed, Gaurav Raj Dwivedi, Giovanna Barrera-Aveleida, Gulnaz Yildirim Koken, Hammed Mogaji, Ikram Ullah, Isabel Baeza, Isabel Wong-Baeza, Iván Galarce-Sosa, Jesús Elías Isidro-Magallán, Juan Carlos Santiago-Hernández, Juan Manuel Serna Velázquez, Kailas Chavan, Ljubo Barbić, Mahaling Bhure, Maja Bogdanić, Malahat Bagirova, Manoj M. Murhekar, Nilam Wavhal, Olaitan O. Omitola, Ozlem Ayse Tosyali, Rajeev Singh, Raphael Deladem Folitse, Rashed Albalawi, Sahar M. Mohammed Jawad, Saidu Kanu, Samira M. Fallatah, Sandeep Chaudhari, Saúl Gómez-Manzo, Serap Yesilkir Baydar, Shahzadi Gulafshan, Shilpshri Shinde, Snježana Židovec-Lepej, Tatjana Vilibić-Čavlek, Uwem Friday Ekpo, Vishnupriya K. Sweety, Vladimir Savić, Vladimir Stevanović, Waqar A. Khan

First published in London, United Kingdom, 2024 by IntechOpen
IntechOpen is the global imprint of INTECHOPEN LIMITED, registered in England and Wales, registration number: 11086078, 167-169 Great Portland Street, London, W1W 5PF, United Kingdom

British Library Cataloguing-in-Publication Data
A catalogue record for this book is available from the British Library

Additional hard and PDF copies can be obtained from orders@intechopen.com

Current Topics in Zoonoses
Edited by Alfonso J. Rodriguez-Morales
p. cm.
Print ISBN 978-1-80356-675-7
Online ISBN 978-1-80356-676-4
eBook (PDF) ISBN 978-1-80356-707-5

For EU product safety concerns:
IN TECH d.o.o., Prolaz Marije Krucifikse Kozulić 3, 51000 Rijeka, Croatia,
info@intechopen.com or visit our website at intechopen.com.

Meet the editor

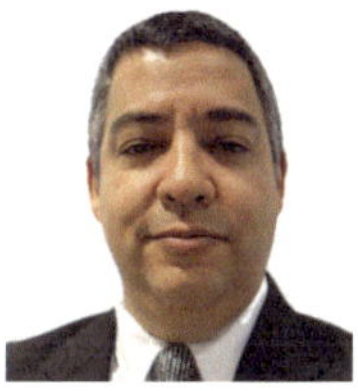

Prof. Alfonso J. Rodríguez-Morales, MD, MSc, DTM&H, DipEd, FRSTM&H(Lon), FFTM RCPS(Glasg), FACE, FISAC, HonDSc, is a senior researcher and faculty at the Faculty of Medicine, Fundación Universitaria Autónoma de las Américas, Pereira, Colombia. He is also a researcher and faculty at the Faculty of Health Sciences, Universidad Científica del Sur, Lima, Peru. In addition, he is a non-resident faculty researcher at the Gilbert and Rose-Marie Chagoury School of Medicine, Lebanese American University, Beirut, Lebanon. Dr. Rodriguez-Morales is an expert in tropical and emerging diseases, particularly in zoonotic and vector-borne diseases, including COVID-19 and mpox, and their occurrence among travellers and migrants. He is the current president of the Latin American Society for Travel Medicine (SLAMVI) and past president of the Colombian Association of Infectious Diseases (ACIN). He is a member of the ACIN's Committee on Tropical Medicine, Zoonoses, and Travel Medicine and its Committee on Adult Vaccines, as well as a member of the council of the International Society for Infectious Diseases (ISID) and a member of the Working Group on Viral Infections (ISAC). Dr. Rodriguez-Morales is a fellow of the International Society for Antimicrobial Chemotherapy (FISAC). He is also editor-in-chief of Travel Medicine and Infectious Diseases. He is a member of the European Society of Clinical Microbiology and Infectious Diseases (ESCMID) and serves on several of the organization's study groups. He was a member of the Technical Working Group of the World Health Organization (WHO) for the Global Research Agenda on Health and Migration and the 3rd Global Consultation on the Health of Migrants and Refugees (co-organized by WHO, UNHCR, and IOM) (2023). He is a current member of the WHO Guideline Development Group (GDG) focused on post covid-19 conditions. Dr. Rodriguez-Morales was recognized as a Highly Cited Researcher by the Web of Sciences-Clarivate in 2022 and 2023.

Contents

Preface

Zoonoses, diseases transmitted from animals to humans, have always been significant in public health. Still, their importance has recently surged, casting a shadow over global health security. The COVID-19 pandemic, caused by the novel coronavirus SARS-CoV-2, is a stark reminder of the devastating potential of zoonotic diseases. Emerging from a likely animal source, possibly bats or pangolins, the SARS-CoV-2 swiftly spread across the globe, triggering unprecedented disruptions to economies, healthcare systems, and daily life. Its rapid transmission highlighted the interconnectedness of human and animal health and the urgency of understanding and mitigating zoonotic threats [1–13]. Beyond COVID-19, numerous other bacterial, fungal, parasitic, and viral zoonotic diseases continue to pose significant challenges. Influenza viruses, including avian and swine flu strains, periodically jump from animals to humans, threatening widespread outbreaks. Ebola virus outbreaks from wildlife reservoirs like bats and primates periodically flare up in African regions, causing considerable morbidity and mortality. Moreover, Zika, West Nile virus, and Lyme disease remind us of the diverse range of pathogens capable of spilling from animals to humans. Deforestation, urbanization, agricultural intensification, and climate change are exacerbating the risk of zoonotic spillover events by altering ecosystems, disrupting wildlife habitats, and bringing humans into closer contact with potentially infectious animals [12–25].

Considering many of these issues, this book presents research and topics related to different zoonotic diseases. The book is organized into four major sections: "Introduction", "Bacterial Zoonoses", "Parasitic Zoonoses", and "Viral Zoonoses".

The commissioning of this book by IntechOpen is partly related to my long commitment to tropical and emerging diseases, especially vector-borne, zoonotic, and neglected tropical diseases. I am a member of the Council of the International Society for Infectious Diseases (ISID), past president of the Colombian Association of Infectious Diseases (Asociación Colombiana de Infectología [ACIN]), as well as member of the Committee on Tropical Medicine, Zoonoses and Travel Medicine of the ACIN. Since 2023, I have been president of the Latin American Society for Travel Medicine (SLAMVI). During 2020 I founded the Latin American Network of Research on COVID-19 (LANCOVID). LANCOVID has contributed to the research on SARS-CoV-2/COVID-19 in Latin America.

Following the same philosophy we used for my eleven previous books with IntechOpen [26–37], this book is not intended to be an exhaustive compilation. Research in zoonoses has become highly dynamic and changing, requiring the most recent available evidence for appropriate diagnostic and, especially, decision-making.

I would like to give a very special thanks to IntechOpen, particularly my Publishing Process Managers Ana Cink and Romina Rovan Bakarčić, Author Service Manager Martina Scerbe, and Commissioning Editor Lucija Tomicic Dromgool, for the opportunity to edit this exciting and important book and for their constant support.

I want to take the appropriate time and space to dedicate this book to my beloved family, which is distributed geographically among Venezuela, Chile, and Colombia (Aurora, Alfonso José, Alejandro, and Andrea, the neurologist). Especially after six marvelous years, I would like to express my feelings of acknowledgment and thanks to Katterine, my beloved wife, who makes every day unique and cares about every aspect of my life. I love her more than anything and am happy to have her lovely existence. I love you more and more every day, from 2018 to eternity.

I would also like to thank my friends and undergraduate and postgraduate students in Colombia, Venezuela, and Latin America. In 2019, I began to work at the Fundacion Universitaria Autonoma de las Americas, Pereira, Risaralda, Colombia, a new "home" that brings me support and trust in my new endeavors in research and teaching. I have to give special thanks in that order to Dr. Maria Monica Murillo, our dean at the Faculty of Medicine, as well as to our former director of the School of Medicine, Dr. Jaime Cardona-Ospina, a long-time friend and fellow, now a Ph.D. student in the United States. I would also like to thank Dr. Percy Mayta-Tristan at Universidad Cientifica del Sur, another prominent supporter and friend of over two decades. I also thank Dr. Samer Saab at the Lebanese American University for welcoming me to this dynamic institution where I may now collaborate as a researcher.

Finally, I hope our readers enjoy this publication as much as I enjoyed putting it together with my talented and knowledgeable collaborators.

**Alfonso J. Rodriguez-Morales MD, MSc, DTM&H, DipEd,
FRSTMH(Lon), FFTM RCPS(Glasg), FACE, FISAC, HonDSc.**
Professor,
Grupo de Investigación Biomedicina,
Faculty of Medicine,
Fundacion Universitaria
Autónoma de las Américas-Institucion Universitaria Vision de las Americas,
Pereira, Risaralda, Colombia

Faculties of Health Sciences and Environmental Sciences,
Universidad Científica del Sur,
Lima, Peru

Gilbert and Rose-Marie Chagoury School of Medicine,
Lebanese American University,
Lebanon

School of Medicine,
Universidad Privada Franz Tamayo,
Cochabamba, Bolivia

References

[1] Bonilla-Aldana DK, Gutierrez-Grajales EJ, Martinez-Arboleda JP, Reina-Mora MA, Trejos-Mendoza AE, Perez-Vargas S, et al. Seroprevalence canine survey for selected vector-borne pathogens and its relationship with poverty in metropolitan Pereira, Colombia, 2020. Parasite Epidemiology and Control. 2022;**17**:e00249

[2] Bonilla-Aldana DK, Rodriguez-Morales AJ. The threat of the spread of SARS-CoV-2 variants in animals. Vet Q. 2021;**41**(1):321-322

[3] Bonilla-Aldana DK, Rodriguez-Morales AJ. Is monkeypox another reemerging viral zoonosis with many animal hosts yet to be defined? Vet Q. 2022;**42**(1):148-150

[4] Bonilla-Aldana DK, Ruiz-Saenz J, Martinez-Gutierrez M, Villamil-Gomez W, Mantilla-Meluk H, Arrieta G, et al. Zero by 2030 and OneHealth: The multidisciplinary challenges of rabies control and elimination. Travel Medicine and Infectious Disease. 2023;**51**:102509

[5] Bonilla-Aldana DK, Trejos-Mendoza AE, Perez-Vargas S, Rivera-Casas E, Munoz-Lara F, Zambrano LI, et al. A systematic review and meta-analysis of bovine brucellosis seroprevalence in Latin America and the Caribbean. New Microbes and New Infections. 2023;**54**:101168

[6] Choudhary P, Shafaati M, Abu Salah MAH, Chopra H, Choudhary OP, Silva-Cajaleon K, et al. Zoonotic diseases in a changing climate scenario: Revisiting the interplay between environmental variables and infectious disease dynamics. Travel Medicine and Infectious Disease. 2024;**58**:102694

[7] Cimerman S, Chebabo A, Cunha CAD, Barbosa AN, Rodriguez-Morales AJ. Human monkeypox preparedness in Latin America - Are we ready for the next viral zoonotic disease outbreak after COVID-19? Brazilian Journal of Infectious Diseases. 2022;**26**(3):102372

[8] Farahat RA, Abdelaal A, Shah J, Ghozy S, Sah R, Bonilla-Aldana DK, et al. Monkeypox outbreaks during COVID-19 pandemic: Are we looking at an independent phenomenon or an overlapping pandemic? Annals of Clinical Microbiology and Antimicrobials. 2022;**21**(1):26

[9] Leon-Figueroa DA, Bonilla-Aldana DK, Pachar M, Romani L, Saldana-Cumpa HM, Anchay-Zuloeta C, et al. The never-ending global emergence of viral zoonoses after COVID-19? The rising concern of monkeypox in Europe, North America and beyond. Travel Medicine and Infectious Disease. 2022;**49**:102362

[10] Montenegro-Idrogo JJ, Bonilla-Aldana DK, Rodriguez-Morales AJ. Risk of human leptospirosis in Colombia: Spatiotemporal analysis and related hydroclimatic factors. Transactions of the Royal Society of Tropical Medicine and Hygiene. 2024

[11] Nishiura H, Ito K, Anzai A, Kobayashi T, Piantham C, Rodriguez-Morales AJ. Relative reproduction number of SARS-CoV-2 Omicron (B.1.1.529) compared with delta variant in South Africa. Journal of Clinical Medicine. 2021;**11**(1)

[12] Ortiz-Martinez Y, Sarmiento J, Bonilla-Aldana DK, Rodriguez-Morales AJ. Monkeypox goes viral:

Measuring the misinformation outbreak on Twitter. Journal of Infection in Developing Countries. 2022;**16**(7):1218-1220

[13] Ortiz-Martinez Y, Zambrano-Sanchez G, Rodriguez-Morales AJ. Monkeypox and HIV/AIDS: When the outbreak faces the epidemic. International Journal of STD & AIDS. 2022;**33**(10):949-950

[14] Poudel S, Ishak A, Perez-Fernandez J, Garcia E, Leon-Figueroa DA, Romani L, et al. Highly mutated SARS-CoV-2 Omicron variant sparks significant concern among global experts - What is known so far? Travel Medicine and Infectious Disease. 2022;**45**:102234

[15] Raut R, Sah R, Dixit K, Rodriguez-Morales AJ, Marco Z, Dhama K, et al. A review of the scientific contributions of Nepal on COVID-19. Current Tropical Medicine Reports. 2021;**8**(4):257-264

[16] Rodriguez-Morales AJ, Barbosa-Quintero ZM, Villamil-Gomez WE. [Is it possible that monkeypox can behave as an opportunistic infection in people living with HIV?]. Revista Chilena de Infectología. 2022;**39**(3):233-237

[17] Rodriguez-Morales AJ, Bonilla-Aldana DK, Risquez A, Paniz-Mondolfi A, Suarez JA. Should we be concerned about Venezuelan hemorrhagic fever? - A reflection on its current situation in Venezuela and potential impact in Latin America amid the migration crisis. New Microbes and New Infections. 2021;**44**:100945

[18] Rodriguez-Morales AJ, Bonilla-Aldana DK, Suarez JA, Franco-Paredes C, Forero-Pena DA, Mattar S, et al. Yellow fever reemergence in Venezuela - Implications for international travelers and Latin American countries during the COVID-19 pandemic. Travel Medicine and Infectious Disease. 2021;**44**:102192

[19] Rodriguez-Morales AJ, Lopardo G, Verbanaz S, Orduna T, Lloveras S, Azenas-Burgoa JM, et al. Latin America: Situation and preparedness facing the multi-country human monkeypox outbreak. Lancet Regional Health – Americas. 2022;**13**:100318

[20] Rodriguez-Morales AJ, Ortiz-Martinez Y, Bonilla-Aldana DK. What has been researched about monkeypox? A bibliometric analysis of an old zoonotic virus causing global concern. New Microbes and New Infections. 2022;**47**:100993

[21] Rosas-Hostos Infantes LR, Paredes Yataco GA, Ortiz-Martinez Y, Mayer T, Terashima A, Franco-Paredes C, et al. The global prevalence of human fascioliasis: A systematic review and meta-analysis. Therapeutic Advances in Infectious Disease. 2023;**10**:20499361231185413

[22] Sah R, Abdelaal A, Reda A, Katamesh BE, Manirambona E, Abdelmonem H, et al. Monkeypox and its possible sexual transmission: Where are we now with its evidence? Pathogens. 2022;**11**(8)

[23] Saydam FN, Erdem H, Ankarali H, El-Arab Ramadan ME, El-Sayed NM, Civljak R, et al. Vector-borne and zoonotic infections and their relationships with regional and socioeconomic statuses: An ID-IRI survey in 24 countries of Europe, Africa and Asia. Travel Medicine and Infectious Disease. 2021;**44**:102174

[24] Silva-Ramos CR, Mejorano-Fonseca JA, Rodriguez-Morales AJ, Hidalgo M, Faccini-Martinez AA. Zoonotic febrile illnesses misdiagnosed

as COVID-19: A review of reported clinical cases. Le Infezioni in Medicina. 2023;**31**(2):151-162

[25] Tazerji SS, Shahabinejad F, Tokasi M, Rad MA, Khan MS, Safdar M, et al. Global data analysis and risk factors associated with morbidity and mortality of COVID-19. Gene Reports. 2022;**26**:101505

[26] Rodriguez-Morales AJ, editor. Current Topics in Tropical Medicine. Croatia: IntechOpen; 2012. ISBN 978-953-51-0274-8. Available from: http://www.intechopen.com/books/current-topics-in-tropical-medicine

[27] Rodriguez-Morales AJ, editor. Current Topics in Public Health. Croatia: IntechOpen; 2013. ISBN 978-953-51-1121-4. Available from: http://www.intechopen.com/books/current-topics-in-public-health

[28] Rodriguez-Morales AJ, editor. Current Topics in Echinococcosis. Croatia: IntechOpen; 2015. ISBN 978-953-51-2159-6. Available from: http://www.intechopen.com/books/current-topics-in-echinococcosis

[29] Rodriguez-Morales AJ, editor. Current Topics in Chikungunya. Croatia: IntechOpen; 2016. ISBN 978-953-51-2595-2. Available from: http://www.intechopen.com/books/current-topics-in-chikungunya

[30] Rodriguez-Morales AJ, editor. Current Topics in Malaria. Croatia: IntechOpen, 2016. ISBN 978-953-51-2790-1. Available from: http://www.intechopen.com/books/current-topics-in-malaria

[31] Rodriguez-Morales AJ, editor. Current Topics in Giardiasis. Croatia: IntechOpen; 2017. ISBN 978-953-51-5260-6. Available from: http://www.intechopen.com/books/current-topics-in-giardiasis

[32] Rodriguez-Morales AJ, editor. Current Topics in Zika. United Kingdom: IntechOpen; 2018. ISBN 978-1-78923-271-4. Available from: https://www.intechopen.com/books/current-topics-in-zika

[33] Rodriguez-Morales AJ, editor. Current Topics in Tropical Emerging Diseases and Travel Medicine. United Kingdom: IntechOpen; 2018. ISBN 978-1-78984-824-3. Available from: https://www.intechopen.com/books/current-topics-in-tropical-emerging-diseases-and-travel-medicine

[34] Rodriguez-Morales AJ, editor. Current Topics in Neglected Tropical Diseases. United Kingdom: IntechOpen; 2019. ISBN 978-1-78923-890-7. Available from: https://www.intechopen.com/books/current-topics-in-neglected-tropical-diseases

[35] Rodriguez-Morales AJ, editor. Current Concepts in Zika Research. United Kingdom: IntechOpen; 2021. ISBN 978-1-83880-876-1. Available from: https://www.intechopen.com/books/current-concepts-in-zika-research

[36] Rodriguez-Morales AJ, editor. Current Topics and Emerging Issues in Malaria Elimination. United Kingdom: IntechOpen; 2021. ISBN 978-1-83968-484-5. Available from: https://www.intechopen.com/books/9528

[37] Rodriguez-Morales AJ, editor. Current Topics in SARS-CoV-2/COVID-19 - Two Years After. United Kingdom: IntechOpen; 2023. ISBN 978-1-80356-234-6. Available from: https://www.intechopen.com/books/11573

Section 1

Introduction

Chapter 1

Introductory Chapter: The Multiple Challenges for the Effective Control of Zoonotic Diseases

Alfonso J. Rodriguez-Morales and D. Katterine-Bonilla-Aldana

1. Introduction

Zoonotic diseases, those that transmit from animals to humans, have been a longstanding threat to public health, manifesting in outbreaks, epidemics, and even pandemics, as recently occurred with the SARS-CoV-2 (severe acute respiratory syndrome coronavirus 2) infection and COVID-19 (Coronavirus disease 2019). Due to their complex nature and myriad challenges, controlling these bacterial, fungal, parasitic, prion, and viral diseases requires a multifaceted approach. From ecological factors to socio-economic dynamics, several interrelated elements contribute to the difficulty in effectively managing zoonotic diseases, requiring multidisciplinary and multisectoral approaches [1–6].

Poverty significantly contributes to the emergence and spread of zoonotic diseases, transmitted between animals and humans. Impoverished communities often live closely with animals, lack access to clean water and healthcare, and engage in risky behaviours like bushmeat hunting. The consequences, such as income loss and limited healthcare, disproportionately affect the poor. To mitigate this, improving living standards and healthcare access and promoting sustainable practices are essential for reducing the prevalence and impact of zoonotic diseases. Understanding and addressing the poverty-zoonoses connection is crucial for safeguarding human and animal health [7–10].

Also, understanding and lessening the impact of zoonotic diseases hinges on environmental factors like habitat destruction, climate change, and biodiversity loss, which are highly relevant in addition to socio-economic factors. Environmental factors greatly influence disease emergence and transmission. For example, deforestation disrupts ecosystems, increasing human-wildlife contact and pathogen spread. Climate change alters disease vector behaviour and range, heightening transmission. Biodiversity loss weakens disease regulation, allowing pathogens to proliferate. Addressing these concerns through conservation, sustainable land management, and climate adaptation is vital for preventing future pandemics and safeguarding public health. Prioritising environmental health fosters a resilient ecosystem-human interface, shielding people and wildlife from infectious disease threats [6, 8, 11, 12].

One of the best examples of recent threats is zoonotic influenza, especially H5N1 [13–16]. Zoonotic H5N1 Influenza, originating in birds, poses a significant public health concern due to its potential to mutate and transmit to humans, causing severe

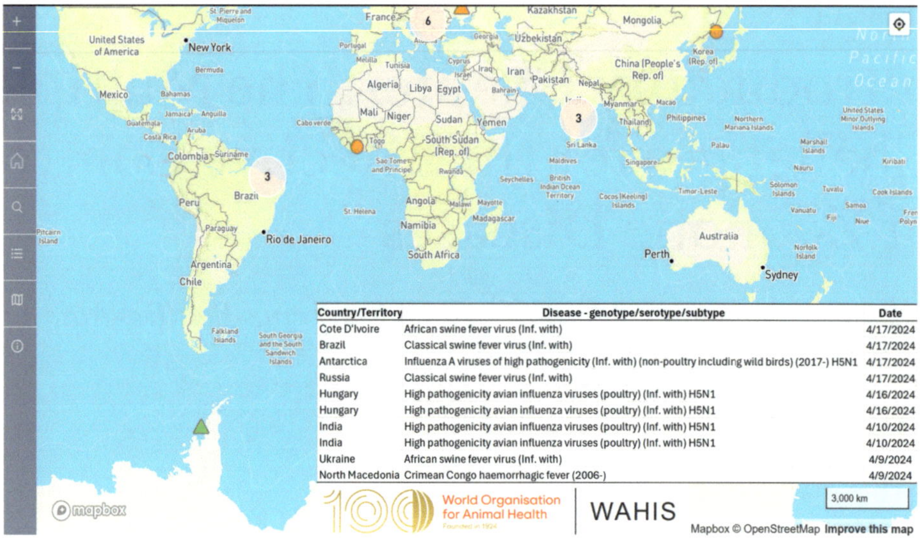

Country/Territory	Disease - genotype/serotype/subtype	Date
Cote D'Ivoire	African swine fever virus (Inf. with)	4/17/2024
Brazil	Classical swine fever virus (Inf. with)	4/17/2024
Antarctica	Influenza A viruses of high pathogenicity (Inf. with) (non-poultry including wild birds) (2017-) H5N1	4/17/2024
Russia	Classical swine fever virus (Inf. with)	4/17/2024
Hungary	High pathogenicity avian influenza viruses (poultry) (Inf. with) H5N1	4/16/2024
Hungary	High pathogenicity avian influenza viruses (poultry) (Inf. with) H5N1	4/16/2024
India	High pathogenicity avian influenza viruses (poultry) (Inf. with) H5N1	4/10/2024
India	High pathogenicity avian influenza viruses (poultry) (Inf. with) H5N1	4/10/2024
Ukraine	African swine fever virus (Inf. with)	4/9/2024
North Macedonia	Crimean Congo haemorrhagic fever (2006-)	4/9/2024

Figure 1.
WAHIS: World animal health information system—Latest animal disease events, April 2024. (https://wahis.woah.org/#/home).

illness and even death. Its ability to cross species barriers heightens the risk of a global pandemic, necessitating vigilance in surveillance, early detection, and rapid response measures. Understanding and monitoring zoonotic H5N1 are crucial to prevent outbreaks, safeguard human health, and mitigate the socio-economic impacts of such a pandemic [17]. Multiple events related to H5N1 Influenza in animals occur in different countries (**Figure 1**).

2. Bacterial zoonoses

Bacterial zoonotic diseases are crucial in public health, agriculture, and ecosystem management (e.g., brucellosis). These diseases, transmitted between animals and humans, pose significant challenges due to their potential for rapid spread and diverse impacts. Understanding and addressing them are essential for several reasons. Bacterial zoonotic diseases can have severe health implications (e.g., leptospirosis). They account for a considerable burden of illness globally, causing symptoms ranging from mild discomfort to life-threatening conditions. Diseases like anthrax, brucellosis, and salmonellosis highlight the diverse range of bacterial pathogens capable of crossing species barriers [3, 18, 19].

These diseases have economic repercussions. Outbreaks can lead to significant losses in agriculture and livestock industries through decreased productivity, trade restrictions, and the costs associated with disease control measures (e.g., bovine tuberculosis). Moreover, human illnesses result in substantial healthcare expenditures and productivity losses [20, 21].

Furthermore, bacterial zoonoses often have complex transmission dynamics influenced by environmental changes, human behaviour, and animal reservoirs. Addressing them requires interdisciplinary approaches integrating veterinary, medical, environmental, and social sciences. Additionally, the interconnected nature of ecosystems and globalisation facilitates the spread of bacterial zoonotic diseases across geographical boundaries. Therefore, effective surveillance, early detection, and rapid response are essential to prevent outbreaks and mitigate their impacts. Then, addressing bacterial zoonotic diseases is critical for safeguarding public health, ensuring food security, and promoting sustainable development in an increasingly interconnected world [3, 22–24].

3. Parasitic zoonoses

Parasitic zoonotic diseases play a crucial role in global health due to their complex transmission dynamics and significant impact on both human and animal populations. These diseases, caused by parasites that can be transmitted between animals and humans, pose serious public health challenges worldwide. The importance of parasitic zoonotic diseases lies in several key aspects. They can lead to substantial morbidity and mortality in humans. Malaria, caused by the *Plasmodium* parasite, and toxoplasmosis, caused by *Toxoplasma gondii*, are prime examples. Malaria is globally distributed, and many aetiological species are now well-known zoonotic [11, 25–27].

Parasitic zoonoses often have economic implications, affecting livestock production, agricultural output, and trade. For example, trichinellosis, caused by the roundworm*Trichinella spiralis*, is a complex disease when humans consume raw or undercooked meat, particularly pork, containing the parasite's larvae. Livestock, such as pigs, can serve as reservoir hosts for *Trichinella*. Trichinellosis can lead to gastrointestinal symptoms initially, followed by more severe manifestations as the larvae migrate and invade various tissues [28, 29]. Even parasites that may not develop into adult forms in humans may cause significant disease, as is the case of toxocariasis, caused by *Toxocara canis* and *Toxocara cati* [30, 31].

Moreover, these diseases highlight the interconnectedness of human, animal, and environmental health. Understanding the ecological factors driving their transmission is crucial for effective prevention and control strategies. Additionally, parasitic zoonoses underscore the importance of One Health approaches, emphasising collaboration between human and veterinary medicine, environmental science, and other disciplines to address health challenges at the human-animal-environment interface [32–35].

4. Viral zoonoses

Viral zoonoses account for a considerable proportion of emerging infectious diseases, such as Ebola, Zika, Mpox, and COVID-19. Their ability to cross species barriers means they can emerge unexpectedly and have devastating consequences. These diseases often highlight the interconnectedness of human, animal, and environmental health, emphasising the importance of a holistic, One Health approach to disease surveillance, prevention, and control [36–40].

Most viral zoonotic diseases can have profound socio-economic impacts, disrupting healthcare systems, causing loss of life, and imposing significant financial burdens on individuals, communities, and governments, as observed during the Zika epidemics in Latin America during 2015–2016 [41–44].

Studying these diseases offers insights into viral evolution, transmission dynamics, and host-pathogen interactions, informing prevention, detection, and response strategies. Recognising the importance of viral zoonotic diseases underscores the need for interdisciplinary collaboration, global cooperation, and proactive measures to mitigate their impact on public health and society.

5. Conclusions

The One Health approach is crucial for managing zoonotic diseases, illnesses transmitted between animals and humans. By recognising the interconnectedness of human, animal, and environmental health, One Health fosters collaboration among various disciplines like medicine, veterinary science, ecology, and public health. This holistic strategy enables early detection, rapid response, and effective control of zoonotic diseases from diverse aetiologies [45, 46].

Implementing One Health principles allows for better surveillance and understanding of disease dynamics at the human-animal-environment interface. It facilitates the identification of emerging pathogens, risk factors, and transmission pathways, leading to proactive measures to prevent outbreaks. Additionally, One Health promotes interdisciplinary research, enabling the development of innovative interventions, such as vaccines, antimicrobial stewardship, and ecosystem management strategies [47, 48].

The One Health approach is essential for safeguarding public health, animal welfare, and environmental sustainability. Addressing health challenges comprehensively enhances resilience to zoonotic diseases, mitigates risks of pandemics, and promotes the well-being of both humans and animals [49, 50].

Author details

Alfonso J. Rodriguez-Morales[1,2,3,4*] and D. Katterine-Bonilla-Aldana[5]

1 Grupo de Investigación Biomedicina, Faculty of Medicine, Fundacion Universitaria Autónoma de las Américas-Institucion Universitaria Vision de las Americas, Pereira, Risaralda, Colombia

2 Faculties of Health Sciences and Environmental Sciences, Universidad Científica del Sur, Lima, Peru

3 Gilbert and Rose-Marie Chagoury School of Medicine, Lebanese American University, Lebanon

4 School of Medicine, Universidad Privada Franz Tamayo, Cochabamba, Bolivia

5 Research Unit, Universidad Continental, Huancayo, Peru

*Address all correspondence to: ajrodriguezmmd@gmail.com

References

[1] Tambo E, El Dessouky AG, Khater EIM. Innovative preventive and resilience approaches against aedes-linked vector-borne arboviral diseases threat and epidemics burden in gulf council countries. Oman Medical Journal. 2019;**34**(5):391-396

[2] Bahrami R, Hashemi D, Aziziraftar SK, Rahimi P. Coronaviruses as the emerging threats for human health: Should we be prepared for the future outbreaks of new coronaviruses? Bratislavské Lekárske Listy. 2020;**121**(10):733-741

[3] Montenegro-Idrogo JJ, Bonilla-Aldana DK, Rodriguez-Morales AJ. Risk of human leptospirosis in Colombia: Spatiotemporal analysis and related hydroclimatic factors. Transactions of the Royal Society of Tropical Medicine and Hygiene. 2024. DOI: 10.1093/trstmh/trae013 [In press]

[4] Bonilla-Aldana DK, Ruiz-Saenz J, Martinez-Gutierrez M, Villamil-Gomez W, Mantilla-Meluk H, Arrieta G, et al. Zero by 2030 and OneHealth: The multidisciplinary challenges of rabies control and elimination. Travel Medicine and Infectious Disease. 2023;**51**:102509

[5] Choudhary P, Shafaati M, Abu Salah MAH, Chopra H, Choudhary OP, Silva-Cajaleon K, et al. Zoonotic diseases in a changing climate scenario: Revisiting the interplay between environmental variables and infectious disease dynamics. Travel Medicine and Infectious Disease. 2024;**58**:102694

[6] Leon-Figueroa DA, Bonilla-Aldana DK, Pachar M, Romani L, Saldana-Cumpa HM, Anchay-Zuloeta C, et al. The never-ending global emergence of viral zoonoses after COVID-19? The rising concern of monkeypox in Europe, North America and beyond. Travel Medicine and Infectious Disease. 2022;**49**:102362

[7] Dell BM, Souza MJ, Willcox AS. Attitudes, practices, and zoonoses awareness of community members involved in the bushmeat trade near Murchison falls National Park, Northern Uganda. PLoS One. 2020;**15**(9):e0239599

[8] Friant S, Paige SB, Goldberg TL. Drivers of bushmeat hunting and perceptions of zoonoses in Nigerian hunting communities. PLoS Neglected Tropical Diseases. 2015;**9**(5):e0003792

[9] Bonilla-Aldana DK, Gutiérrez-Grajales EJ, Martínez-Arboleda JP, Reina-Mora MA, Trejos-Mendoza AE, Pérez-Vargas S, et al. Seroprevalence canine survey for selected vector-borne pathogens and its relationship with poverty in metropolitan Pereira, Colombia, 2020. Parasite Epidemiology and Control. 2022;**17**:e00249

[10] Torres-Torres J, Martinez-Portilla RJ, Espino YSS, Estrada-Gutierrez G, Solis-Paredes JM, Villafan-Bernal JR, et al. Comorbidity, poverty and social vulnerability as risk factors for mortality in pregnant women with confirmed SARS-CoV-2 infection: Analysis of 13 062 positive pregnancies including 176 maternal deaths in Mexico. Ultrasound in Obstetrics & Gynecology. 2022;**59**(1):76-82

[11] Saydam FN, Erdem H, Ankarali H, El-Arab Ramadan ME, El-Sayed NM, Civljak R, et al. Vector-borne and zoonotic infections and their relationships with regional and socioeconomic statuses: An ID-IRI

survey in 24 countries of Europe, Africa and Asia. Travel Medicine and Infectious Disease. 2021;**44**:102174

[12] Bonilla-Aldana DK, Rodriguez-Morales AJ. Is monkeypox another reemerging viral zoonosis with many animal hosts yet to be defined? The Veterinary Quarterly. 2022;**42**(1):148-150

[13] Bonilla-Aldana DK, Aguirre-Florez M, Villamizar-Pena R, Gutierrez-Ocampo E, Henao-Martinez JF, Cvetkovic-Vega A, et al. After SARS-CoV-2, will H5N6 and other influenza viruses follow the pandemic path? Le Infezioni in Medicina. 2020;**28**(4):475-485

[14] Priyanka KR, Chopra H, Choudhary OP, Bonilla-Aldana DK, Rodriguez-Morales AJ. The re-emergence of H3N2 influenza: An update on the risk and containment. New Microbes New Infections. 2023;**53**:101147

[15] Ahmad F, Haque S, Tawil S, Husni R, Bonilla-Aldana DK, Montenegro-Idrogo JJ, et al. Avian influenza spillover to humans: Are we prepared to deal with another potential pandemic? Travel Medicine and Infectious Disease. 2023;**55**:102634

[16] Rodriguez-Morales AJ, Bonilla-Aldana DK, Paniz-Mondolfi AE. Concerns about influenza H5N8 outbreaks in humans and birds: Facing the next airborne pandemic? Travel Medicine and Infectious Disease. 2021;**41**:102054

[17] Chaudhary RK, Ananthesh L, Patil P, Mateti UV, Sah S, Mohanty A, et al. System biology approach to identify the hub genes and pathways associated with human H5N1 infection. Vaccines (Basel). 2023;**11**(7):1269

[18] Bonilla-Aldana DK, Rivera-Casas E, Moreno-Ramos E, Barboza JJ, Salas-Matta LA, Rodriguez-Morales AJ. Mapping bovine brucellosis in Colombia with geographical information systems, 2009-2019 - implications for OneHealth. New Microbes New Infections. 2024;**56**:101197

[19] Bonilla-Aldana DK, Trejos-Mendoza AE, Perez-Vargas S, Rivera-Casas E, Munoz-Lara F, Zambrano LI, et al. A systematic review and meta-analysis of bovine brucellosis seroprevalence in Latin America and the Caribbean. New Microbes New Infections. 2023;**54**:101168

[20] Rodriguez-Morales AJ, Castañeda-Hernández DM. Bacteria: Mycobacterium bovis. In: Reference Module in Food Science. Boston: Elsevier; 2019

[21] Bonilla-Aldana DK, Jiménez-Diaz SD, Lozada-Riascos C, Silva-Cajaleon K, Rodríguez-Morales AJ. Mapping bovine tuberculosis in Colombia, 2001-2019. Veterinary Sciences. 2024;**11**(5):220. DOI: 10.3390/vetsci11050220

[22] Cardenas R, Sandoval CM, Rodriguez-Morales AJ, Franco-Paredes C. Impact of climate variability in the occurrence of leishmaniasis in northeastern Colombia. The American Journal of Tropical Medicine and Hygiene. 2006;**75**(2):273-277

[23] Cardenas R, Sandoval CM, Rodriguez-Morales AJ, Vivas P. Zoonoses and climate variability. Annals of the New York Academy of Sciences. 2008;**1149**:326-330

[24] Herrera-Martinez AD, Rodriguez-Morales AJ. Potential influence of climate variability on dengue incidence registered in a western pediatric hospital of Venezuela. Tropical Biomedicine. 2010;**27**(2):280-286

[25] Rodriguez-Morales AJ, Paniz-Mondolfi AE, Faccini-Martínez ÁA, Henao-Martínez AF, Ruiz-Saenz J, Martinez-Gutierrez M, et al. The constant threat of zoonotic and vector-borne emerging tropical diseases: Living on the edge. Frontiers in Tropical Diseases. 2021;**2**:676905

[26] Taha AM, Nguyen D, Montenegro-Idrogo JJ, Rodriguez-Morales AJ. Malaria vaccine development in Mali: A step towards transmission-blocking strategies. The Lancet Infectious Diseases. 2024;**24**(4):e207-e2e8

[27] Rodriguez-Morales AJ. Malaria: An eradicable threat? The Journal of Infection in Developing Countries. 2008;**2**(01):001-002

[28] Echeverry DM, Henríquez A, Oyarzún-Ruiz P, Silva-de la Fuente MC, Ortega R, Sandoval D, et al. First record of Trichinella in *Leopardus guigna* (Carnivora, Felidae) and *Galictis cuja* (Carnivora, Mustelidae): New hosts in Chile. PeerJ. 2021;**9**:e11601

[29] Gajadhar A, Konecsni K, Scandrett B, Buholzer P. Validation of a new commercial serine protease artificial digestion assay for the detection of *Trichinella larvae* in pork. Food and Waterborne Parasitology. 2018;**10**:6-13

[30] Bonilla-Aldana JL, Espinosa-Nuñez AC, Bonilla-Aldana DK, Rodriguez-Morales AJ. *Toxocara cati* infection in cats (*Felis catus*): A systematic review and meta-analysis. Animals (Basel). 2024;**14**(7):1022

[31] Bonilla-Aldana DK, Morales-Garcia LV, Ulloque Badaracco JR, Mosquera-Rojas MD, Alarcón-Braga EA, Hernandez-Bustamante EA, et al. Prevalence of Toxocara eggs in Latin American parks: A systematic review and meta-analysis. Le Infezioni in Medicina. 2023;**31**(3):329-349

[32] Rodriguez-Morales AJ, Patino-Cadavid LJ, Lozada-Riascos CO, Villamil-Gomez WE. Mapping Zika in municipalities of one coastal department of Colombia (Sucre) using geographic information systems during the 2015-2016 outbreak: Implications for public health and travel advice. International Journal of Infectious Diseases. 2016;**48**:70-72

[33] Bonilla-Aldana DK, Holguin-Rivera Y, Perez-Vargas S, Trejos-Mendoza AE, Balbin-Ramon GJ, Dhama K, et al. Importance of the One Health approach to study the SARS-CoV-2 in Latin America. One Health. 2020;**10**:100147

[34] Rodriguez-Morales AJ, Schlagenhauf P. Zoonoses and travel medicine: "one world--one health". Travel Medicine and Infectious Disease. 2014;**12**(6 Pt A):555-556

[35] Cabrera M, Leake J, Naranjo-Torres J, Valero N, Cabrera JC, Rodriguez-Morales AJ. Dengue prediction in Latin America using machine learning and the One Health perspective: A literature review. Tropical Medicine and Infectious Disease. 2022;**7**(10):322

[36] Cimerman S, Chebabo A, Cunha CAD, Barbosa AN, Rodriguez-Morales AJ. Human monkeypox preparedness in Latin America - are we ready for the next viral zoonotic disease outbreak after COVID-19? The Brazilian Journal of Infectious Diseases. 2022;**26**(3):102372

[37] Silva-Ramos CR, Mejorano-Fonseca JA, Rodriguez-Morales AJ, Hidalgo M, Faccini-Martinez AA. Zoonotic febrile illnesses misdiagnosed

as COVID-19: A review of reported clinical cases. Le Infezioni in Medicina. 2023;**31**(2):151-162

[38] Eser-Karlidag G, Chacon-Cruz E, Cag Y, Martinez-Orozco JA, Gudino-Solorio H, Cruz-Flores RA, et al. Features of Mpox infection: The analysis of the data submitted to the ID-IRI network. New Microbes New Infections. 2023;**53**:101154

[39] Swed S, Bohsas H, Patwary MM, Alibrahim H, Rakab A, Nashwan AJ, et al. Knowledge of mpox and its determinants among the healthcare personnel in Arabic regions: A multi-country cross-sectional study. New Microbes New Infections. 2023;**54**:101146

[40] Al-Kassab-Cordova A, Ulloque-Badaracco JR, Benites-Zapata VA, Sah R, Rodriguez-Morales AJ. Facing Mpox (former Monkeypox) in Latin America: The example of Peru and its vulnerable healthcare system. Vaccines (Basel). 2022;**11**(1):10

[41] Rodriguez-Morales AJ. Zika: The new arbovirus threat for Latin America. Journal of Infection in Developing Countries. 2015;**9**(6):684-685

[42] Patino-Barbosa AM, Medina I, Gil-Restrepo AF, Rodriguez-Morales AJ. Zika: Another sexually transmitted infection? Sexually Transmitted Infections. 2015;**91**(5):359

[43] Martinez-Pulgarin DF, Acevedo-Mendoza WF, Cardona-Ospina JA, Rodriguez-Morales AJ, Paniz-Mondolfi AE. A bibliometric analysis of global Zika research. Travel Medicine and Infectious Disease. 2016;**14**(1):55-57

[44] Sabogal-Roman JA, Murillo-Garcia DR, Yepes-Echeverri MC, Restrepo-Mejia JD, Granados-Alvarez S, Paniz-Mondolfi AE, et al. Healthcare students and workers' knowledge about transmission, epidemiology and symptoms of Zika fever in four cities of Colombia. Travel Medicine and Infectious Disease. 2016;**14**(1):52-54

[45] Sánchez CA, Venkatachalam-Vaz J, Drake JM. Spillover of zoonotic pathogens: A review of reviews. Zoonoses and Public Health. 2021;**68**(6):563-577

[46] Ellwanger JH, Byrne LB, Chies JAB. Examining the paradox of urban disease ecology by linking the perspectives of urban One Health and ecology with cities. Urban Ecosystem. 2022;**25**(6):1735-1744

[47] Mader R, Damborg P, Amat JP, Bengtsson B, Bourély C, Broens EM, et al. Building the European antimicrobial resistance surveillance network in veterinary medicine (EARS-Vet). Euro Surveillance. 2021;**26**(4):2001359

[48] Sleeman JM, DeLiberto T, Nguyen N. Optimization of human, animal, and environmental health by using the One Health approach. Journal of Veterinary Science. 2017;**18**(S1):263-268

[49] Diller ER, Williamson L. Supporting One Health for pandemic prevention: The need for ethical innovation. Journal of Bioethical Inquiry. 2023;**20**(3):345-352

[50] Aggarwal D, Ramachandran A. One Health approach to address zoonotic diseases. Indian Journal of Community Medicine. 2020;**45**(Suppl. 1):S6-s8

Section 2

Bacterial Zoonoses

Chapter 2

The Socio-Economic Impact of Brucellosis Outbreaks among Large and Small Ruminant under Extensive Nomadic Management System in Sierra Leone

Saidu Kanu

Abstract

Livestock, particularly ruminants, are vital for resource-poor rural farmers in Sierra Leone, serving as a primary source of income and fulfilling socio-cultural roles. In addition to being a valuable protein source, livestock offer an opportunity to escape poverty. However, the transhumance nomadic extensive system, reliant on natural resources, poses challenges for ruminant production, including disease outbreaks like Brucellosis. A sero-prevalence study in Falaba and Koinadugu districts found a 33.3% infection rate, primarily affecting female small ruminants (90% of cases out of 135). Among the 150 confirmed cases, 66% were pregnant, and 25% experienced abortion. Implementing integrated prevention and control measures through the One Health strategy is crucial to combat the disease effectively. At present, the One Health approach is being used for the control of Brucellosis and hopefully, all stakeholders will appreciate the new dispensation in the control and prevention of many animal diseases in the country.

Keywords: brucellosis, sero-prevalence, nomadic, transhumance, one health

1. Introduction

Sierra Leone is a small country located along the west coast of Africa, with an estimated population of approximately 8,908,040 and an annual growth rate of 2.41% [1]. Agriculture is the mainstay of the economy, contributing between 45 and 50% of the Gross Domestic Product (GDP). However, livestock only contribute minimally to the GDP, estimated at 3.15%, compared to crops which contribute about 35.2%. This discrepancy is due to the fact that most agricultural development initiatives have been focused on the crop sector [2].

Livestock populations in Sierra Leone are estimated at 546,881 for cattle, 812,906 for goats, 427,667 for sheep, 1,956,650 for chickens, and 217,497 for pigs [3]. The herd size for small ruminants (goats and sheep) varies between 10 and 20 heads, tethered under a semi-free range system. However, the numbers can significantly increase from 50 to 100 when reared together with cattle. Livestock production, particularly large ruminants (cattle), is dominated by transhumance nomadic pastoralists from neighboring Guinea and other countries in the sub-region. Transhumance refers to the use of grassland grazing for livestock production [4]. These migrant pastoralists do not hold land title rights and depend on local landowners to lease them a place to rear their livestock. The traditional communal land ownership often creates social tension between nomadic livestock farmers and crop farmers, as strayed livestock can destroy crops and endanger the livelihoods of crop farmers.

Sierra Leone's animal health delivery services face challenges due to poor diagnostic infrastructure, inadequately trained personnel, and inadequate logistics for rapid response to animal disease outbreaks (**Figure 1**). The country is a hotspot for the outbreaks of several transboundary zoonotic diseases. In 2018, an outbreak of Foot-and-Mouth Disease (FMD) was reported in Kambia and Port Loko districts. In 2020, a Brucellosis outbreak was reported in Falaba and Koinadugu districts, and in 2022, Anthrax outbreaks were reported in Port Loko and Kambia districts, followed by Bombali district in 2023. Endemic diseases in the country include Peste des petit ruminants (PPR), Newcastle disease (NCD), Fowl pox, and contagious pustular dermatitis.

Livestock production in Sierra Leone is a key source of livelihood, especially for resource-poor rural farmers, and contributes 8.2% to the Agricultural Gross Domestic Product [2]. Livestock production is well integrated into the socio-cultural practices of many traditional societies in the country. Besides providing a readily available source of animal proteins, livestock play a critical role in the fulfillment of many socio-cultural traditions. For example, sheep are often slaughtered during the feast

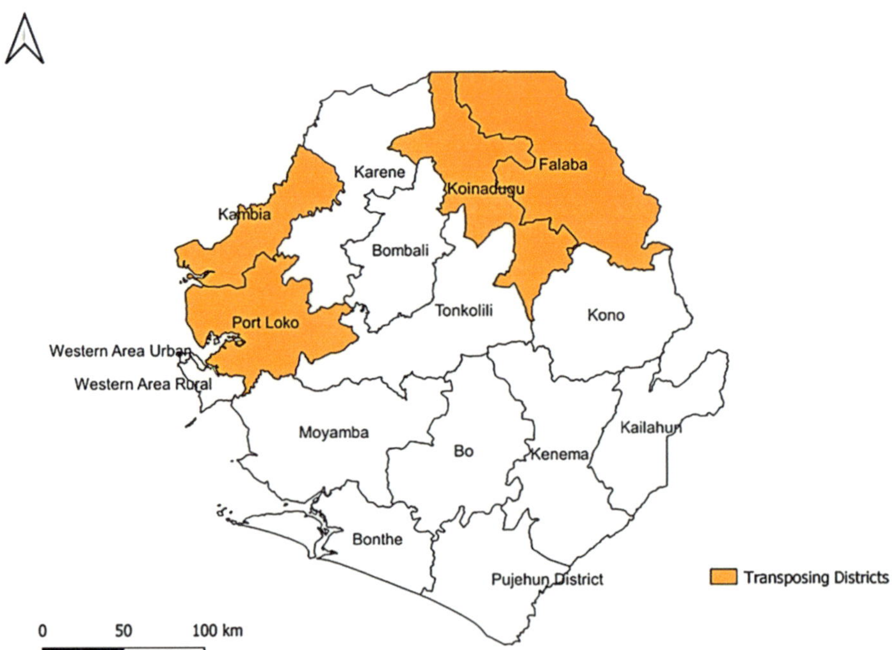

Figure 1.
Map of Sierra Leone indicating four districts affected by animal diseases outbreaks. Source: Livestock and veterinary services division, epidemiological unit, Ministry of Agriculture and food security.

of Edul Ada to fulfill an important Muslim religious rite. Livestock such as cattle, goats, or sheep are also offered as part of matrimonial bride packages. Livestock are required for other social functions, including initiations and the practices of secret societies such as Wunde, Poro, and Bondo. Livestock also contribute significantly to poverty reduction among resource-poor rural farming communities. Small ruminants (goats and sheep), local poultry, and large ruminants (cattle) can be easily traded and converted into cash, which can be used to finance developmental initiatives such as school fees and medical bills. Traditionally, the number of herds owned by farmers determines their societal hierarchy and influence in making important decisions for their communities.

In rural Sierra Leone, livestock production is predominantly under traditional management systems and is characterized by transhumance and nomadic practices. These nomadic pastoralists are mainly migrants from neighboring Guinea and other countries in the sub-region, such as Mali and Burkina Faso. The transhumance production system involves nomads or pastoralists crossing the border from neighboring countries during specific times, usually during the dry season, in search of pastures and to market their livestock at the International Livestock Trading Center in Gbindi, Koinadugu district. This migration pattern faces several challenges, including conflicts with crop farmers and other indigenous livestock farmers, leading to heightened conflicts between livestock grazers and crop farmers. There is also a risk of introducing transboundary zoonotic diseases. Nomadic pastoralists are constantly seeking production resources, such as land, water, and pastures, which are also of interest to crop farmers. This conflict of interest is now a major source of tension between the major agricultural players in the country. The escalation of grazers-farmer conflicts is a subject of concern as it may have a direct effect on food and nutrition security, threatening the national security of the country.

2. Status of animal health delivery services and brucellosis in Sierra Leone

2.1 Animal health delivery services and status of brucellosis

Sierra Leone is a hotspot for many transboundary zoonotic diseases (**Table 1**). As recently as 2014, an Ebola outbreak was reported in the sub-region of West Africa, including Guinea, Liberia, and Sierra Leone. In 2018, there was an outbreak of FMD in the northwestern part of the country, and in 2020, Brucellosis was reported in Koinadugu and Falaba districts, while Anthrax was reported again in 2021 in Port Loko and Kambia districts. The West African region is highly active in the circulation of various transboundary and priority zoonotic diseases (PZDs) such as PPR, NCD, FMD, viral hemorrhagic fevers (VHFs) like Lassa fever, Ebola, and Marburg, as well as rabies [2].

The animal health delivery services, under the Livestock and Veterinary Services Division of the Ministry of Agriculture and Food Security, are severely limited in terms of diagnostic facilities and trained and qualified human resources. In rural areas, animal health services are provided by the staff of the Ministry of Agriculture and Food Security. However, due to a lack of trained and qualified personnel, trained Community Animal Health Workers (CAHWs) are also complementing the efforts of the Ministry. In extreme and desperate situations in remote and inaccessible rural areas, traditional livestock farmers reportedly resort to self-administration of animal health services.

No	Disease	Category
1	PPR	TAD
2	Rinderpest	TAD
3	Foot-and-mouth disease	TAD
4	African swine fever	TAD
5	Trypanosomiasis	TAD
6	Hemorrhagic septicemia	TAD
7	Contagious bovine pleuro-pneumonia	TAD
8	Black quarter	TAD
9	Bovine tuberculosis	Zoonosis
10	Brucellosis	Zoonosis
11	Anthrax	Zoonosis
12	Rabies	Zoonosis
13	Highly pathogenic avian influenza	Zoonosis
14	Viral hemorrhagic fevers (Ebola, Marburg, Lassa fever, Rift Valley fever, Crimean Congo fever)	Zoonosis
15	Salmonellosis	Zoonosis
16	Plague	Zoonosis

Source: Livestock and Veterinary Services Division of the Ministry of Agriculture and Food Security Of Sierra Leone. TAD = Transboundary Animal Diseases.

Table 1.
List of priority transboundary and zoonotic diseases in Sierra Leone.

2.2 Status of brucellosis under nomadic and transhumance production systems in Sierra Leone

Brucellosis is one of the neglected reportable zoonotic diseases of public health concern, causing significant economic losses in traditional livestock production systems in Africa. The disease primarily affects livestock, including cattle, goats, sheep, and pigs, but it can also infect other animals and wildlife. The etiology of Brucellosis is a gram-negative, non-motile, non-sporing, rod-shaped, facultative, and aerobic intracellular cocobacilli. Infection with Brucellosis leads to serious economic losses due to abortion, reproductive failure, sterility, and reduced milk production in affected animals [5]. The etiology is shed in large numbers in the animal's urine, milk, placental fluid, and other fluids.

Brucellosis in animals can result in various reproductive problems, such as abortion, stillbirths, reduced fertility, and decreased milk production. These effects cause significant economic losses for livestock farmers and negatively impact the overall productivity of animal agriculture. Moreover, infected animals serve as reservoirs for the bacteria, perpetuating the disease within herds and posing a risk of transmission to humans.

In Sierra Leone, the nomadic production system takes the form of communal grazing, where healthy, sick, and susceptible animals converge, increasing the risk of infection for healthy ones. Infected animals or aborted fetuses and fluids can contaminate the pasture, and healthy animals that feed on such pastures can easily become infected. Furthermore, communal grazing also provides opportunities for communal mating. If a bull mates with an infected cow with Brucellosis, it can infect susceptible healthy cows or heifers during their next mating. As a result, Brucellosis has become endemic in most communal grazing herds, and the disease continues to persist, especially in areas with poor animal health delivery services and surveillance systems, along with unchecked cross-border livestock trade.

Brucellosis is a prioritized zoonotic disease in Sierra Leone. Its first detection in the country dates back to 1966 [6, 7], but official reports of outbreaks were not made until 2020, when cases were identified in the Koinadugu and Falaba districts. During the 2020 outbreaks, the estimated prevalence of Brucellosis among goats and sheep in these districts was 38.3% for goats and 33.3% for sheep. The laboratory-confirmed cases of Brucellosis between 2019 and 2020 were estimated at 36.8%. It is important to note that these figures do not indicate the absence of the disease in susceptible herds but rather highlight the lack of an animal disease surveillance system, limited diagnostic facilities, and insufficient staff to effectively diagnose and respond to animal diseases.

To enhance disease reporting, the FAO's Emergency Center for Transboundary Animal Diseases (ECTAD) Project, with support from United States Agency for International Development (USAID) under the Global Health Security Agenda (GHSA), established the Integrated Animal Health Disease Surveillance and Reporting System (IADSR) and facilitated the creation of the Epidemiology Unit at the Livestock and Veterinary Services Division (LVSD).

A comprehensive report on the sero-prevalence of Brucellosis among cattle at the Njala and Newton production facilities concluded that the disease is enzootic in semi-intensive production systems, with a prevalence rate of 75% [8]. In the same year, a suspected outbreak of Brucellosis was investigated in the Koinadugu and Falaba districts, which are located in the northern part of the country bordering Guinea. The results revealed a high sero-prevalence (90%) among females (n = 135) aged 1–2 years, with a prevalence of 10% (n = 15) among heifers. Out of the 150 confirmed cases, 66% were pregnant, and 25% resulted in abortions [7]. Additionally, 50 cattle imported from neighboring Guinea succumbed to the disease before testing, indicating the potential for transboundary introduction of the disease in the sub-region.

3. Brucellosis and its impact on public health in Sierra Leone

3.1 Public health risk along the livestock value chain

Brucellosis poses risks at various stages of the livestock value chain, from production to consumption. It is crucial to address these risks at each stage by promoting awareness and implementing best practices to minimize disease transmission and protect both animal and human health. The different stages of the livestock value chain include:

i. Animal acquisition: When introducing new animals into a herd or farm, there is a risk of introducing Brucella-infected animals. Purchasing animals from unknown or untrusted sources increases the likelihood of bringing in infected animals that can spread the disease to the existing herd.

ii. Animal movement: The movement of infected animals between farms, markets, or slaughterhouses can contribute to the spread of Brucellosis. Infected animals shedding the Brucella bacteria in their urine, milk, placental fluid, and other body fluids can contaminate the environment, feed, and water sources, making it easier for healthy animals to become infected.

iii. Breeding and reproduction: Brucellosis can be transmitted through mating or artificial insemination. If a bull or ram carrying the Brucella bacteria mates with a susceptible female, the infection can be transmitted. Additionally, infected animals may experience reproductive issues such as abortions, stillbirths, or reduced fertility, which can lead to further spread of the disease.

iv. Handling and milking: During the milking process, Brucellosis can be transmitted from infected animals to humans. Contaminated milk or milk products can pose a risk of infection if consumed without proper pasteurization. Direct contact with infected animals' bodily fluids, such as through wounds or mucous membranes, also presents a risk of transmission.

v. Slaughter and meat processing: Infected animals can carry Brucella bacteria in their lymph nodes, organs, and reproductive tissues. Improper handling and slaughter practices, as well as inadequate meat inspection and processing, can lead to the contamination of meat products with Brucella. Consuming undercooked or raw meat from infected animals can result in human infection [9].

vi. Consumption: Consumption of unpasteurized milk, cheese, or other dairy products made from infected animals can pose a direct risk of Brucellosis transmission to humans. Additionally, consuming contaminated meat or meat products without proper cooking can also lead to human infection. Brucellosis is a well-documented zoonotic disease and a major public health concern worldwide. However, in Africa, particularly in Sierra Leone, the disease has been long neglected, and associated risks and health factors are not routinely ascertained [6, 10].

A mapping and analysis of the livestock value chain, particularly for ruminants (cattle, goats, and sheep), in Sierra Leone, as shown in **Figure 2**, provides a better understanding of the stakeholders at risk.

Stage 1: At the production stage, farmers, including cowboys who care for the animals during grazing, women who milk the cows, and household family members who participate in animal production, are at risk of contracting the disease. They

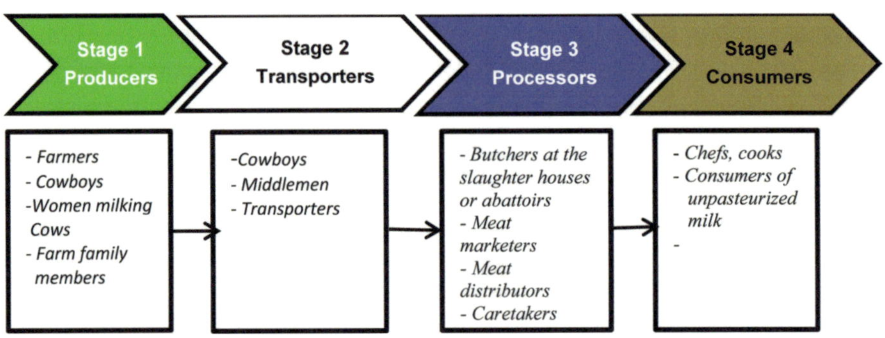

Figure 2.
Schematic representation of stakeholders at risk of contracting brucellosis along the ruminant value chain in Sierra Leone.

come into direct contact with infected animals or their products, such as feces, urine, or milk, which may carry a high concentration of the etiology.

Stage 2: This stage involves the transportation of live animals from remote production sites to the market. Animals are often trekked for miles to reach transportation centers where they are loaded onto trucks and vans for their final destinations. The key players involved are cowboys, middlemen, and farmers themselves. These individuals are also at high risk of contracting the disease because they come into direct contact with the animals and their waste products.

Stage 3: The processing stage encompasses several stakeholders, including caretakers at livestock holding facilities, butchers at abattoirs and slaughterhouses, and meat marketers and distributors. They are all at high risk of contracting Brucellosis. Their jobs require them to come into direct contact with live and slaughtered animals, as well as the meat and waste products. In Sierra Leone, these meat processors are rarely seen wearing any form of personal protective equipment (PPE) at all stages of processing. The fact remains that they are simply not aware of the associated risks of contracting zoonotic diseases from infected animals.

Stage 4: The consumer stage is the final stage of the ruminant value chain. Meat is processed in restaurants in various forms, and there is a possibility of serving undercooked meat. Meanwhile, chefs, cooks, and other individuals involved in meal preparation could also be at risk.

3.2 Public health risk from traditional consumption practices

Extended literature reviews have indicated that 4% of the global foodborne disease burden and 12% of the animal-source disease burden are attributed to dairy products [11–13]. The consumption of raw or unpasteurized milk is a subject of discussion and is influenced by people's knowledge and the rules and regulations governing the consumption of such products. Some people consume raw milk because they believe it enhances the nutritive value of the product and preserves the original taste. However, raw milk may contain complex microbiological components that pose serious health risks. Pathogens such as Campylobacter, Cryptosporidium, *E. coli*, Listeria, Brucella, and Mycobacterium can be present in raw milk.

In Sierra Leone, the custom of consuming unpasteurized milk is prevalent. Pasteurization, a process that involves heating milk to a specific temperature to kill harmful bacteria, including Brucella, is not routinely carried out. Consequently, raw unpasteurized milk remains untreated and may contain pathogens, including Brucella. Therefore, consuming raw milk increases the risk of Brucellosis infection. Pasteurization is a crucial step in ensuring the safety of milk and dairy products. It effectively kills harmful bacteria, including Brucella, thereby reducing the risk of foodborne illnesses. Pasteurization is widely recommended as a preventive measure to eliminate or reduce the transmission of Brucellosis and other pathogens.

The process of collecting and processing milk is often unhygienic. Women in traditional cattle production facilities are responsible for milking the cows. Ideally, before collection, the teats of the udder should be thoroughly cleaned to minimize the chances of contamination. However, in traditional cattle production systems, milk is directly harvested from cows with little consideration for hygiene. The fat is then extracted from the milk using crude methods and subjected to fermentation. The fermented unpasteurized milk is sold to the public for consumption. Personal conversations with people who consume raw milk indicate a lack of knowledge and understanding about the risks associated with consuming such products.

Health authorities, such as the World Health Organization (WHO) and the Centers for Disease Control and Prevention (CDC), strongly advise against consuming raw milk due to the associated health risks, including the transmission of Brucellosis. They recommend consuming only pasteurized milk and dairy products.

Public awareness campaigns play a crucial role in educating individuals about the risks of consuming raw milk and the importance of pasteurization. It is important to inform consumers about the potential health consequences and promote safe milk consumption practices.

3.3 Public health risk from antimicrobial resistant (AMR) Brucella parasites and one health interventions

Antimicrobial resistance (AMR) is a significant public health concern that leads to treatment failures, prolonged hospitalizations, and high mortality rates among humans. It is estimated that in 2019, 1.27 million deaths were directly attributed to drug resistance, and projections indicate that by 2050, annual deaths could reach 10 million [14]. A recent report highlighted that if substantive efforts are not made to contain this threat, 10 million deaths and a loss of 100 trillion USD in the world's economic outputs could be attributed to AMR by 2050 [15].

Livestock play a crucial role in many impoverished countries, particularly in Africa, where they hold a unique socio-cultural niche. Resistant strains of bacteria in terrestrial and aquatic animals can worsen animal performance, which, in turn, affects the livelihoods of poor rural African communities. Approximately 1.3 billion people rely on livestock for their livelihood, and over 20 million people depend on aquaculture [16]. Livestock contribute significantly to the development and transmission of zoonotic antibacterial-resistant parasites, including Brucellosis. Infected animals can act as reservoirs for the transmission of resistant strains to humans through direct contact, consumption of contaminated animal products (such as unpasteurized milk and cheese), or inhalation of contaminated aerosols. This can lead to treatment challenges, more severe illness, and potentially higher mortality rates among affected individuals.

Antibiotics are commonly used in the treatment of Brucellosis in both animals and humans. However, the development of antibiotic resistance in Brucella parasites can render standard treatment protocols ineffective. This poses a challenge in managing and controlling Brucellosis infections, resulting in prolonged illness, increased treatment costs, and potential treatment failures. Moreover, with the emergence of antibiotic resistance, the range of effective antibiotics for treating Brucellosis becomes limited. This reduction in treatment options can make it more difficult to achieve successful outcomes in infected animals and individuals.

A situation analysis report on antimicrobial use and resistance in the food and agricultural sector in Sierra Leone was conducted in 2021. Key findings indicate that methods for quantifying antimicrobial use in animals have not been developed, and the use of antimicrobials is undocumented. An estimated 74.1% of farmers use antimicrobials as growth promoters. Antimicrobials are also used as chemoprophylactic or chemotherapeutic drugs. Tetracycline (51.3%, n = 421), amoxicillin (18.4%, n = 151), ampicillin (11.8%, n = 97), and penicillin (5.9%, n = 48) are among the most commonly used antibiotics by livestock farmers. Approximately 60% of livestock farmers lack knowledge about antibiotics, and 27% disclose using antibiotics for treating infections without providing details about the name and description of the infection they treated. This underscores the fact that antimicrobials are haphazardly used in livestock production without an adequate understanding of their impact on generating resistant zoonotic parasites [17]. People consuming meat with a high burden of AMR parasites are at a high risk of contracting these parasites.

There is limited information available regarding people diagnosed with Brucellosis parasites, but this does not imply that such cases do not exist. The Livestock and Veterinary Services Delivery Unit of the Ministry of Agriculture and Food Security faces significant resource and capacity constraints in terms of human resources, diagnostic capabilities, and surveillance systems. In remote and inaccessible livestock production systems, local farmers often administer animal health services as a last resort to address desperate situations. Under such conditions, the proliferation of resistant Brucella parasites is extensive and can be easily transmitted to vulnerable and susceptible populations.

The emergence of antibiotic-resistant Brucellosis highlights the importance of a One Health approach that recognizes the interconnectedness of animal, human, and environmental health. Collaboration between veterinary and human healthcare professionals, as well as agricultural and environmental stakeholders, is essential in monitoring and managing the spread of antibiotic-resistant strains and implementing effective control measures. To mitigate the impact of antibiotic-resistant Brucella parasites, responsible and judicious use of antibiotics is crucial. This includes proper diagnosis, appropriate prescription, adherence to treatment protocols, and the promotion of alternative disease control strategies, such as vaccination and improved biosecurity measures. Lastly, regular surveillance of Brucellosis cases, including monitoring for antibiotic resistance, is vital for detecting and tracking the emergence and spread of resistant strains. This information can guide treatment protocols, inform public health interventions, and support the development of targeted control strategies.

3.4 The One Health approach

The One Health strategy plays a crucial role in the control and prevention of Brucellosis in both animals and public health. The One Health approach recognizes the interconnectedness of human, animal, and environmental health and promotes collaboration between multiple sectors to address health issues comprehensively [18]. The One Health strategy contributes to the control and prevention of Brucellosis through several key measures:

- Early detection and surveillance: One Health emphasizes the importance of active surveillance systems to promptly detect Brucellosis cases in animals and humans. This involves regular monitoring of livestock, wildlife, and humans in high-risk areas to identify infected individuals and trace the sources of infection.

- Integrated control measures: The One Health approach promotes integrated control measures that encompass both animal and human health [18]. This includes implementing vaccination programs for livestock, wildlife, and pets to prevent the spread of Brucellosis. Additionally, coordinated efforts are made to improve animal health management practices, such as hygiene, biosecurity, and proper waste disposal, which can help to reduce the transmission of Brucella bacteria.

- Collaboration and information sharing: One Health encourages collaboration among various stakeholders, including veterinarians, physicians, epidemiologists, public health officials, and policymakers. Sharing information and expertise across disciplines facilitates a better understanding of Brucellosis transmission dynamics, risk factors, and control strategies. This collaboration enhances surveillance, diagnostics, and treatment protocols for both animals and humans.

- Public awareness and education: The One Health approach recognizes the importance of public awareness and education in preventing Brucellosis. Raising awareness about the disease, its transmission routes, and preventive measures can help to reduce the risk of infection in both animal handlers and the general public. Education programs target livestock owners, hunters, farmers, and other individuals at higher risk of exposure to Brucellosis.

- Research and innovation: The One Health strategy emphasizes the need for continued research and innovation in the field of Brucellosis prevention and control. This includes developing improved diagnostic tools, vaccines, and treatment options for animals and humans. Research efforts focus on understanding the epidemiology of the disease, identifying risk factors, and evaluating the effectiveness of control strategies [18].

Sierra Leone has adopted the One Health (OH) approach with a vision of creating a healthy Sierra Leone where people and animals coexist in a safe environment, achieved through effective One Health collaboration. The One Health approach in Sierra Leone is guided by the concept of effective collaboration and integration through multidisciplinary and multisectoral engagement for the health of people, animals, and the environment. The country has established a One Health coordination structure, which is currently being tested. This approach has helped to overcome weak and ill-capacitated health delivery systems by enabling the prevention, prediction, detection, and response to health emergencies. The organizational structure ensures that decisions are made at higher political levels, thereby ensuring political will that is then cascaded to units responsible for coordinating the entire process.

The countries in the Mano River Union sub-region (Guinea, Liberia, Sierra Leone, and Ivory Coast) continue to face growing threats from zoonotic diseases. Weak health delivery systems, poor coordination of efforts, and mistrust among key stakeholders have exacerbated this problem, leading to inadequate response initiatives during disease outbreaks. In 2014, the sub-region experienced the devastating Ebola pandemic, followed by the COVID-19 outbreak in 2020. The experiences gained from these outbreaks, particularly the Ebola outbreak, laid the foundation for the establishment of the One Health platform.

This shift in the approach to disease outbreak response brought together other key players and institutions, such as the Ministry of Health and Sanitation, Ministry of Agriculture and Food Security, and Ministry of the Environment and Climate Change, to collaborate and pool resources for effective surveillance and response to disease outbreaks. Brucellosis is among the PZDs in Sierra Leone, and outbreaks of alarming proportions will receive the attention and response of the One Health platform for appropriate action.

DOI: http://dx.doi.org/10.5772/intechopen.114278

4. Control and prevention strategies

4.1 Prevention and control of brucellosis in animals

Prevention and control of Brucellosis among ruminants in extensive free-range systems pose significant challenges. This is exacerbated by the constant influx of sick livestock from across the border, increasing the likelihood of infecting local herds. Furthermore, the movement of herds in communal grazing lands allows for direct contact and transmission through mating and natural instincts. However, concerted efforts and strategies must be implemented to establish effective prevention and control measures. The best approach is to adopt an integrated strategy for controlling and preventing the disease, which includes the following measures:

1. *Mass vaccination of susceptible herds:* Vaccinating enzootic areas can help to reduce the infection burden. For small ruminants, a vaccination schedule of at least every 6 months for three consecutive periods should be followed, including the vaccination of kids and lambs. It's important to note that vaccination, when combined with proper husbandry practices, is more likely to achieve successful prevention and control of Brucella infections [19].

2. *Laboratory-based surveillance:* Both active and passive surveillance are essential for effective prevention and control measures. Passive surveillance is usually carried out by CAHWs who closely collaborate with local livestock farmers. They act as frontline personnel, identifying disease outbreaks and reporting them to the relevant authorities. During the 2020 Brucellosis outbreak, CAHWs were in the field to assess the nature and magnitude of the outbreak. Subsequently, active surveillance was initiated, and veterinarians were dispatched to collect samples, which were then sent to the Central Veterinary Laboratory at Teko in Makeni. Confirmed cases were identified, and prevalence and disease incidence were determined. Necessary prevention and control measures, such as herd movement restrictions, quarantine, selective testing, and slaughter, were implemented.

3. *Community-based actions:* Nomadic pastoralist farmers, known for their constant movements in search of pasture and water, contribute to the rapid spread of Brucellosis among vulnerable herds. Local authorities, including chiefs, village heads, and heads of livestock associations, play a crucial role in Brucellosis control. In Sierra Leone, Livestock bye-laws were developed and enforced in several communities where livestock are reared. These bye-laws prohibit livestock farmers from moving animals without prior approval from local authorities, and all livestock farmers are obligated to vaccinate their herds. Such bye-laws significantly reduce the spread of Brucellosis, as observed in the Falaba and Koinadugu districts.

4. *Training and sensitization of stakeholders:* Knowledge is essential in combating Brucellosis, as lack of knowledge can lead to misinformation and rumors. Training frontline Animal Health Workers is crucial, particularly in safe sample collection, community engagement, and proper transportation of samples. It is important to sensitize farmers and other stakeholders to understand the risks associated with handling Brucella-infected animals. Raising awareness among livestock farmers will foster cooperation in managing the outbreak.

5. *Strengthening point of entry border posts:* The ruminant livestock industry in Sierra Leone is largely influenced by migrants from Guinea and neighboring countries like Mali, Ivory Coast, and Burkina Faso. These transhumance nomadic migrants constantly move with their livestock in search of pasture and markets, following specific routes to cross international borders. Strengthening point of entry (PoE) posts by equipping them with basic testing equipment and establishing adequate quarantine facilities can help to prevent the introduction of sick animals into the country.

6. *Use of protective equipment:* In the ruminant value chain analysis, it is important to identify stakeholders at risk of contracting the disease. Farmers, transporters, processors, marketers, and even cooks are at risk if proper preventive measures are not taken. The use of PPE will prevent direct contact between farmers and other stakeholders along the value chain and sick animals or their products (meat, feces, urine, aborted placentas, or fetuses).

4.2 Prevention and control of brucellosis in humans

Brucellosis is a well-documented zoonotic disease that can cause severe illness in humans. It has been noted that humans can contract the disease from infected animals or contaminated animal products. The most common ways of contracting Brucellosis include consuming raw dairy products contaminated with Brucella, inhaling air contaminated by Brucella, and coming into contact with the blood or body fluids of infected animals [20]. In Sierra Leone, many people have contracted the disease due to ignorance and traditional cultural practices. To prevent and control the occurrence and spread of Brucellosis, the following measures are essential:

1. *Pasteurization of milk:* The consumption of raw, unpasteurized milk is a common practice in Sierra Leone. The public and other stakeholders must be educated about the risks associated with consuming unpasteurized milk. Additionally, traders in fresh milk should be taught simple techniques of pasteurization and other value-addition methods to increase their income.

2. *Strengthening and enforcing ante- and post-mortem inspection of meat and animal products:* Conducting ante- and post-mortem inspections of meat animals and their products is crucial in safeguarding consumers from contracting Brucellosis. This can be achieved through the presence of adequate facilities and trained personnel who can effectively perform these inspections.

3. *Use of personal protective equipment (PPE):* Individuals who handle meat, fluids, and other animal products infected with Brucella are at risk of contracting the disease. Butchers in abattoirs and slaughterhouses are particularly exposed to the disease and should wear effective PPE to protect themselves.

4. *Public sensitization and education:* Many people are unaware of the risks involved in dealing with Brucella-infected animal products. Mass sensitization campaigns aimed at educating the public about basic prevention and control measures can help to curb human infections.

5. *The One Health approach:* The One Health approach is gaining recognition among health workers and policymakers. This approach is particularly suitable for

low-income countries with limited facilities and infrastructure for effective and rapid response to outbreaks. In Sierra Leone, the Ministry of Health is closely collaborating with the Livestock and Veterinary Division of the Ministry of Agriculture and Food Security, allowing the Livestock Division to benefit from the facilities and experiences of the Ministry of Health [21].

5. Conclusions

Brucellosis, a priority animal disease with public health implications, has been a neglected issue in Sierra Leone, resulting in significant economic losses for farmers. Despite its detection in 1966, insufficient efforts have been made to control and prevent the disease among livestock. As a consequence, Sierra Leone continues to experience sporadic outbreaks of Brucellosis, leading to substantial economic losses and deepening poverty among rural livestock farmers. The persistence of Brucellosis poses a significant challenge to the development of the livestock sector, particularly within the nomadic extensive free-range system, primarily for ruminants. The complexity of the prevention and control measures is further compounded by this system.

However, the introduction of the One Health approach has revitalized efforts for the control and prevention of Brucellosis. This approach promotes collaboration across sectors and disciplines, facilitating prompt detection and response to Brucellosis outbreaks. Currently, all endeavors are concentrated on effectively controlling and preventing the disease in Sierra Leone. It is hoped that through the implementation of this new approach, Brucellosis outbreaks will be minimized, allowing farmers to reap the economic benefits associated with their livestock.

Acknowledgements

My profound appreciation to Dr. Sahr Raymond Gborie of the Epidemiological Unit at the Livestock and Veterinary Services Division of the Ministry of Agriculture and Food Security for drawing the map of Sierra Leone. Let me conclude by thanking my students at the Faculty of Agriculture and Food Security for improving my internet connectivity.

Conflict of interest

There is no conflict of interest in this piece of academic work. It has been written to improve the knowledge of my students and other users who may find it useful.

Author details

Saidu Kanu
Dean of Faculty of Agriculture and Food Sciences, University of Makeni, Makeni, Sierra Leone

*Address all correspondence to: saidukanu2020@gmail.com

References

[1] World Bank. Sierra Leone Population. Trading Economics. 2023. Available from: tradingeconomics.com/sierra-leone/population-total-wb-data.html [Accessed: May 20, 2023]

[2] Statistics Sierra Leone. Report on the 2021 and 2022 Real Gross Domestic Product (RGDP) Figures at 2006 Prices. Sierra Leone: National Accounts Section; 2022

[3] Kwaku Agyemang. Sierra Leone National Livestock Sample Survey. Sierra Leone: FAO; 2017

[4] Racloz V, Schelling E, Chitnis N, Roth F, Zinsstag J. Persistence of brucellosis in pastoral systems. Revue Scientifique Et Technique De L Office International Des Epizooties. Revue Scientifique Et Technique. Apr 2013;**32**(1):61-70

[5] Lokamar PN, Kutwah MA, Atieli H, Gumo S, Ouma C. Socio-economic impacts of brucellosis on livestock production and reproduction performance in Koibatek and Marigat regions, Baringo County, Kenya. BMC Veterinary Research. 2020;**16**:61. DOI: 10.1186/s12917-020-02283-w

[6] Suluku R, Nyandeboh JPJ, Moiforay S. One Health Approach to Control Brucellosis in Sierra Leone. Budapest, Hungary: Intechopen; 2019. DOI: 10.5772/intechopen.82378

[7] Massaquoi M, Elduma AH, Hakizimana JL, Kamara K, Gebru GN. Investigation of brucellosis outbreak in cattle in Koin adugu district, Sierra Leone, march 2021. Journal of Applied Veterinary Sciences. 2021, 2022;**7**(3):30-34. Available from: https://javs.journals.ekb.eg

[8] Sesay ME, Kanu EM, Bagla VP, Norman PE. Prevalence of Brucella abortus in cattle in the Njala and Newton ranches of Sierra Leone using serological analysis. Animal and Veterinary Sciences. 2021;**9**(6):191-195. DOI: 10.11648/j.avs.20210906.15. Available from: http://www.sciencepublishinggroup.com/j/avs

[9] Zinsstag J. Brucellosis Surveillance and Control: A One Health Case Study. Switzerland: Cabi Digital Library; 2023. DOI: 10.1079/onehealthcases.2023.0004

[10] Gashaw Adane Erkyihun, Fikru Regassa Gari, and Gezahegne Mamo Kassa. Bovine Brucellosis and its Public Health Importance in Ethiopia. China CDC: Zoonoses; 2022

[11] de Klerk JN, Robinson PA. Drivers and Hazards of Consumption of Unpasteurised Bovine Milk and Milk Products in High-Income Countries. 2022. DOI: 10.7717/peerj.13426

[12] Baron-Epel O, Obeid S, Kababya D, Bord S, Myers V. A health promotion perspective for the control and prevention of brucellosis *(Brucella melitensis)*; Israel as a case study. PLoS Neglected Tropical Diseases. 2022;**16**(9):e0010816. DOI: 10.1371/journal.pntd.0010816 [Accessed: May 20, 2023]

[13] Grace D, Wu F, Havelaar A. Foodborne diseases from dairy products in developing countries: Review of causes and health and economic implications. Journal of Dairy Science. Nov 2020;**103**(11):9715-9729. DOI: 10.3168/jds.2020-18323

[14] Medina M-J, Legido-Quigley H, Hsu LY. Antimicrobial Resistance in One Health. United States of America: Global Health Security; 2020

[15] Jiang T, Chen X-S. Outcome impacts due to pathogen-specific antimicrobial resistance: A narrative review of published literature. Open Access. International Journal of Environmental Research and Public Health. 21 Feb 2020;**17**(4):1395. DOI: 10.3390/ijerph17041395

[16] WOAH. Antimicrobial Resistance. 2023. Available from: https://www.woah.org/en/what-we-do/global-initiatives/antimicrobial-resistance/ [Accessed: May 18, 2023]

[17] FAO. Situation Analysis of Antimicrobial Use and Resistance in the Food and Agriculture Sector in Sierra Leone. Sierra Leone: FAO; 2022

[18] Charypkhan D, Rüegg SR. One Health evaluation of brucellosis control in Kazakhstan. PLoS ONE. 2022;**17**(11):e0277118. DOI: 10.1371/journal.pone.0277118

[19] Dadar M, Tiwari R, Sharun K, Dhama K. Importance of brucellosis control programs of livestock on the improvement of one health. Veterinary Quarterly. Dec 2021;**41**(1):137-151. DOI: 10.1080/01652176.2021.1894501. PMID: 33618618; PMCID: PMC7946044

[20] Libers A. What is Brucellosis? Symptoms, Causes, Diagnosis, Treatment, and Prevention. Everyday health; 2023. Available from: https://www.everydayhealth.com/brucellosis/guide/

[21] Ghanbari MK, Gorji HA, Behzadifar M, Sanee N, Mehedi N, Bragazzi NL. One Health Approach to Tackle Brucellosis: A Systematic Review. Tropical Medicine and Health. Open Access; 2020

Chapter 3

Brucellosis as a Multisystem Disease

Abdelrahman Mokhtar, Rashed Albalawi and Samira M. Fallatah

Abstract

Brucellosis, one of the common zoonotic diseases all over the world, is still underdiagnosed. Under diagnosis is mostly due to certain concepts that should be revised especially in endemic areas. First of all, in endemic areas especially raw milk consuming communities, it is not logic to consider brucellosis only in certain occupations, while the whole community is exposed through utilization of non-pasteurized dairy products. Unawareness about the protean manifestations of brucellosis and its ability to affect almost every system in the body from heal to crown is another problem that needs orientation. Brucellosis now is one of the great imitators like SLE and TB. Chronic brucellosis can present by different manifestations even in the absence of fever and with low serum antibody titers. So, physicians in endemic areas should be aware by the usual and unusual presentations of brucellosis and should consider brucellosis in the differential diagnosis of almost every unexplained medical problem until proved otherwise.

Keywords: fever, osteoarticular, brucella hepatitis, brucella pancreatitis, neurobrucellosis, gonadal infection, endocarditis, and hematopoiesis

1. Introduction

Brucellosis is a common zoonotic disease. After routine screening of domestic livestock and application of animal vaccination programs, in industrialized countries, it became rare [1, 2].

In many endemic regions, about 500,000 incident cases of human brucellosis reported per year. Yet, because of the poor infrastructure and the inefficient notification systems, the true incidence is estimated to be 5,000,000 to 12,500,000 cases annually [3].

The variable and non-specific clinical presentations of brucellosis in human being yields great diagnostic difficulties [4].

The clinical picture has changed, in developing countries, because patients used to take antibiotics for any fever on their own initiative, or at the suggestion of the pharmacist. This has reduced the blood culture yield, making the diagnosis of brucellosis more difficult [5].

The course of the disease, may be: *Acute brucellosis,* characterized by: asthenia, headache, undulant fever, profuse sweating, hot flushes, myalgia, arthralgia, testicular pain in men, enlarged liver and spleen (approximately 50–60% of cases), dyspepsia, diarrhea, nausea, vomiting, constipation, and anorexia. The acute phase may end in death (in rare situations), recovery or passing into a sub-acute or chronic form.

Sub-acute brucellosis, this refers to relapsing patients, usually after incomplete or partial antibiotic treatment. The clinical picture is more protean and may present as fever of unknown origin. The symptoms are generally milder, and localized infection can be seen. *Chronic brucellosis,* the organism can remain at a low replication rate for a long time, and under favorable conditions again, it infects other cells and start new replicative cycles. Lymph nodes, spleen, lungs, and the reproductive organs, mammary glands and joints, are well-known target organs. All these organs allow brucella replication and may contribute to its persistence [6].

Chronic brucellosis, usually present by psychoneurosis, sweating, and weight loss. Fever is not a must, and the agglutinins may be undetected; So, it resembles chronic fatigue syndrome. Localization can be seen in tissues, like bone, joints, cerebrospinal fluid, liver, kidneys, spleen, or skin. Localization may be the main presentation of systemic infection or may be the only manifestation of a chronic infection [4, 5].

Because of its non-specific clinical features, slow growth rate in the blood culture, and the complexity of its serodiagnosis, the timely and accurate diagnosis of human brucellosis is still challenging [7]. In the coming pages we will review the clinical presentation of brucellosis in different body systems.

2. Review of the body systems

2.1 Musculoskeletal and rheumatologic manifestations of brucellosis

The most common complication of brucellosis is reported to be osteoarticular involvement. It can mimic rheumatologic diseases. This may cause misdiagnosis and lead to malpractice [8].

Sacroiliitis, spondylitis, arthritis, osteomyelitis, tenosynovitis, and bursitis all were reported. The spine is the usual targeted site in the elderly, while in young the sacroiliac joints and knee arthritis predominate [9].

Gotuzzo et al. [10] retrospectively analyzed 304 cases of brucellosis. Articular manifestations were detected in 33.8% of patients. The most frequent pattern was sacroiliitis, then peripheral arthritis, manifested either as a single large lower extremity joint or as an asymmetric pauciarthritis. Mixed arthritis was a combination of the first two. Spondylitis was the least common, and significantly with more prolonged duration of symptoms (chronic course), affecting elder than young, with less frequent fever and malaise. It also tends to be destructive [10].

Mimicking rheumatic disorders was not only on the clinical level but also increased rates of positive RF (Rheumatoid Factor), anti-CCP; and decreased 25OHD levels in brucella seropositive patients were reported. So, in endemic areas it was recommended to consider brucellosis in the differential diagnosis of patients with rheumatologic manifestations even in the presence of autoimmune markers [8].

Spinal brucellosis is defined as involvement of the vertebral column, interspinal spaces and/or paraspinal areas (**Figure 1**) [11].

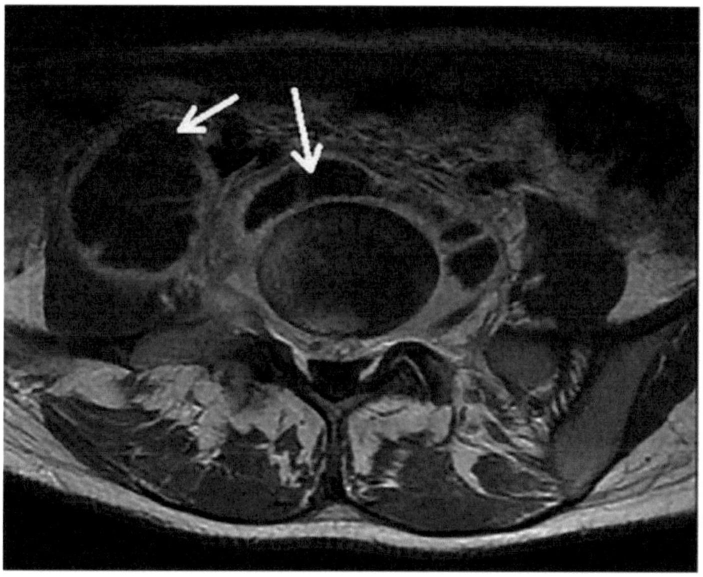

Figure 1.
Magnetic resonance imaging (MRI) of the lumbar spine revealed findings consistent with circumscribed spinal brucellosis complicated by lumbar spondylodiscitis, epidural abscess and large right-sided paraspinal abscess extended from L4 to the sacrum.

Spondylitis or vertebral osteomyelitis is inflammation and infection of vertebrae. It may affect lumbar (60%), sacral (19%) and cervical vertebrae (12%) [12]. Spondylodiscitis (simultaneous inflammation of vertebrae and disc) and discitis (intervertebral disc infected without spondylitis) were also reported [13].

To diagnose vertebral involvement during brucellosis, routine clinical and laboratory assessments are not always sufficient. More advanced imaging techniques such as bone scintigraphy, computed tomography (CT), or magnetic resonance imaging (MRI) are required [14]. Predominant lymphocyte infiltration, new bone formation, epitheloid granuloma lesions on the ventral sides of the vertebral bodies, no, or very mild, vertebral body deformation, no abnormal paraspinal soft tissue signal, no intraosseous or paraspinal abscesses, and thin and irregular abscess walls, all these features (histopathological and MRI) are more suggestive of brucella spondylitis than pyogenic or the more destructive tuberculous varieties [15]. Osteomyelitis or destructive arthritis were encountered in few cases. The lumbosacral region is the most frequently involved region, while the thoracic and cervical regions were less likely to be affected [16].

On the other hand, the midthoracic spine, vertebral destruction with gibbus deformity, disk collapse, and paraspinal abscesses all were more frequent with tuberculous spondylitis [17].

Definite diagnosis of brucellosis is established by clinical manifestations and the isolation of brucella species from blood or bone marrow cultures. In the absence of bacteriologic confirmation, a positive serology for brucella is needed for definite diagnosis [15].

In comparison with spondylarthritis, Wang et al. [18] found that, the average disease duration of brucellosis patients was shorter than that of spondylarthritis patients, especially for the axial forms (5 months vs. 87 months, $P = 0.001$).

History of animal contact (59.09%) and more frequent elevation of temperature, should alert physicians to consider brucellosis. In addition, low back pain (LBP) of brucellosis patients was generally less improved with exercise. The pain presented as persistent LBP, and was associated with higher rate of walking difficulties. Myalgia was another major musculoskeletal manifestation and seen in nearly half (45.45%) of brucellosis patients. Additionally, HLA-B27 was usually negative in cases with brucellosis [18].

Apart from the spinal affection, the sacroiliac (SI) joints are the most commonly reported especially in acute brucellosis and may be associated with spinal brucellosis. Patients may present with hip or low back pain, mimics acute low back pain of lumbar disc herniation and the back pain may radiate into thigh however, chronic sacroiliitis is associated with chronic back pain [7]. Both unilateral and bilateral affection were reported [19]. Sacroiliitis was also simultaneously seen with dactylitis, olecranon bursitis, humerus osteomyelitis and iliac muscle abscess, and with other systemic diseases, like endocarditis, pyelonephritis and thyroiditis [20–23].

Peripheral skeleton involvement is less frequent than vertebral among patients with brucellosis. Arthralgia, enthesopathy, osteomyelitis, arthritis, bursitis, tendonitis, and tenosynovitis (**Figures 2** and **3**) [24] were all reported. Knee (**Figures 4** and 5) [25], hip, and ankle joints are among the most common peripheral regions affected. Shoulders, wrists, elbows, interphalangeal and sternoclavicular joints may also be involved [13].

In addition, brucellosis, in endemic areas should be in the differential diagnosis of some soft tissue syndromes like bursitis and plantar fasciitis [26, 27].

Bursitis could be the presenting feature of brucellosis. Brucella bursitis usually lacks local inflammatory signs and fever [28]. Most patients have prolonged symptoms from few months to many years with the exception of few cases presented acutely. Culturing the bursal aspirate usually prove the diagnosis. Serological detection of brucella infection via standard tube agglutination (STA) test has been reported to exhibit a sensitivity of 84.6%. However, lacking a detectable immune response has been frequently recognized in patients with localized disease [29].

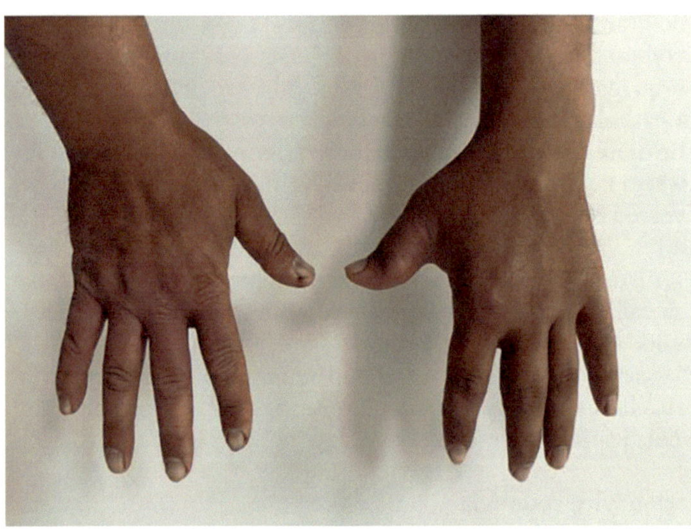

Figure 2.
Isolated diffuse thickening of the left hand without any arthralgia.

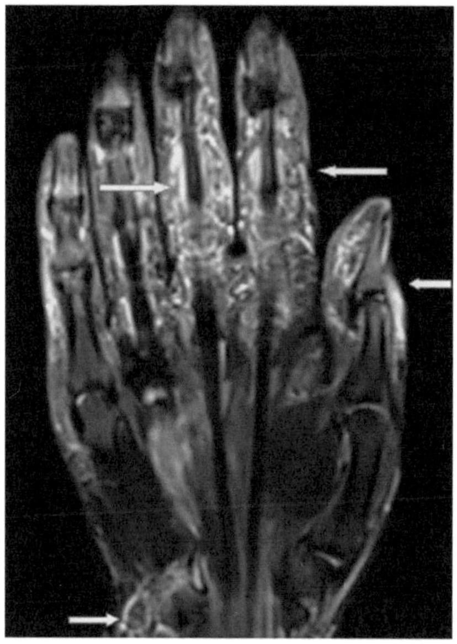

Figure 3.
Tenosynovitis of the flexor tendon sheaths, synovitis of the intercarpal, and 2–3 metacarpophalangeal joints and medullary bone marrow edema of the capitatum were detected in the magnetic resonance imaging of the hand in ***Figure 2****.*

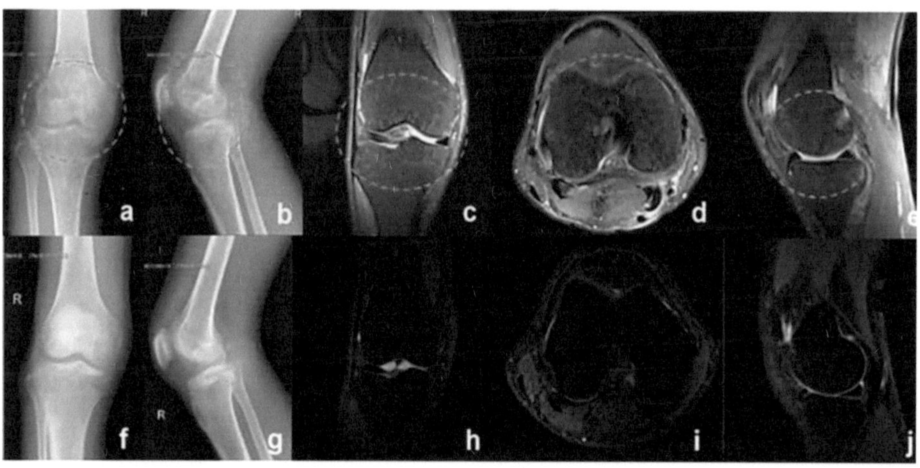

Figure 4.
X-ray images showed multiple cystic low density areas (blue circle) of distal right femur and proximal tibia (a, b). PDWI (proton density weighted image) sequence of MRI showed effusion and synovial thickening of the right knee joint, and subchondral bone marrow edema (blue circle) of the distal femur and proximal tibia (c–e). Post-treatment X-ray images showed the low density area was significantly reduced (f, g). Post-treatment PDWI sequence of magnetic resonance images indicated the high signal area of bone marrow edema had disappeared (h–j).

2.2 Gastrointestinal manifestations of brucellosis

Ingestion of non-pasteurized milk and/or raw animal products are the main sources for infection in endemic areas. So, gastrointestinal (GI)manifestations of brucellosis are variable from mild chronic symptoms up to emergency presentation in rare cases [30].

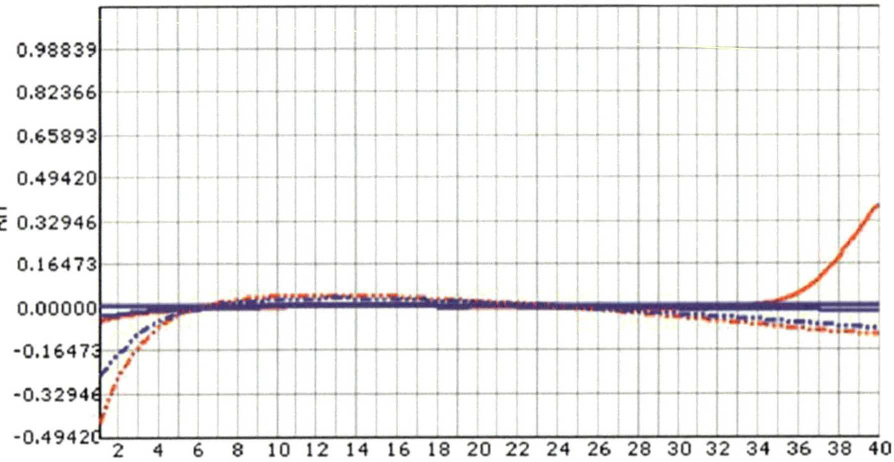

Figure 5.
Results of the synovial aspiration from the inflammed knee in ***Figure 4****. The real-time PCR of purulent joint synovial fluid of right knee showed that there was Brucella melitensis in the synovial fluid. DNA content of Brucella melitensis (solid red line) increased in 35 cycles.*

Upper GI manifestations like anorexia. Nauseas and vomiting are frequently reported up to hematemesis in rare cases associated with thrombocytopenia [31].

Abdominal pain with different clinical modalities and different underlying lesions has been reported in association with brucellosis e.g. abdominal visceral pain due to hepatitis [32], cholecystitis [33], terminal ileitis, colitis [34, 35] and occasionally oophoritis in females [36] has been described in the literature.

Acute abdominal pain due to acute pancreatitis [37], and acute bowel ischemia secondary to brucella induced vasculitis has been also reported [38]. Abdominal pain due to inflammatory peritonitis is another possibility which may occur in patients with liver cirrhosis (spontaneous bacterial peritonitis)or rarely as a direct peritoneal infection without cirrhosis [39]. Pain is not only visceral, but also abdominal wall pain in combination with fever and severe low back pain has been reported [40].

Lower GI symptoms like chronic diarrhea may also be a feature of brucellosis and so in endemic areas, it should be ruled out before immunosuppressive therapy in cases diagnosed as IBD (inflammatory bowel disease) [41].

Hepatic and splenic involvement with both hepatomegaly and splenomegaly are frequently encountered in brucellosis. Hepatomegaly may be documented in 15–20% of cases. Meanwhile, derangement of liver biochemistry is usually minor. Granulomatous hepatitis, diffuse hepatitis without granuloma, focal necrosis and rarely liver abscess (brucelloma) have been rarely reported [42]. Radiologically, two main patterns were recognized; solitary abscesses involving liver (**Figure 6**) and multiple smaller abscesses, with frequent splenic affection, and absence of calcifications characterize the second pattern [43, 44].

Brucella can stimulate collagen deposition, leading to scar formation, chronic fibrosis or cirrhosis. On the other hand, it is possible that brucellosis can trigger decompensation, in pre-existing cirrhosis [45].

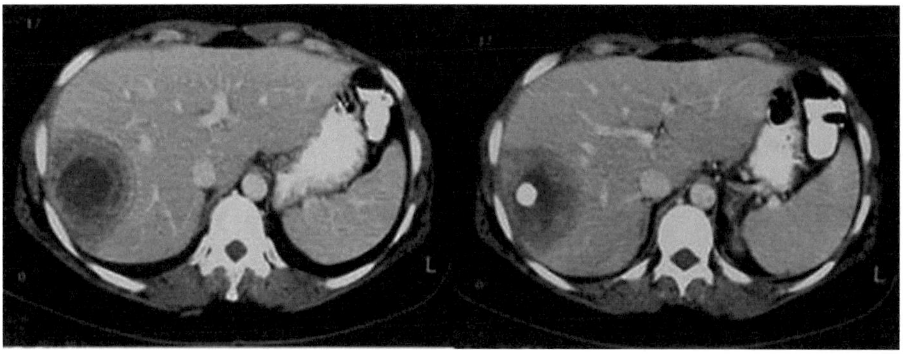

Figure 6.
A liver abscess is seen on contrast CT in a patient with brucellosis.

2.3 Cardiovascular manifestations of brucellosis

Cardiovascular complications of brucellosis may include endocarditis, pericarditis and mycotic aneurysms involving the brain, aorta, and other vessels [46].

Cardiac affection is generally rare accounting for less than 2% of patients with brucellosis, yet frequently fatal. The incidence of endocarditis due to brucellosis ranges from 0.7 to 10.9% of endocarditis cases worldwide, mainly in Mediterranean countries.

Brucella endocarditis is a life-threatening infection accounting for the majority of mortality related to brucellosis (80%) [47]. Mortality from brucella endocarditis was found to be increased 47-fold in presence of associated pericardial effusion and 25-fold in association with congestive heart failure that developed after brucella endocarditis [46].

Almost 75% of brucella endocarditis involves the aortic valve (**Figure** 7) [48]. It may lead to abscess formation in the aortic root. The mitral valve is less frequently

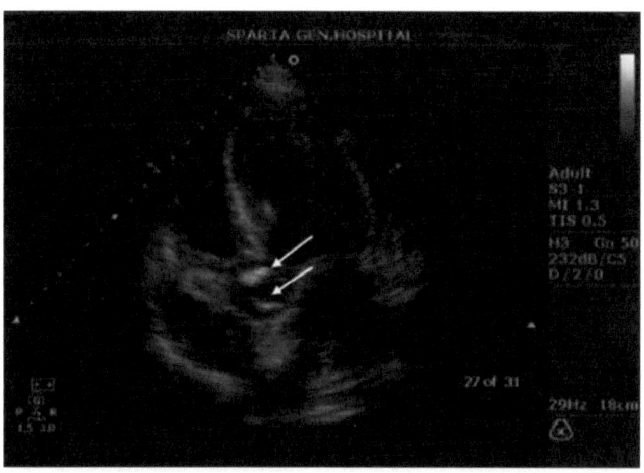

Figure 7.
A transthoracic echocardiogram performed on a patient with brucellosis: The white arrows point to the thickened aortic valves. This thickening is secondary to vegetations.

affected unless diseased. Pre-existing valve disease predisposes to valve involvement. Prosthetic valve endocarditis due to brucellosis has also been reported [49].

Diagnosis of brucella endocarditis requires a high index of suspicion especially in endemic areas, in cases with history of Contact with livestock and endocarditis with negative blood cultures [50].

In 1960, Perry and Belter published their interesting study included 44 patients died from fatal brucellosis and they concluded that, the usual cause of death during brucellosis was endocarditis. In some instances myocarditis and pericarditis were evident. Most patients die from valve deformity and congestive heart failure rather than from sepsis or embolism. Tissue examination revealed micro-abscesses within valve cusps, the destruction of the commissures, and the nodular, calcific nature of the deformity indicate that this is a chronic bacterial endocarditis. There was nothing in the lesions to suggest a hypersensitivity reaction; and eosinophils were lacking [51]. Mortality drops from 32.7% in the medical treatment only group, to 6.7% when surgery is combined to the medical treatment [52]. Fibrosis, hyalinization, and calcification were more frequently seen in brucella endocarditis than endocarditis caused by other bacteria. Most patients died because of valve deformity and congestive heart failure, which were hard to treat with medicine only [53].

Patients should be followed up by an infectious disease specialist in the first 6 months after surgery, during which the risk of relapse is high. After 6 months, a continued follow-up with a cardiologist is more appropriate [54]. In almost 40% of the cases blood culture came negative. So, the diagnosis of brucella prosthetic valve endocarditis and its complications is mainly echocardiographic. Despite occasional recovery with antibiotics alone, adding surgery to medical treatment is the most efficient therapeutic approach, yielding significant decrease in mortality [55].

Idiopathic pericardial effusion or myocarditis, even in the absence of concomitant endocarditis are other potential complications of brucellosis. Lacking of routine thorough echocardiographic studies in patients with brucellosis may explain the underestimation of isolated affection of pericardium or myocardium in the absence of concomitant endocarditis. So, in endemic areas, brucellosis should be considered in the differential diagnosis of disorders that affect the pericardium or myocardium even in the absence of concomitant endocarditis [56]. The occurrence of isolated myocarditis has been seen in endemic areas. Pulmonary edema and interstitial pneumonia due to brucella myocarditis, which was treated successfully has been reported by Jubber and associates in 1990 [57]. A 35-year-old female patient, found to have both myocarditis and pneumonia associated with effusion both pericardial and pleural was reported, with bilateral pleural thickening and pleural adhesion. Etiologically, next-generation sequencing, revealed brucella-related myocarditis and pneumonitis, with good response to anti- brucellosis antibiotics. When appropriate cultures are negative, next-generation sequencing to identify pathogens was recommended by the authors [58]. Timely diagnosis of brucella-related myocarditis and administration of appropriate antibiotic therapy can be life saving [59].

2.4 Haematologic manifestations of brucellosis

In the course of human brucellosis, anemia, leucopenia, thrombocytopenia and pancytopenia were all frequently reported [60]. In one series, anemia, leukopenia and thrombocytopenia were found in 74, 45, and 39.5% of cases respectively [61]. Associated increased and normal bone marrow cellularity ruled out bone marrow failure as a cause. The most common findings in the bone marrow evaluation were histiocytic hemophagocytosis and granulomas. Brucellosis was also, concurrently diagnosed with hematological malignancies in extremely rare cases in which the leukemic infiltrate was the cause of pancytopenia [62]. Hypersplenism, autoimmune hemolysis or alteration of iron metabolism secondary to infection are other possible mechanisms [63].

Brucellosis is unique in that it often manifests as a febrile pancytopenia in contrast to the leukocytosis and neutrophilia with bandemia that usually seen with bacteremia. Though, no specific hematological findings could be used to diagnose brucellosis. Yet, certain findings should alert the physician to the possibility of brucellosis especially in endemic areas e.g. Leukopenia with relative lymphocytosis [64], leucocytosis with relative lymphopenia [65], and eosinopenia that has been suggested as an early finding even before the serology became positive [66].

Brucellosis-induced cytopenia has no specific discriminating features from non-infectious etiologies, and therefore, brucellosis is frequently misdiagnosed as a primary hematologic disease or malignancy. However, with treatment of the underlying brucellosis hematologic manifestations usually resolves. So, brucellosis, should be in the differential diagnosis of any case of cytopenia, especially if living in, or exposed to, endemic areas [67].

Hemolysis, is another potential presentation of brucellosis, though rare yet, still brucellosis should be in the differential diagnosis as an underlying trigger for any case of hemolysis, especially those living in areas where brucellosis is endemic. Microangiopathic hemolytic anemia (MAHA) is the most common presentation (DIC, TTP and HUS) [8]. However, the literature revealed few reports about brucella presenting with Coombs-positive AIHA [68, 69].

In addition to DIC that can occur as a feature of sepsis in acute brucellosis venous or arterial thrombotic insults were rarely reported. The reported cases include abdominal artery thrombosis, popliteal artery aneurysm, deep vein thrombosis, portal vein thrombosis and cerebral vein thrombosis [70].

2.5 Skin manifestations in brucellosis

Patients may primarily present with cutaneous lesions in about 3–14% of cases with brucellosis in some series. Papulonodular lesions, erythema nodosum-like lesions, maculopapular eruptions, and contact urticaria were all frequently reported [71].

An inflammatory process in the dermis, such as perivascular and periadnexal lymphohistiocytic infiltrates and focal granulomatous lesions usually detected during histologic examination. These findings are similar to those found in the liver and bone marrow biopsies in brucellosis patients [72].

Vasculitic lesions, petechiae, purpura (in case of thrombocytopenia), liquefactive panniculitis, subcutaneous abscesses, chronic ulcerations, recurrent epidermal cyst, palmar erythema and livedo reticularis were rarely reported.

Such cutaneous lesions are not specific to brucellosis and so, brucellosis should be kept in mind in the differential diagnosis of such lesions especially in endemic areas and when the epidemiologic history of the patient is risky for such a zoonotic infection [71].

The cutaneous lesions were reported in every phase of the disease and regress with anti-brucella treatment. So, in acute brucellosis the presentation will be associated with fever, while fever may not be present in chronic brucellosis. Direct inoculation of the bacteria into the skin, deposition of immune complexes, hypersensitivity phenomena, and invasion of the skin via a hematogenous route are suggested scenarios for skin involvement in brucellosis. So, the clinician in endemic area should always keep in mind that a skin rash could represent a rare manifestation of this relatively common infectious disease [73].

The role of infectious diseases in urticaria (and angioedema) has been discussed for more than a century. Resolution of urticaria with eradication of the infection was clearly evident; however, a causal relationship with underlying or precipitating infection is difficult to establish. Among trigger factors, brucellosis should be in the differential diagnosis especially in endemic areas. Eradication of the infection could in fact lead to the resolution of urticaria [74].

2.6 Neurological manifestations of brucellosis (neurobrucellosis)

Nervous system involvement is either due to direct damage of nervous tissue or indirectly, via the production of endotoxins and immune response that are triggered by the presence of the bacteria in the human body [75]. The neurological presentation usually includes meningitis, meningoencephalitis, and encephalitis [76, 77]. Different varieties of meningovascular complications are also frequently described (mycotic aneurysms, ischemic strokes, and subarachnoid hemorrhages, etc.). Intracranial hypertension due to the arachnoid drainage system affection has been described [78]. Sensorineural hearing loss due to vestibulocochlear nerve affection is the commonest feature of cranial nerve involvement [79]. Spinal cord can also be affected; myelitis [80] and transverse myelitis [81] were reported. Spinal cord or spinal root compression can be the presentation of abscess or granuloma caused by neurobrucellosis [78].

Peripheral nervous system involvement occurs in 7% of neurobrucellosis [82]; Acute, subacute, and chronic polyradiculoneuropathies can occur. The clinical presentation may mimic Guillain-Barré Syndrome [82, 83].

Other complications, as psychiatric symptoms, are rare; the most commonly observed are depression, personality changes, euphoria, and psychosis [84].

Central nervous system involvement in brucellosis may be seen at every stage of the illness, even long after the convalescence phase. In some case reports from endemic area neurobrucellosis progresses gradually 3 months after the occurrence of the first symptom. Ataxia occurring months after the beginning of the first symptoms (post-infectious cerebellar ataxia) was also seen. So, clinicians should keep in mind that similar to tuberculosis, these manifestations may also develop due to brucellosis [79]. Epilepsy, is another suggested sequela [85, 86].

Because of the lack of pathognomonic signs and symptoms, clinical suspicion plays a key role in endemic areas. Compatible clinical picture as in (**Figures 8** and **9**) [87], inflammatory spinal fluid analysis and evidence of brucella infection in CSF or blood are the main clues to diagnose. CSF cultures being the reference standard for the diagnosis yet, are often negative. So, high titers of brucella antibodies in serum or CSF detected by various agglutination tests are still the most frequent supportive test for the diagnosis in practice [88].

2.7 Respiratory manifestations of brucellosis

Though pulmonary involvement is rare yet, in endemic areas, brucellosis should always be considered as a potential causative agent in patients with pulmonary symptoms [89].

The most frequent symptom of lung involvement is non-productive cough. Dry cough can be seen in 10 to 33% of patients. Respiratory airways are responsible for such symptoms in less than half of patients with abnormalities in the chest X-ray [90].

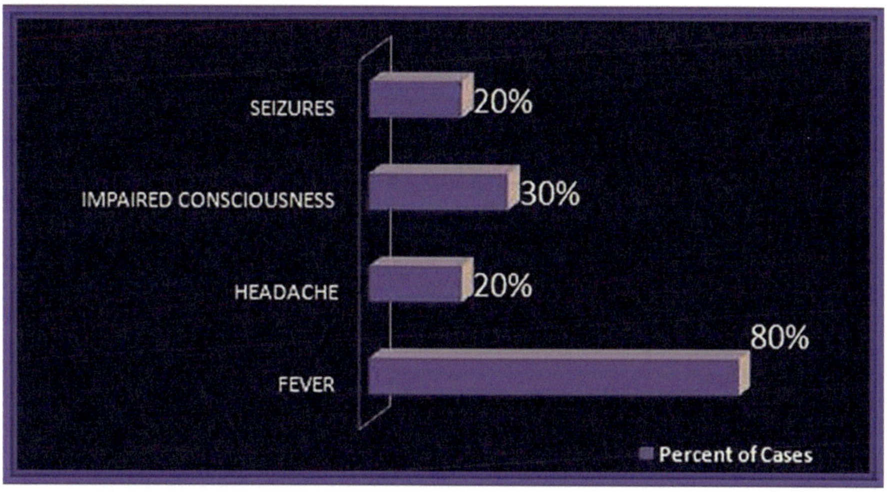

Figure 8.
Clinical presentation of Neurobrucellosis (Part 1).

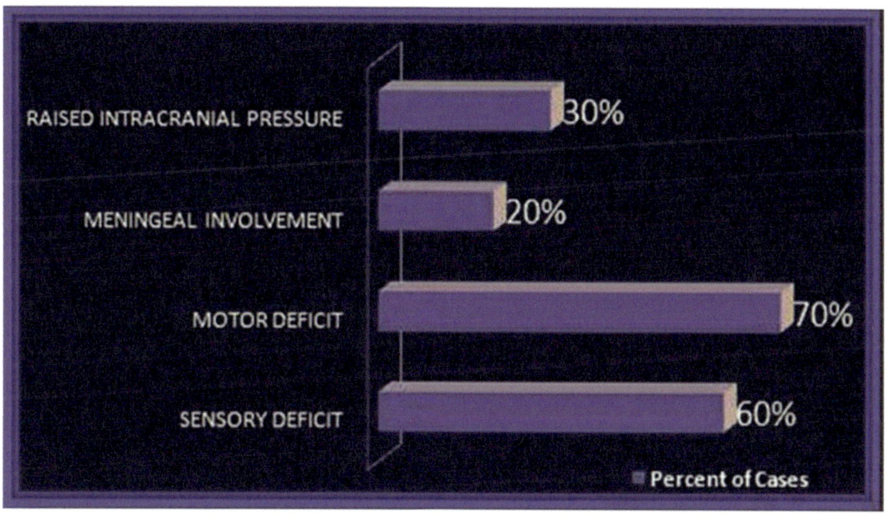

Figure 9.
Clinical presentation of Neurobrucellosis (Part 2).

Objective features of respiratory involvement are only present in around 1% of patients however, some authors from endemic areas reported 7%. Pneumonia, bronchopneumonia, pleural effusion with a predominance of monocytic or lymphocytic infiltrates, and paroxysmal dry cough all were reported. Less frequently, empyema, granulomas and solitary nodules, interstitial pneumonia, hilar and paratracheal lymphadenopathy, and even pneumothorax have all been described [91, 92].

Neither clinical features nor chest radiography revealed specific findings in brucellosis with pulmonary involvement. Respiratory culture yield was very low, with none of sputum samples and only 10% of pleural effusion samples showing positive results in some series [93, 94].

Unless the clinicians identify epidemiologic risk and clinical features of brucellosis and then request specific serologic and culture methods to confirm the diagnosis, they will miss brucellosis as the underlying etiology.

A delay for about 1 month before the recognition of brucella pneumonia is usual, and concurrent rheumatologic symptoms are present in almost half of patients. Neutrophilia is uncommon, but many patients have mildly raised transaminase levels and thrombocytopenia. The clinician should request specific serologic and culture tests required for the diagnosis of brucella once clinically suspected [94].

2.8 Genitourinary manifestations of brucellosis

Approximately 2–20% of brucellosis cases involve the genitourinary system. Epididymo-orchitis or orchitis is the most common manifestation, followed by cystitis, tubo-ovarian abscess in females, and prostatitis in males [95]. Suggestive epidemiologic history, seasonal pattern in endemic areas, gradual onset, longer duration all are suggestive points in the history. Undulatory fever with periods of apyrexia, variable local features from minimal to florid inflammation, with no associated lower urinary tract symptoms and no serious leukocytosis in the blood picture, with failure of response to empiric antibiotics in a case of epidedimo-orchitis all will suggest brucella epidedimo-orchitis rather than non-specific epidedimo-orchitis. High clinical suspicion, together with imaging diagnostic tools and microbiologic studies contribute to the reduction of unnecessary orchiectomies [96].

Involvement of the prostate gland may mimic cancer [97] and also Tubo-Ovarian brucellosis in females may mimic ovarian tumors [36].

The hazards of the female reproductive system in patients with brucellosis include pregnancy disorders at various times, intrauterine fetal death, as well as endometritis, oophoritis, mastitis, placentitis, and causeless abortions [98]. Neither the serum agglutination titer, nor the clinical type of the disease show any correlation with the occurrence of abortion [99]. Mastitis and breast abscess due to brucellosis, though rare, is another reported hazard for women infected with brucellosis [100]. Again in areas where ingestion of unpasteurized milk and milk products is common brucellosis as a potential etiologic agent, should be considered for any breast mass or abscess [101].

Kidneys (glomerulonephritis, pyelonephritis) are rarely involved [102]. Hematuria, dysuria, and hydronephrosis are rare. Medical history of consumption of non-pasteurized dairy products is important for diagnosis, otherwise it may be overlooked easily [103].

2.9 Occular manifestations of brucellosis

Eye involvement may be serious with grave complications, so early consideration and recognition can lead to prompt treatment and might prevent blindness from severe ocular damage [104]. Uveitis, neuritis, optic neuritis, papilledema, keratitis, and more-diverse ocular and neurological presentations associated with brucellosis have been reported [105]. Ocular features might also involve dacryoadenitis, conjunctivitis, episcleritis, keratitis, iritis, iridocyclitis, neuroretinitis, retinitis, chorioiditis, panuveitis, pars planitis, and hyalitis [106].

Optic nerve involvement in brucellosis is part of neurobrucellosis and it usually involves both optic nerves [107]. Rarely, premacular hemorrhage may be seen in the context of brucella endocarditis [108].

Ophthalmic brucellosis may present by injection, blurred vision, eye pain, lacrimation, double vision, foreign body sensation, cotton-wool lesions, exudative retinal detachment, and retinal hemorrhage [106]. Diagnosis of ocular brucellosis mainly depends on culture and serology of blood and intraocular fluids [109].

A thorough ophthalmic examination for features of eye involvement, has been recommended in endemic areas for any case of brucellosis whether they have ophthalmic symptoms or not [106].

2.10 Other unusual presentations of brucellosis

In addition to systemic manifestations reported above, daily reports from endemic areas describe more unusual presentations of this endemic disease. Septic shock is one of the rare presentations of brucellosis [110]. Case reports about febrile neutropenia in patients with known malignancies proved to be another unusual presentation of brucellosis. SO, it should be considered in the differential diagnosis of febrile neutropenia in patients with cancer, particularly in endemic countries [111].

Infective thyroiditis due to brucellosis has been also noticed in endemic areas (**Figure 10**) [112]. So, the authors concluded that particularly in brucella-endemic regions, when mass formation on neck area is encountered, brucella induced abscess should be considered.

Brucella infection of prosthetic devices includes breast implants [113]. Prosthetic joints, prosthetic heart valves, and one case of an infected pacemaker has been reported [114]. Spontaneous fracture due to brucella osteomyelitis is another unusual presentation [115].

Severe pharyngitis [116], abdominal; mesenteric and retroperitoneal lymphadenopathies, mimicking lymphoma has also, been reported. So in communities endemic in brucellosis; the diagnosis of brucellosis should be considered in any long duration fever even in the absence of a typical clinical presentation [117].

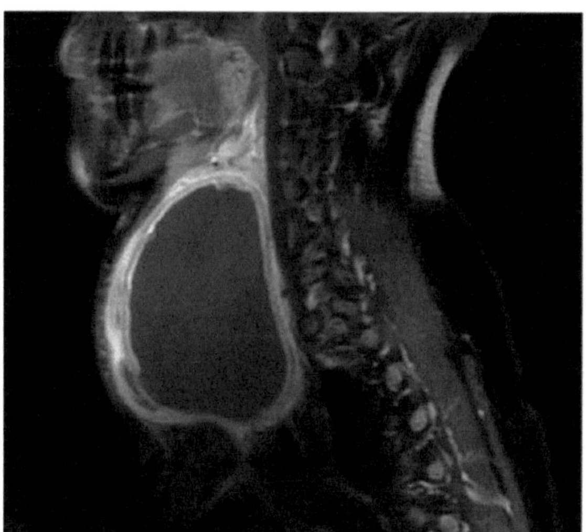

Figure 10.
Giant thyroid abscess related to postpartum brucella infection. On MRI, a cystic mass lesion, approximately 10.5 × 8.5 × 7 cm, thick-walled, slightly hyperintense on T1-oriented images, and hyperintense on T2-oriented images, with peripheral contrast following intra-venous contrasting material injection, containing thin septa, attracted attention.

3. Summary and conclusion

The WHO has recognized brucellosis as one of the NZD (Neglected zoonotic Diseases).

Brucella infection is often not recognized due to failure of most of the health care givers to realize that; the classic acute febrile illness with non-specific symptoms, may yield a multisystem disease with localized suppurative complications in at least one third of cases.

Sticking to the traditional picture of the febrile illness in a farmer or a worker with direct exposure to animals stands behind failure to diagnose a lot of serious complicated brucella cases in the community.

A new look to this endemic disease is urgently needed, especially in endemic areas and raw milk consuming communities, taking in consideration the following points:

1. In communities known to be endemic in brucellosis and known to consume non-pasteurized milk (like, the middle east and Sud America); all the community are exposed, regardless of job, culture or socioeconomic status.

2. Considering brucellosis only in febrile patients is another pitfall especially in presence of positive epidemiologic history (residency or recent travel to endemic area or recent consumption of raw milk product). In chronic, localized or complicated brucellosis the temperature is usually normal i.e. absence of fever does not exclude brucellosis.

3. The characteristic symptom of brucellosis is that no characteristic symptom. So, oriented physician with high index of suspicion is vital for early screening, diagnosis and treatment.

4. Awareness about, the possible presentation of brucellosis that can face each physician in his specialty (e.g. The ear specialist about Brucellosis as a possible cause of sensory neural hearing loss & the ophthalmologist for brucellosis as a potential cause of uveitis, etc.) is mandatory.

To conclude: Brucellosis is an infectious disease with protean clinical presentation. Fever and musculoskeletal manifestations are the commonest clinical manifestations. The disease however can involve any organ, as mentioned above. Therefore, brucellosis should be considered in the differential diagnosis of any compatible clinical scenario, particularly in areas where brucellosis is endemic.

Author details

Abdelrahman Mokhtar[1]*, Rashed Albalawi[2] and Samira M. Fallatah[3]

1 Mansoura University – Egypt and Consultant of Internal Medicine, King Salman Military Hospital, Tabuk, Saudi Arabia

2 Department and Consultant of Infectious Disease, King Salman Military Hospital, Tabuk, Saudi Arabia

3 King Salman Military Hospital, Tabuk, Saudi Arabia

*Address all correspondence to: abdelrahman_mokhtar_7@outlook.com

References

[1] Pappas G, Papadimitriou P, Akritidis N, Christou L, Tsianos V. The new global map of human brucellosis. The Lancet Infectious Diseases. 2006;**6**:91-99. DOI: 10.1016/S1473-3099(06)70382

[2] Mancini F, Bella A, Graziani C, Marianelli C, Mughini-Gras L, Pasquali P, et al. Trends of human brucellosis in Italy, 1998-2010. Epidemiology & Infection. 2014;**142**:1188-1195. DOI: 10.1017/S0950268813002227

[3] Giambartolomei V, Delpino M. Immunopathogenesis of hepatic brucellosis. Frontiers in Cellular and Infection Microbiology. 2019;**9**:423. DOI: 10.3389/fcimb.2019.00423

[4] Galińska E, Zagórski J. Brucellosis in humans – Etiology, diagnostics, clinical forms. Annals of Agricultural and Environmental Medicine. 2013;**20**(2):233-238. DOI: 10.4103/0974-2727.72149

[5] Doganay M, Aygan B. Human brucellosis: An overview. International Journal of Infectious Disease. 2003;**7**:173-182

[6] González-Espinoza G, Arce-Gorvel V, Mémet S, Gorvel J. Brucella: Reservoirs and niches in animals and humans. Pathogens. 2021;**10**:186. DOI: 10.3390/pathogens10020186

[7] Christopher S, Umapathy L, Ravikumar L. Brucellosis: Review on the recent trends in pathogenicity and laboratory diagnosis. Journal of Laboratory Physicians. 2010;**2**(2):56-60. DOI: 10.4103/0974-2727.72149

[8] Cuzdan N, Duran A, Atik T. Serological interpretation of rheumatic manifestations in brucellosis. Journal of the College of Physicians and Surgeons–Pakistan. 2022;**32**(4):503-509. DOI: 10.29271/jcpsp.2022.04.503

[9] Tali ET. Spinal infections. European Journal of Radiology. 2004;**50**(2):120-133. DOI: 10.1016/j.ejrad.2003.10.022

[10] Gotuzzo E, Alarcón G, Bocanegra T, Carrillo C, Guerra J, Rolando I, et al. Articular involvement in human brucellosis: A retrospective analysis of 304 cases. Seminars in Arthritis and Rheumatism. 1982;**12**(2):245-255. DOI: 10.1016/0049-0172(82)90064-6

[11] Farrokhi MR, Mousavi SR. Spinal brucellosis with large circumscribed paraspinal and epidural abscess formation: A case report. British Journal of Neurosurgery. 2021;**35**(6):714-718. DOI: 10.1080/02688697.2020.1789557

[12] Bozgeyik Z, Aglamis S, Bozdag PG, Denk A. Magnetic resonance imaging findings of musculoskeletal brucellosis. Clinical Imaging. 2014;**38**:719-723. DOI: 10.1016/j.clinimag.2014.04.007

[13] Esmaeilnejad-Ganji S, Esmaeilnejad-Ganji S. Osteoarticular manifestations of human brucellosis: A review. World Journal of Orthopedics. 2019;**10**(2):54-62. DOI: 10.5312/wjo.v10.i2.54

[14] Koubaa M, Maaloul I, Marrakchi C, Lahiani D, Hammami B, Mnif Z, et al. Spinal brucellosis in south of Tunisia: Review of 32 cases. The Spine Journal. 2014;**14**(8):1538-1544. DOI: 10.1016/j.spinee.2013.09.027

[15] Li T, Liu T, Jiang Z, Cui X, Sun J. Diagnosing pyogenic, brucella and tuberculous spondylitis using histopathology and MRI: A retrospective

study. Experimental Therapy Medicine. 2016;**12**(4):2069-2077. DOI: 10.3892/etm.2016.3602

[16] Al-Shahed M, Sharif H, Haddad M, Aabed M, Sammak B, Mutairi M. Imaging features of musculoskeletal brucellosis. Radiographics. 1994;**14**(2): 333-348. DOI: 10.1148/radiographics.14.2.8190957

[17] Sharif H, Aideyan O, Clark D, Madkour M, Aabed M, Mattsson T, et al. Brucellar and tuberculous spondylitis: Comparative imaging features. Radiology. 1989 May;**171**(2):419-425. DOI: 10.1148/radiology.171.2.2704806

[18] Wang Y, Gao D, Ji X, Zhang J, Wang X, Jin J, et al. When brucellosis met the assessment of spondyloarthritis international society classification criteria for spondyloarthritis: A comparative study. Clinical Rheumatology. 2019;**38**(7):1873-1880. DOI: 10.1007/s10067-019-04481-w

[19] Gheita T, Sayed S, Azkalany G, El Fishawy H, Aboul-Ezz M, Shaaban M, et al. Subclinical sacroiliitis in brucellosis. Clinical presentation and MRI findings. Zeitschrift für Rheumatologie. 2015;**74**:240-245. DOI: 10.1007/s00393-014-1465-1

[20] Mamalis I, Panagopoulos M, Papanastasiou D, Bricteux G. Sacroilitis and osteomyelitis of the humeral bone due to *Brucella melitensis* in an adolescent. Revue Médicale de Liège. 2008;**63**:742-745

[21] Turan H, Serefhanoglu K, Karadeli E, Timurkaynak F, Arslan H. A case of brucellosis with abscess of the iliacus muscle, olecranon bursitis, and sacroiliitis. International Journal of Infectious Diseases. 2009;**13**:e485-e487 10.1016/j.ijid.2009.02.002

[22] Acar A, Turhan V, Diktaş H, Oncül O, Cavuşlu S. A case of brucellosis complicated with endocarditis, pyelonephritis, sacroileitis and thyroiditis. Mikrobiyoloji Bülteni. 2009;**43**:141-145

[23] Batmaz I, Tekin R, Sariyildiz M, Deveci O, Cevik R. A case of brucellosis with simultaneous dactylitis and sacroiliitis. Journal of Medical Cases. 2012;**3**:304-307. DOI: 10.4021/jmc701w

[24] Elmas A, Ulutaş F. Peripheral arthritis and tenosynovitis in a patient with brucellosis. Cureus. 2023;**15**(2):e35292. DOI: DOI10.7759/cureus.35292

[25] Wang J, Zhang Q. Early diagnosis and treatment of acute brucellosis knee arthritis complicated by acute osteomyelitis: Two cases report. BMC Infectious Diseases. 2022;**22**:430. DOI: 10.1186/s12879-022-07392-5

[26] Guiral J, Reverie D, Carrero P. Iliopsoas bursitis due to *Brucella melitensis* infection-a case report. Acta Orthopaedica Scandinavica. 1999;**70**(5):523-524. DOI: 10.3109/17453679909000995

[27] Seçilmiş Y, Hüsrevoğlu F, Yucel D, Öztürk MA. Plantar fasciitis and bone marrow edema in brucellosis. The Journal of Pediatrics. 2017;**183**:200. DOI: 10.1016/j.jpeds.2016.12.073

[28] Traboulsi R, Uthman I, Kanj SS. Prepatellar *Brucella melitensis* bursitis: Case report and literature review. Clinical Rheumatology. 2007;**26**(11):1941-1942. DOI: 10.1007/s10067-007-0565-6

[29] Almajid F. A rare form of Brucella bursitis with negative serology: A case report and literature review. Case Reports Infectious Diseases. 2017;**2017**:9802532. DOI: 10.1155/2017/9802532

[30] Madkour M, Madkour's Brucellosis. 2nd edition. Springer-Verlag Berlin Heidelberg; 2001. 150 p. DOl: 10.1007/978-3-642-59533-2

[31] Baldane S, Sivgin S, Alkan TS, Kurnaz F, Pala C, Keklik M, et al. An atypical presentation of brucellosis in a patient with isolated thrombocytopenia complicated with upper gastrointestinal tract bleeding. Case Reports in Medicine. 2012;**2012**:473784. DOI: 10.1155/2012/473784. Epub 2012 Oct 18. PMID: 23118764; PMCID: PMC3483866

[32] Williams R, Crossley K. Acute and chronic hepatic involvement of brucellosis. Gastroenterology. 1982;**83**:455-458

[33] Speiser L, Hsieh L, Huang SS, Bittencourt C, Forthal D. Brucellosis presenting as cholecystitis: A case report and literature review. Open Forum Infectious Diseases. 15 Jul 2019;**6**(10):ofz334. DOI: 10.1093/ofid/ofz334. PMID: 31660329; PMCID: PMC6765347

[34] Correa A, Zamora I. Brucella terminal ileitis: A rare cause of intestinal obstruction. International Journal of Research in Medical Sciences. 2021;**9**:2831-2834. DOI: 10.18203/2320-6012.ijrms20213429

[35] Stemer E, Levy N, Potasman I, Jaffe M, Boss J. Brucellosis as a cause of severe colitis. American Journal of Gastroenterology. 1991;**86**:917-919

[36] Seoud M, Kanj S, Habli M, Araj G, Khalil A. Brucella pelvic Tubo-ovarian abscess mimicking a pelvic malignancy. Scandinavian Journal of Infectious Diseases. 2003;**35**(4):277-278. DOI: 10.1080/00365540310005396

[37] Berber I, Erkurt M, Yetkin F, Unlu S, Yılmaz S, Bentli R, et al. A rare disease in the differential diagnosis of acute pancreatitis: Acute brucellosis. Internal Medicine. 2014;**53**:2401-2404. DOI: 10.2169/internalmedicine.53.2510

[38] Wang M, Zhu Q, Yang Q, Li W, Wang X, Liu W, et al. Intestinal brucellosis associated with celiac artery and superior mesenteric artery stenosis and with ileum mucosa and submucosa thickening: A case report. Medicine (Baltimore). Jan 2017;**96**(2):e5893. DOI: 10.1097/MD.0000000000005893. PMID: 28079834; PMCID: PMC5266196

[39] Güçlü M, Yakar T, Habeoğlu M. Sponatneous bacterial peritonitis and chylothorax related to brucella infection in a cirrhotic patient. European Journal of General Medicine. 2007;**4**:201-204

[40] Altunçekiç Yildirim A, Kurt C, Çetinkol Y. Brucellosis with rare complications and review of diagnostic tests: A case report. Journal of Medical Case Reports. 2022;**16**:492. DOI: 10.1186/s13256-022-03702-2

[41] Ben Salah R, Frikha F, Kallel R, Boudawara T, Bahloul Z. Un exceptional cause of lymphocytic colitis: Brucellosis. Hematology and Medical Oncology. 2017;**2**:1-2. DOI: 10.15761/HMO.1000134

[42] Moignea F, Vitry T, Gérômeb P, Vinurel N, Ducerfd C, Rodee A, et al. Necrotizing pseudotumoral hepatic brucelloma: Imaging-pathologic correlation. Diagnostic and Interventional Imaging. 2016;**97**:243-246. DOI: 10.1016/j.diii.2014.08.007

[43] Heller T, Bélard S, Wallrauch C, Carretto E, Lissandrin R, Filice C, et al. Patterns of Hepatosplenic Brucella abscesses on cross-sectional imaging: A review of clinical and imaging features. The American Journal of Tropical Medicine and Hygiene. 2015;**93**:761-766. DOI: 10.4269/ajtmh.15-0225

[44] Jin M, Fan Z, Gao R, Li X, Gao Z, Wang Z. Research progress on

complications of Brucellosis. Frontiers in Cellular and Infection Microbiology. 2023;**13**:1136674. DOI: 10.3389/fcimb.2023.1136674

[45] Koruk S, Erdem H, Koruk I, Erbay A, Tezer-Tekce Y, Erbay A, et al. Management of Brucella endocarditis: Results of the Gulhane study. International Journal of Antimicrobial Agents. 2012;**40**(2):145-150. DOI: 10.1016/j.ijantimicag.2012.04.009

[46] Chourmouzi D, Boulogianni G, Kalomenopoulou M, Kanellos I, Drevelegas A. Brucella liver abscess; imaging approach, differential diagnosis, and therapeutic management: A case report. Cases Journal. 2009;**2**:7143. DOI: 10.4076/1757-1626-2-7143

[47] Elfadil O, Al-Amri K, Al-Wahaibi K, Osman A, Al-Wahshi Y. Fatal Brucella endocarditis in a middle-aged male: Lessons on diagnostic and therapeutic challenges. SN Comprehensive Clinical Medicine. 2021;**3**:210-212. DOI: Doi.org/10.1007/s42399-020-00669-3

[48] Shawky H. Brucella endocarditis. Heart Views. 2006;**7**:111-114. Available from: https://www.heartviews.org/text.asp?2006/7/3/111/63924

[49] Tammiraju I. A review of Brucella endocarditis. Indian Journal of Cardiovascular Diseases in Women. 2021;**6**:256-260. DOI: 10.1055/s-0041-1742212

[50] Raju IT, Solanki R, Patnaik AN, Barik RC, Kumari NR, Gulati AS. Brucella endocarditis - a series of five case reports. Indian Heart Journal. Jan-Feb 2013;**65**(1):72-77. DOI: 10.1016/j.ihj.2012.12.017. Epub 2013 Jan 2. PMID: 23438616; PMCID: PMC3860836

[51] Peery T, Belter F. Brucellosis and heart disease. II. Fatal brucellosis: A review of the literature and report of new cases. The American Journal of Pathology. 1960;**36**(6):673-697

[52] Keshtkar-Jahromi M, Razavi SM, Gholamin S, Keshtkar-Jahromi M, Hossain M, Sajadi MM. Medical versus medical and surgical treatment for brucella endocarditis. The Annals of Thoracic Surgery. 2012;**94**(6):2141-2146. DOI: 10.1016/j.athoracsur.2012.07.006

[53] Li X, Wang T, Wang Y, Xie S, Tan W, Li P. Short- and long-term follow-up outcomes of patients with Brucella endocarditis: A systematic review of 207 Brucella endocarditis cases. Bioengineered. 2021;**12**(1):5162-5172. DOI: 10.1080/21655979.2021.1962683

[54] Pettersson B, Coselli S, Hussain T, Griffin B, Blackstone H, Gordon M, et al. AATS surgical treatment of infective endocarditis consensus guidelines. The Journal of Thoracic and Cardiovascular Surgery. 2017;**153**(6):1241-1258.e29. DOI: 10.1016/j.jtcvs.2016.09.093

[55] Taamallah K, Hammami F, Gharsallah H, Koubaa M, Ben Jemaa M, Fehri W. Brucella prosthetic valve endocarditis: A systematic review. Journal of the Saudi Heart Association. 2021;**33**(3):Article 3. DOI: 10.37616/2212-5043.1257

[56] Gatselis N, Konstantinos P, Makaritsis K, Gabranis I, Stefos A, Karanikas K, et al. Unusual cardiovascular complications of brucellosis presenting in two men: Two case reports and a review of the literature. Journal of Medical Case Reports. 2011;**5**:22. Available from: http://www.jmedicalcasereports.com/content/5/1/22

[57] Jubber S, Gunawardana R, Lulu R. Acute pulmonary edema in Brucella myocarditis and interstitial pneumonitis. Chest. 1990;**97**(4):1008-1009. DOI: 10.1378/chest.97.4.1008

[58] He Y, Wei C, Yun S, Wei J, Pu Z, Dai P. A case report of rare complication of brucellosis infection: Myocarditis and pneumonitis. The Journal of International Medical Research. 2023;**51**(3):3000605231163818. DOI: 10.1177/03000605231163818

[59] Bhatty S, Kumar P, Javed B, Zafar A. A rare presentation of brucellosis as myocarditis. Cureus. 2020;**12**(11):e11345. DOI: 10.7759/cureus.11345

[60] Albushra Y, Ahmed A. Rare presentation of brucellosis. Journal of Bacteriology and Parasitology. 2013;**2013**:5. DOI: 10.4172/2155-9597.S5-006

[61] Crosby E, Liosa L, Micro Quesada M, Carillo C, Gotuzzo E. Hematologic changes in brucellosis. The Journal of Infectious Diseases. 1984;**150**:419-424. DOI: 10.1093/infdis/150.3.419

[62] Sari I, Altuntas F, Hacioglu S, Kocyigit I, Sevinc A, Sacar S, et al. A multicenter retrospective study defining the clinical and hematological manifestations of brucellosis and pancytopenia in a large series: Hematological malignancies, the unusual cause of pancytopenia in patients with brucellosis. American Journal of Hematology. 2008;**83**:334-339. DOI: 10.1002/ajh.21098

[63] Ajlouni M, Shaker K. Hematological manifestation of human brucellosis. Qatar Medical Journal. 1998;**1**(2):41-43. DOI: 10.5339/qmj.1998.2.15

[64] Chang C, Beutler BD, Ulanja MB, Uche C, Zdrnja M. Brucellosis presenting with febrile pancytopenia: An atypical presentation of a common disease and review of brucellosis. Case Reports in Infectious Diseases. 4 Jan 2021;**2021**:2067570. DOI: 10.1155/2021/2067570. PMID: 33489391; PMCID: PMC7801079

[65] Balın ŞÖ, Tartar AS, Akbulut A. The predictive role of haematological parameters in the diagnosis of osteoarticular brucellosis. African Health Science. 2018;**18**(4):988-994. DOI: 10.4314/ahs.v18i4.19

[66] Jiao P, Chu W, Ren G, Hou J, Li Y, Xing L. Expression of eosinophils be beneficial to early clinical diagnosis of brucellosis. International Journal of Clinical and Experimental Medicine. 2015;**8**(10):19491-19495

[67] Kaya S, Elaldi N, Deveci O, Eskazan A, Bekcibasi M, Hosoglu S. Cytopenia in adult brucellosis patients. Indian Journal of Medical Research. 2018;**147**(1):73-80. DOI: 10.4103/ijmr.IJMR_542_15

[68] Meena DS, Sonwal VS, Rohila AK, Meena V. Acute brucellosis presenting as an autoimmune hemolytic anemia. Case Reports in Infectious Diseases. 25 Oct 2018;**2018**:1030382. DOI: 10.1155/2018/1030382. PMID: 30498608; PMCID: PMC6222226

[69] Eskazan A, Dal M, Kaya S, Dal T, Ayyildiz O, Soysal T. Two cases of autoimmune Hemolytic Anemia secondary to brucellosis: A review of Hemolytic disorders in patients with brucellosis. Internal Medicine. 2014;**53**:1153-1158. DOI: 10.2169/internalmedicine.53.0936

[70] Koçak S, Dikmetaş C, Dündar Z, Erdemir E, Keşli R. Acute deep venous thrombosis associated with acute brucellosis: A case report. JAEMCR. 2012;**3**:118-120. DOI: 10.5505/jaemcr.2012.96967

[71] Korkmaz P, Kartal E. Skin manifestations associated with brucellosis. EMJ Dermatology. 2016;**4**(1):119-125

[72] Milionis H, Christou L, Elisaf M. Cutaneous manifestations in brucellosis:

Case report and review of the literature. Infection. 2000;**28**:124-126

[73] Metin A, Akdeniz H, Buzgan T, Delice I. Cutaneous findings encountered in brucellosis and review of the literature. International Journal of Dermatology. 2001:434-438. DOI: 10.1046/j.1365-4362.2001.01237.x

[74] Rudenko M. The role of infection and autoimmunity in Urticaria and angioedema as a common entity. EMJ Allergy Immunology. 2021;**6**(1):79-85. DOI: DOI/10.33590/emjallergyimmunol/20-00148

[75] Bouferraa Y, Bou Zerdan M, Hamouche R, Azar E, Afif C, Jabbour R. Neurobrucellosis: Brief review. The Neurologist. 2021;**26**(6):248-252. DOI: 10.1097/NRL.0000000000000348

[76] Mahajan S, Sharma A, Kaushik M, Raina R, Sharma S, Banyal V. Neurobrucellosis: An often forgotten cause of chronic meningitis. Tropical Doctor. 2016;**46**(1):54-56. DOI: 10.1177/0049475515592571

[77] Dreshaj S, Shala N, Dreshaj G, Ramadani N, Ponosheci A. Clinical manifestations in 82 neurobrucellosis patients from Kosovo. Mater Sociomedicine. 2016;**28**(6):408-411. DOI: 10.5455/msm.2016.28.408-411

[78] Soares C, Angelim A, Brandão C, Santos R, Mehta R, Silva M. Neurobrucellosis: The great mimicker. Revista da Sociedade Brasileira de Medicina Tropical. 2022;**55**:e05672021. DOI: 10.1590/0037-8682-0567-2021

[79] Sengoz G, Yasar K, Yildirim F, Nazlican O. Sensorineural hearing loss in neurobrucellosis. Neurosciences. 2008;**13**(3):299-301. Available from: http://nsj.org.sa/content/13/3/299

[80] Gündüz T, Tektürk P, Yapıcı Z, Kürtüncü M, Somer A, Törün S, et al. Characteristics of isolated spinal cord involvement in neurobrucellosis with no corresponding MRI activity: A case report and review of the literature. Journal of Neurological Science. 2017;**372**:305-306. DOI: 10.1016/j.jns.2016.11.076

[81] Krishnan C, Kaplin A, Graber J, Darman J, Kerr D. Recurrent transverse myelitis following neurobrucellosis: Immunologic features and beneficial response to immunosuppression. Journal of Neurovirology. 2005;**11**(2):225-231. DOI: 10.1080/13550280590922801

[82] Abuzinadah A, Milyani H, Alshareef A, Bamaga A, Alshehri A, Kurdi M. Brucellosis causing subacute motor polyradiculopathy and the pathological correlation of pseudomyopathic electromyography: A case report. Clinical Neurophysiology Practice. 2020;**5**:130-134. DOI: 10.1016/j.cnp.2020.05.003

[83] Alanazi A, Al Najjar S, Madkhali J, Al Malik Y, Al-Khalaf A, Alharbi A. Acute brucellosis with a Guillain-Barre syndrome-like presentation: A case report and literature review. Infectious Disease Report. 2021;**3**(1):1-10. DOI: 10.3390/idr13010001

[84] Shah I, Kawoos Y, Sanai B, Rabyang S, Banday D. Neurobrucellosis presenting as acute psychosis. Journal of Neuroscience in Rural Practice. 2018;**9**(4):644-646. DOI: 10.4103/jnrp.jnrp_16_18

[85] Alnaji A. Dormant and subclinical bacterial infections of brain may Be the cause behind all epilepsies including that due to post-traumatic or associated with space occupying lesion SOL. Journal of Neurology and Experimental

Neuroscience. 2017;**2017**. DOI: 10.29011/JNNS-125. 100025

[86] Yilmaz M, Ozaras R, Ozturk R, Mert A, Tabak F, Aktuglu Y. Epileptic seizure: An atypical presentation in an adolescent boy with neurobrucellosis. Scandinavian Journal of Infectious Diseases. 2002;**34**(8):623-625. DOI: 10.1080/00365540210147561

[87] Tarfarosh S, Manzoor M. Neurological manifestations of brucellosis in an Indian population. Cureus. 2016;**8**(7):e684. DOI: 10.7759/cureus.684

[88] Dar W, Wani M, Mir F, Asimi R, Yaqoob A, Raina A, et al. Isolated neurobrucellosis-characteristic clinical and laboratory features. Acta Neurologica Belgica. 2022;**122**(6):1469-1475. DOI: 10.1007/s13760-020-01573-2

[89] Hatipoglu C, Bilgin G, Tulek N, Kosar U. Pulmonary involvement in brucellosis. The Journal of Infection. 2005;**51**(2):116-119. DOI: 10.1016/j.jinf.2004.10.004

[90] Mutlu P, Mirici N, Hunerel O. Lung involvement in brucellosis. Journal of Lung, Pulmonary and Respiratory Research. 2017;**4**(2):63-65. DOI: 10.15406/jlprr.2017.04.00124

[91] García-Rodriguez A, García-Sánchez J, Muñoz Bellido J, de Ortiz Tabla V, Barbero J. Review of pulmonary brucellosis: A case report on brucellar pulmonary empyema. Diagnostic Microbiology and Infectious Disease. 1988;**11**(1):53-60

[92] Patel P, Al-Suhaibani H, Al-Aska A, Kolawole T, Al-Kassimi F. The chest radiograph in brucellosis. Clinical Radiology. 1988;**39**(1):39-41. DOI: 10.1016/S0009-9260(88)80336-2

[93] Pappas G, Bosilkovski M, Akritidis N, Mastora M, Krteva L, Tsianos E. Brucellosis and the respiratory system. Clinical Infectious Diseases. 2003;**37**(7):e95-e99. DOI: 10.1086/378125

[94] Erdem H, Inan A, Elaldi N, Tekin R, Gulsun S, Ataman-Hatipoglu C, et al. Respiratory system involvement in brucellosis: The results of the Kardelen study. Chest. 2014 Jan;**145**(1):87-94. DOI: 10.1378/chest.13-0240

[95] Batirel A, Regmi S, Singh P, Mert A, Konety B, Kumar R. Urological infections in the developing world: An increasing problem in developed countries. World Journal of Urology. 2020;**38**(11):2681-2691. DOI: 10.1007/s00345-020-03120-3

[96] Papatsoris A, Mpadra F, Karamouzis M, Frangides C. Endemic brucellar epididymo-orchitis: A 10-year experience. International Journal of Infectious Diseases. 2002;**6**(4):309-313. DOI: 10.1016/s1201-9712(02)90166-9

[97] Karabakan M, Akdemir S, Akdemir A, Erkmen A, Kayabas U. A rare case of prostatic brucellosis mimicking prostate cancer. Urology Journal. 2014;**11**(6):1987-1988

[98] Otaraeva B, Tsallagova L, Bazaev V, Fidarov F. Brucellosis: Problems of female and male organs. International Transaction Journal of Engineering, Management, & Applied Sciences & Technologies. 2022;**13**(8):1-11. Available from: http://TUENGR.COM/V13/13A8I.pdf. DOI: 10.14456/ITJEMAST.2022.156

[99] Kurdoglu M, Cetin O, Kurdoglu Z, Akdeniz H. The effect of brucellosis on Women's health and reproduction. International Journal of Women's Health and Reproduction Sciences. 2015;**3**(4): 176-183. DOI: 10.15296/ijwhr.2015.38

[100] Gurleyik E. Breast abscess as a complication of human brucellosis. The Breast Journal. 2006;**12**(4):375-376. DOI: 10.1111/j.1075-122X.2006.00281.x

[101] Nemenqani D, Yaqoob N, Khoja H. Breast brucellosis in Taif, Saudi Arabia: Cluster of six cases with emphasis on FNA evaluation. Journal of Infection in Developing Countries. 2009;**3**(4):255-259. DOI: 10.3855/jidc.121

[102] Alfouzan W, Al-Sahali S, Sultan H, Dhar R. Classical presentation of acute pyelonephritis in a case of brucellosis. Case Reports in Nephrology and Dialysis. 2016;**6**(2):83-88. DOI: 10.1159/000446393

[103] Ibrahim A, Awad R, Shetty S, Saad M, Bilal N. Genito-urinary complications of brucellosis. British Journal of Urology. 1988;**61**(4):294-298. DOI: 10.1111/j.1464-410x.1988.tb13960.x

[104] Rolando I, Olarte L, Vilchez G, Marina M, Otero L, Paris M, et al. Ocular manifestations associated with brucellosis: A 26-year experience in Peru. Clinical Infectious Diseases. 2008;**46**(9):1338-1345. DOI: 10.1086/529442

[105] Puig S, Heatley J, Arenas F, Guerrero IG. Ocular complications in brucellosis. American Journal of Ophthalmology. 1953;**36**(5):675-689. DOI: 10.1016/0002-9394(53)90310-9

[106] Ghasemi R, Meraat H, Pahlevan A. A review on ophthalmic manifestations of brucellosis and reporting a case of ophthalmic brucellosis. Iranian Red Crescent Medical Journal. 2011;**13**(5):352-353

[107] Adibelli F, Altinbay D. Low vision aid for a patient with the optic neuropathy due to neuro-brucellosis. International Journal of Ophthalmology and Clinical Research. 2018;**5**:96. DOI: 10.23937/2378-346X/1410096

[108] Sahin O, Pelit A, Turunc T, Akova Y. Ophthalmoparesis, papillitis and premacular hemorrhage in a case with endocarditis: A rare presentation of brucellosis. Indian Journal of Ophthalmology. 2010;**58**(5):164-166. DOI: 10.4103/0301-4738.60098

[109] Sahin O. Ocular Manifestations of Brucellosis. In: Updates on Brucellosis. London, UK: InTech; 2015. DOI: 10.5772/61475

[110] Haran M, Agarwal A, Kupfer Y, Seneviratne C, Chawla K, Tessler S. Brucellosis presenting as septic shock. BMJ Case Reports. 2011;**2011**: bcr1220103586. DOI: 10.1136/bcr.12.2010.3586

[111] Darazam I, Imanzade F, Rabiei M, Shokouhi S, Erdem H. Brucellosis in patients with neoplasm: A research article. 2021. DOI: 10.21203/rs.3.rs-191086/v1.LicenseCCBY4.0

[112] Akdemir Z, Karaman E, Akdeniz H, Alptekin C, Arslan H. Giant thyroid abscess related to postpartum brucella infection. Case Reports in Infectious Diseases. 2015;**2015**. Article ID 646209, 3 pages. DOI: 10.1155/2015/646209

[113] Estagnasié C, Surgers L, Berdugo K, Monnier-Cholley L, Schmidt M, Meynard J, et al. Recurrence of brucellosis on breast implants. Infectious Diseases. Mar 2023;**53**(2):104644. DOI: 10.1016/j.idnow.2023.01.004

[114] de la Fuente A, Sanchez JR, Uriz J, et al. Infection of a pacemaker by *Brucella melitensis*. Texas Heart Institute Journal. 1997;**24**(2):129-130

[115] Luc M, Armingeat T, Pham T, Legré V, Lafforgue P. Chronic Brucella infection of the humerus diagnosed after a spontaneous fracture. Joint, Bone, Spine. 2008;**75**(2):229-231. DOI: 10.1016/j.jbspin.2007.04.024

[116] Zachou K, Papamichalis PA, Dalekos GN. Severe pharyngitis in stockbreeders: An unusual presentation of brucellosis. Occupational Medicine (London). 2008;**58**(4):305-307. DOI: 10.1093/occmed/kqn020

[117] Massoud M, Kerbage F, Antoun L, Merhi R, Hallit S, Hallit R. Brucellosis: A lymphoma-like presentation. Asian Pacific Journal of Tropical Medicine. 2017;**10**(8):833-834. DOI: 10.1016/j.apjtm.2017.07.025

Chapter 4

Perspective Chapter: Zoonosis – Brucellosis a Clinically Relevant Bacterial Disease

Shahzadi Gulafshan, Rajeev Singh, Manoj M. Murhekar and Gaurav Raj Dwivedi

Abstract

In 2020–2022, infectious diseases were the major causes of infection and death globally. Many viral and bacterial diseases are starting to emerge/reemerge frequently. The zoonotic infections were reported to be dominant in a few decades. Now the holistic one-health approach is the need of the hour to tackle the emerging and reemerging pathogens by extensive and heedless use of antimicrobials, lack of novel antimicrobials, and unavailability of appropriate vaccines increased the severity of pathogens. Brucellosis is a well-known zoonotic disease also called undulant fever, Malta fever, Mediterranean fever, etc. Many components of the genus Brucella will be discussed in this chapter, namely pathogenesis, genes/proteins responsible for diseases in animal and humans, available treatment options, drug resistance phenomenon, etc.

Keywords: Brucella, zoonosis, one health, virulence factor, human brucellosis, antimicrobial resistance

1. Introduction

In developing and underdeveloped world, communicable diseases are the key cause of illness and death. Among the wide range of infectious diseases, bacterial infectious diseases are concerned due to prevalence of the drug resistance [1]. After the Industrial Revolution, about 350 infectious emerging/reemerging pathogens evolved since 1940 [2]. The majority of these events are linked with animals [3]. Recently, accelerated climatic, demographic, and technological changes due to anthropogenic activities have transformed the risks associated with infectious diseases [4]. Due to limited treatment options, these resistant bacteria put an extra burden and cost and boost infection severity many times [5]. Gram-negative bacteria are one of the major cause of neglected tropical diseases [6].

Human brucellosis poses serious challenges for scientists and clinicians to understand the pathogenic mechanisms of Brucella spp., identification of severity markers for disease progression, regimen for treatment, and developmental progress of advanced treatment arsenals [7]. Brucellosis is a zoonotic disease that manifests systemic symptoms by involving several organs [8]. Major causes of infection were reported to be consumption of raw dairy products and occupational contact. Brucella, a gram-negative coccobacillus reported as a slow grower *in vitro* [9]. Six species of brucella are so far reported to cause infection in humans [10]. With the backdrop of neglected tropical diseases and a traditional biological weapon make these bacteria a serious health issue [8]. It was the subject of vast bioweapon research topics in the past and a category B pathogens [8]. This book chapter was conceptualized on the prevalent strain, epidemiology, virulence, pathogenesis, genes/proteins responsible for diseases in animals and humans, available treatment options, drug resistance phenomenon, etc. This book chapter summarizes current knowledge of the pathogenic mechanisms, therapeutic options, and the situation of developing countries regarding human brucellosis.

2. Zoonosis

Nature has created the planet in such a way that the health of all the creatures, that is, humans, animals, and environment are linked with the health of each other [11]. The interaction among them is not always of benefit but also has some negative influences on animals, plants, environment as well as on humans. Zoonoses are a great example of this. Etymologically, the word zoonosis has been picked up from the Greek dictionary and is made up of the union of two words, that is., zoon, which means animal, and nosos, meaning disease or illness or unwellness [12].

Zoonoses are those diseases in humans that are acquired by direct or indirect communication with infected animals [13]. In other words, zoonoses are the diseases that are gifted from infected wild animals to human in order to interfere or grab their natural habitat (as these animals are the natural home for various pathogens and these pathogens rarely cause diseases in them). The pathogens responsible for zoonosis could either be bacteria, viruses, protozoa, or parasites [3].

Humans can screw up with these pathogens either by direct contact, indirect contact, or through vectors. When a person gets infected after contact with the blood, saliva, urine, mucous, feces, or other fluids of infected animal, then it is considered as direct transmission of disease, for example, Ebola virus disease (EVD) [14]. Person can fall for zoonotic disease even after not having any direct interaction with infected animals but living in the area where infected animals live or contact with fomites are other means of infection. Besides this, zoonoses also transmit from the consumption of food that is derived from the infected animals, for example, milk, milk products, and meat, which is called foodborne zoonosis, for example, brucellosis [4]. Many vectors, such as mosquitoes, fleas, mites, and ticks, play a crucial role in the transmission of diseases from animals to other animals and human, for example, Japanese encephalitis, plague, scrub typhus, etc. [15–17].

3. Concept of one health

One health is a collaborative, multisectoral, and transdisciplinary approach and is built to collaborative work of all disciplines of health (human, animal, and environment) only for the sake of health regardless of their disciplines to attain an optimal yield of health [18]. According to one health approach, the health of human has a direct link with the health of animals and their shared environment. In other words, the healthier the animal and environment are, the healthier humans will be (**Figure 1**).

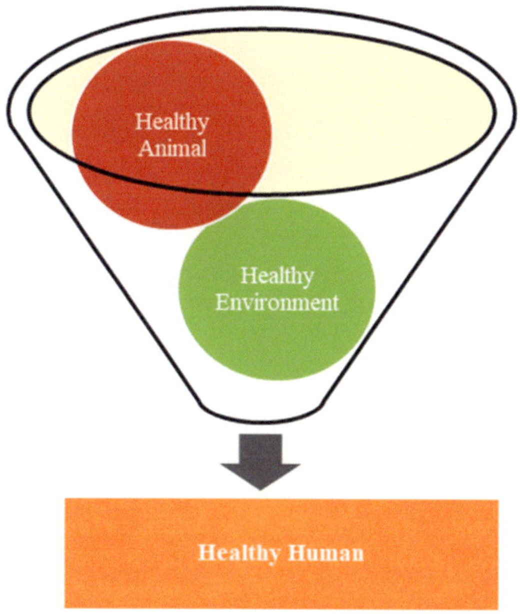

Figure 1.
One health concept.

About 1415 species of pathogens have so far been identified by researchers that are causing diseases in human beings. Of those 1415, 868 (61%) are zoonoses and 75 (12%) are emerging infectious diseases (EIDs). EIDs are cases of infectious diseases with a significant increment of their incidence in past two decades [19, 20]. According to WHO, among all the emerging infectious diseases, 75% are zoonotic in nature. Besides emerging infectious diseases (EIDs), reemerging infectious diseases (REIDs) are also reported as a threat to human beings. REIDs are pathogenic diseases with a sudden rise after a significant decline in infections [21].

4. Brucellosis

Brucellosis, a zoonosis, which is transmitted directly or indirectly to humans by infected animals. Many names have been given in the past to the diseases on the basis of the name of the place where it was endemic, or whom it is infecting, that is, animal or human, or on the name of any event that was going at that time or on the name of its discoverer. These names are remittent fever (body temperature above normal all day), undulant fever (wave pattern body temperature, that is, sudden rise and fall), Mediterranean fever, Maltese fever, Gibraltar fever, Crimean fever, goat fever, and Bang's disease [9].

5. Genus Brucella

Brucellae are gram-negative, non-capsulated, aerobic, intracellular, and nonmotile bacteria. They are very small in size (0.5–0.7 × 0.6–1.5 μm) and coccobacillus in shape [22]. Brucella cells do not have plasmids instead, they possess two circular

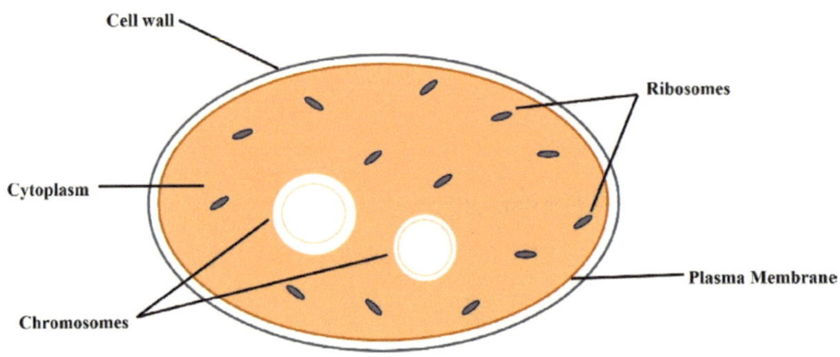

Figure 2.
A typical Brucella cell.

chromosomes of different sizes. The larger chromosome is of 2.1 Mb and the smaller one is of 1.2 Mb. Hence, they are known to have 3.3 Mb average genome size (**Figure 2**). The members of the genus Brucella belong to the family Brucellaceae, class α-proteobacteria and order Rhizobiales. Morphologically, they are non-flagellated and cannot move but, in some species, genome sequencing has confirmed the presence of flagellar genes. Functionally, the flagellum is known for the motility of the organism but here in the genus Brucella they act as a virulence factor [23–25].

Sir David Bruce had discovered the bacteria in the eighteenth century but in reality, the genus Brucella came into existence in the early nineteenth century. To know, what made this journey too long, it is necessary to contemplate its historical background.

6. Journey of Brucella

Marston, a British army physician of Malta Island, in 1859 segregated a Mediterranean remittent fever from other different prevalent fevers. When Sir David Bruce (pathologist and microbiologist) was in his service at Malta, a British soldier died due to Malta fever. He then started his study on patients who were died with Malta fever in the year 1866–1867. During this period, he successfully isolated an organism from the spleen of the cadaver and established a relation between this organism and Marston's described fever in 1887 [26]. Because the bacteria seem very small and round in shape so Bruce's assistant, Surgeon Captain Matthew Louis Hughes named the organism *Micrococcus melitensis* and to disease undulant fever [27]. But the source of the bacteria was still hidden and it was first described by the Maltese scientist and archeologist Themistocles Zammit in 1905. According to him the bacteria causing Malta fever in Maltese is actually coming from the consumption of infected goat milk [28].

On the other hand, in 1897, independent of Bruce work, Danish veterinarian Bernhard Bang, isolated rod-shaped bacteria that were causing a spontaneous abortion in cows and named the disease Bang's disease. He classified the bacteria as bacillus. This was another species of Brucella known as *Brucella abortus* [29].

In 1906, Alice C. Evans, a bacteriologist in America, during her study on the etiological agent of Bang's disease, she realized there was no difference between Bruce's cocci and bang's bacillus. Then she finds they are neither coccus nor bacillus, that is, they are not two different organisms but one coccobacillus. Evans then changed the bacteria's name from Micrococcus to Brucella in 1920 in the honor of Bruce's work [30].

Scientists have discovered a total of 12 species in genus Brucella till date [31]. All of them have some definite host with whom they reside and spread disease. Moreover, some species also have biovars. Biovars are the subdivision of the species in which strains of a species differ biochemically and physiologically from each other. *B. melitensis, B. abortus,* and *B. suis* contain 3, 7, and 5 biovars, respectively. Earlier, *B. abortus* was known to have 8 biovars but later it was found that the biovar 7 is actually the combination of the biovar 3 and 5. Hence, they are now considered to have only 7 biovars [32].

Prior, it was known that terrestrial mammals are the only reservoir of this bacteria. However, it is also infecting aquatic mammals was came to light in 1994 when one of its strains was found in the aborted fetus of a marine bottlenose dolphin (*Tursiops truncatus*). Afterward, many other species were isolated from the marine mammals [33, 34]. The details of the Brucella species known till date are given below.

i. *Brucella melitensis:* They are distributed globally and are highly pathogenic for humans. Sheep and goats are their usual host. However, they can also infect camels and cattle. *Brucella melitensis* has three biovars. In isolation, species form smooth colony on a culture plate that defines bacteria possess a smooth type of Lipopolysaccharide (LPS) [31].

ii. *Brucella abortus:* Infection caused by *B. abortus* differs from other species because it has the capability to become chronic. Cattles are their preferred host but they can also infect other mammals such as camel, Bison, horse, and elk. *B. abortus* contains seven biovars. Their pathogenicity to humans is high but less than *B. melitensis*. Along with the respiratory or oral route, *B. abortus* can also transmit through arthropods like ticks. They are also distributed worldwide [35].

iii. *Brucella suis:* It was discovered in 1929 by Huddleson and is the first strain that was used as a biological weapon in 1952 in the United States [8, 10]. They are divided into five biovars, that is, 1 to 5. All biovars are highly specific to their host. Biovars 1 and 3 are concerned with infecting humans and are highly pathogenic and virulent. However, biovar 2 has nothing to do with human infection. Biovars 1, 2, and 3 are known to infect members of the family Suidae. Moreover, Biovar 2 is also known to infect Hares along with Suidae [36].

iv. *Brucella ovis:* This species was first found in New Zealand by M. B. Buddle while searching for the cause of abortion and epididymitis in ovine or sheep and named the organism as *B. ovis* in 1956. Sheep are their preferred host and organisms are responsible for epididymitis in them. They are non-pathogenic to humans and have no biovars. Members of the species have rough LPS makes them less virulent. Stable flies (*Stomoxys calcitrans*) are another source of transmission of infection [37].

v. *Brucella neotome*: It was first isolated from desert wood rats (*Neotoma lepida*) in the United States of America (USA) in year 1957. Earlier, it was known that they do not infect humans and are non-pathogenic like some other species. Later, after about 60 years, its zoonotic nature was revealed. At present, no biovars have been discovered for this species [38].

vi. *Brucella canis:* This strain was first isolated from aborted tissues of Beagle (a breed of dog) and vaginal discharge of canines in the year between 1966 and 1967. However, *B. canis* is a common cause of brucellosis in dogs but in a small proportion of cases other species, such as *B. melitensis, B. abortus*, or *B. suis,* have also been seen for causing the disease. Disease in dogs is concerned with the reproductive disorder while in humans it is concerned with febrile syndrome and/or with some organ manifestation [39].

vii. *Brucella ceti:* They are the first Brucella strain known to infect aquatic animals. It was first isolated in 1994 from aborted fetus of a bottlenose dolphin [33]. They specifically infect members of the infraorder cetacea (whales, dolphins, and porpoises).

viii. *Brucella pinnipedialis:* Another brucella strain from the Scottland was discovered in the same year in which *B. ceti* was discovered from the stranded harbored seal (*Phoca vitulina*) and was named *B. pinnipedialis* [40].

ix. *Brucella microti:* It was first isolated in the late twentieth century from common voles (*Microtus arvalis*) in South Moravia, Czech Republic [41]. Unlike other species, it lives in soil [42].

x. *Brucella inopinata:* It was first recognized in the women with breast transplants showing symptoms of brucellosis. A Brucella strain ($BO1^T$) was isolated from her breast transplant wound in the year 2010 and was called *B. inopinata* [43].

xi. *Brucella papionis:* Two strains (F8/08-60(T) and F8/08-61) were discovered in the year 2014 for the first time in primates (baboons) that were facing stillbirth and named *B. papionis* [44].

xii. *Brucella vulpis:* Two isolates (strains F60T and F965) in the year 2016 from the mandibular lymph node of red fox (*Vulpes vulpes)* were discovered in Austria. Hence, they were named *B. vulpis* [45].

7. Epidemiology

Brucellosis is distributed almost every corner of the earth but it is commonly found in Mediterranean countries, the Middle East, India, Mexico, Central Asia, and Central and South America. Brucellosis is a notifiable disease in most of countries (**Figure 3**) [46]. The prevalence of infection with *B. melitensis* has the highest prevalence in the world than other species. The incidence of Brucella cases in developing countries is comparably higher than in developed countries due to poor health infrastructure, unprotected farm practices, etc. According to the data analysis of the incidence of brucellosis 2017, Kenya, Yemen, Syria, and Greece are ranked 1st, 2nd, 3rd, and 4th, respectively. However, Sweden, Finland, Germany, the United Kingdom, and Belgium are Brucella-free countries but they still report few cases [47, 48].

Any person can get infected with bacteria but people at higher risk are those who live in direct exposure to animals due to their occupation. This includes veterinarians, slaughterhouse workers, meat packers, laboratory workers, and animal hunters.

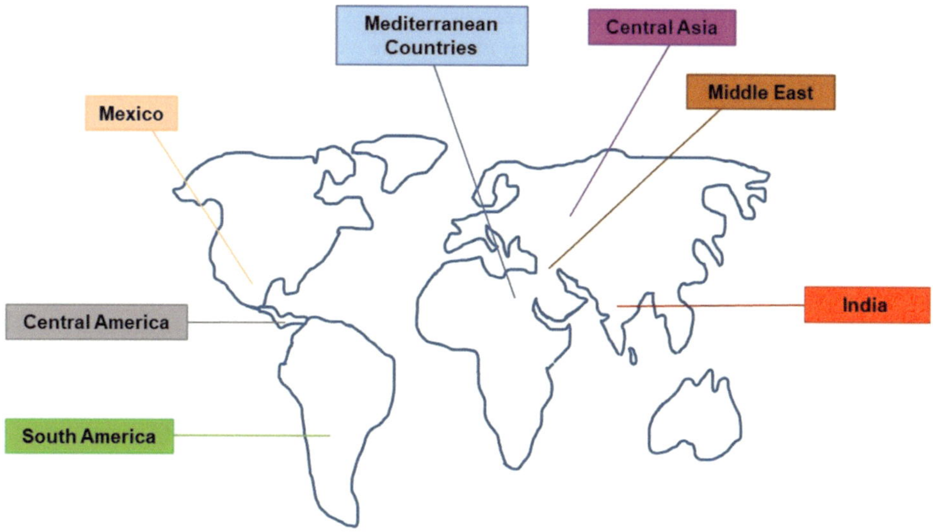

Figure 3.
Brucella endemic areas.

Transmission among humans with a human is rare but possible. A breastfeeding mother can pass the infection to their child, an infected blood or tissue donor to its accepter. Moreover, sexual transmission is extremely rare but cases like this also exist [49].

8. Clinical expressions

Brucellar infection in animals is associated with sterility and abortion. However, in humans, brucellosis can represent with simple flu-like illness (fever, malaise, fatigue, joint and back pain, etc.) to severe organ manifestation. Hepatic abscess (hepatic brucelloma), spinal brucellosis, neuro-brucellosis, myocarditis, pneumonitis, and ocular involvement are the other complications that have been seen in chronic brucellar infection [50–54]. Among 12, only 4 species, that is, *B. melitensis, B. suis, B. abortus,* and *B. canis* are responsible for the above-described complication in humans and the rest of them do not infect humans but their respective animal hosts.

The mortality rate due to brucellosis is very low but the rate of infection is really high. The infectious dose of brucellosis is very low and varies between 10 and 100 bacteria. However, the time taken by bacteria to show first symptom after getting infected (incubation period) is very high, that is, 5 days to 6 months but the average period is between two and 4 weeks [55].

9. Virulence factor

Virulence is concerned with the ability of the organism that define its destructiveness. Brucella has several virulence factors that help them to invade the host cell, causing illness, and to protect them from the host immune response. The reported virulence factors of this pathogen are lipopolysaccharide (LPS), base excision repair (BER), cyclic β-1-2-glucans (CβG), superoxide dismutase (SOD) and catalase, type

IV secretion system (T4SS), cytochrome oxidase, urease, alkyl hydroperoxide reductase (AhpC, AhpD), BvrR/BvrS system, nitric oxide reductase (NorD), and *Brucella* virulence factor A (BvfA) [56–62].

9.1 Lipopolysaccharide (LPS)

Being the weak inducer of the host inflammatory response, Brucellar LPS plays a major role in virulence [63]. In gram-negative bacteria, lipid A, O-antigen, and core sugar are the three components of LPS. Two structural variants of Brucella were reported based on the structure of LPS. The first one is smooth strains of Brucella which possess a complete LPS structure with O-antigen chain and the other one carries LPS which does not possess O-antigen chain and is called a rough strain of bacteria [64].

The structure of LPS of brucellae differs from the LPS of other gram-negative bacteria and thus their LPS is regarded as nonclassical LPS which is less pyrogenic in nature when compared to other classical types of LPS-bearing bacteria (e.g., enterobacteria). The presence of diaminoglucose in place of glucosamine and longer acyl group in lipid A made the brucellar LPS unconventional [65]. Also, in Brucella, lipid A does not connect to the core by ester and amide bonds but by amide bonds.

The structure of S-LPS of the smooth strain of Brucella composed of.

I) Lipid A (two types aminoglycose, fatty acids besides β-hydroxymiristic acid); II), the core which is made up of quinovosamine, glucose, and mannose and III) O-chains with 4-formamido-4,6-dideoxymannose. However, R-LPS of Brucella strain contains every content as smooth strain except O-chain [48, 65, 66].

9.2 Reactive oxygen and nitrogen-based regulators

9.2.1 Superoxide dismutase (SOD) and catalase

When Brucella enters to reside into the macrophage cell, the macrophages then start producing reactive oxygen intermediates (ROIs). These oxygen intermediates (hydrogen peroxide, superoxide, and hydroxyl radical) are extremely destructive in nature. They can stop bacterial replication or even kill the bacteria. Enzymes, superoxide dismutase (SOD), and catalase are produced by Brucella to get protection against ROIs. SOD is a metalloenzyme. Some species of Brucella contain two types of SOD (SodA and SodC). SodA is cytoplasmic and contains Mn as cofactor. Whereas, SodC is periplasmic and contains Cu, Zn as cofactor. SOD converts superoxide into hydrogen peroxide and oxygen. However, catalase is responsible for the breakdown of hydrogen peroxide into water and oxygen [48, 67].

9.2.2 Alkyl hydroperoxide reductase (AhpC, AhpD)

These enzymes are used by the bacteria as a defense system for the detoxification of reactive oxygen and nitrogen, which facilitates their survival in the environmental stress produced by the host immune system [68, 69].

9.2.3 Nitric oxide reductase (NorD)

It is another mechanism of the bacteria that saves them from the scarcity of oxygen in the macrophage cell. NorD is a defensive enzyme of the organism against nitric oxide (NO) toxicity (innate immune response to the infection). Nitric oxide metabolizes by the bacteria in the presence of any four types of reductases, that is, Nar–nitrate reductase, Nir–nitrite reductase, Nos–nitrous oxide reductase, and Nor–nitric oxide reductase into nitrous oxide (N2O) that favors their establishment inside the cell [48, 70].

9.2.4 Cytochrome bd oxidase

Brucellae are aerobes which means oxygen is a necessary condition for their growth but there is a scarcity of oxygen in macrophage cells (targeted host cells). Cytochrome bd oxidase functions to manage oxygen shortage inside the host cell and makes the intracellular environment suitable for their multiplication [48].

9.3 Type IV secretion system (T4SS)

Type IV secretion systems (T4SS), a channel of large protein complexes that transport proteins and protein-DNA complexes across the cell membrane. The T4SS of Brucella *in vivo* neither help them in invasion, infection dissemination, and in developing early infection but they are meant for the persistence of infection [71].

9.4 Cyclic β-1-2-glucans (CβG)

Synthesis of Cyclic β-1-2-glucans is another strategy of Brucella to protect themselves from the host defense mechanism and to make their persistence for a long duration. Functionally, CβG prevents the fusion of phagosome to lysosome and in this way Brucella saves them from acidic, microbicidal, and hydrolytic activity of lysosome [72].

9.5 Urease

Urease is a metalloenzyme that works for the protection of bacteria when it enters the body through the digestive route. The high acidic environment of the digestive tract can cause trouble in their survival. Hence, by using the enzyme urease, they decompose urea to ammonium and carbonic acid, which raises the pH of the surrounding to make the environment suitable for their existence until they enter into the target cells. Almost every species of Brucella produces urease except *B. ovis* [61, 73].

9.6 *Brucella* virulence factor A (BvfA)

BvfA is very unique and only found in the genus Brucella but is essentially required for the virulence of *B. suis*. It is a small periplasmic protein that is used to establish an intracellular replication niche [74].

9.7 Base excision repair (BER)

The damage in the DNA of the bacteria due to oxidation in the macrophage cells, is fixed by base excision repair (BER) with the help of the enzyme exonuclease III [48, 57].

9.8 BvrR/BvrS system

BvrR/BvrS, the two-component regulatory system of Brucella controls cell invasion and their survival inside the host cell. It prevents phagosome fusion to lysosome, which enables them to replicate. This system is essential for the virulent nature of *B. abortus* [75].

10. Pathogenesis

Microorganisms that enter the host have to fight with various protective mechanisms of the host. In the case of Brucella, when they enter the phagocytes they have to meet with several unpleasant ambience and then some (10%) who win the fight for survival (initial phase of infection) linger rest die [71]. However, brucellae possesses several strategies to evade from host defense system.

Brucella can infect diverse categories of cells, whether they are professional phagocytes (macrophages and dendritic cells), nonprofessional phagocytes (placental trophoblast and epithelial cells), or other blood cells like RBCs and other WBCs. However, Brucella does not replicate inside RBCs and lymphocytes but they play a role in bacterial dispersal [76]. Brucellae expertise in the survival and multiplication inside the macrophages capacitate them to cause chronic infection and persisting complications [72].

The process of brucellar infection starts with the adherence of bacterial cells to the host cell and ends with the dispersal of bacteria in other organs of the host body. Brucella has many adhesion proteins called adhesins that assist them in the process of adherence with the host cell. It has been observed that brucellae holds several different adhesin molecules for different host cell types [77]. The adhesins of Brucella, their respective host cell types and the receptors used by the bacteria are mentioned in **Table 1**.

Adhesins of Brucella	Host cell type	Host receptor types
SP29	Red blood cell (RBC)	Sialic acid-containing proteins
SP41	Epithelial cell (HeLa)	
BigA	Madin-Darby canine kidney (MDCK) and Caco-2 cells	Immunoglobulin-like protein
BigB	Epithelial HeLa cells	
BmaC	Epithelial (HeLa, A549), Synoviocytes, Osteoblasts	Fibronectin, type I collagen
BmaA	Epithelial (HT 29, Caco.2), Synoviocytes, Osteoblasts, Trophoblasts	Fibronectin, type I collagen
BmaB	Synoviocytes, Osteoblasts, Trophoblasts	Fibronectin
Bp26	Obscure	Type I collagen, vitronectin, fibronectin
BtaE	Epithelial (HeLa, A549)	Fibronectin, hyaluronic acid
BtaF	Epithelial (HeLa, A549)	Fibronectin, hyaluronic acid, fetuin, type I collagen

Table 1.
List of brucellar adhesins and their respective host cell type and receptors.

After the adherence, internalization takes place. Brucella uses a zipper-like mechanism to enter inside the macrophage cell. Internalization of smooth or virulent Brucella species occurs through the lipid rafts present on the macrophage cell. On the other hand, internalization of rough or avirulent species does not occur through lipid rafts but normally by the process of phagocytosis hence they get connected rapidly with the lysosome resulting destruction of the bacteria which shows that lipid raft is a necessary condition for the survival of early stage of bacteria in the host cell [78, 79].

Internalization results in wrapping of the bacteria in a vesicle. This wrapped structure is now called phagosomes or Brucella-containing vacuoles (BCV).

Normally, phagocytes engulfed bacteria to destroy them with the help of lysosome but brucellae prefers to reside and grow inside macrophages. In the process of invasion, several Toll-like receptors (TLRs) provide security to the organism from cytokines by checking the intracellular signaling associated with the activation of transcription of nuclear factor kappa B ($NF\text{-}_kB$) [48, 71].

At first, the 5 minutes old BCVs fuse with early endosomes and form early BCV (eBCV), which is marked by early endosomal antigen 1 (EEA1), Rab5 (GTP-binding protein), and transferrin receptor (TfR) marker. Brucella perpetuates fusion with late endosomes to form late BCVs, which is characterized by the markers lysosomal-associated membrane proteins (LAMP1), RILP, and Rab7 [80].

The avirulent one, that is, Brucella strain with R-LPS will now merge with lysosome to form phagolysosome (**Figure 4A**). Lysosomes contain reactive oxygen species (ROS), nitric oxide (NO), and antimicrobial peptides which are released inside the phagolysosome to destroy the invading bacteria [48, 63, 81].

Contrary to this the virulent Brucella strains (with S-LPS) resist fusion with lysosome by secreting a lysozyme-like protein (muramidase) coded by SegA gene. This SegA protein prevents eBCVs from becoming late BCVs and its encounter with lysosome by changing intracellular trafficking [82]. Moreover, brucellar T4SS plays an important role in keeping away the BCVs from the host immune response. The early BCVs now interact with the endoplasmic reticulum (ER) to form replicative BCVs (rBCV) which are characterized by several ER markers, namely calnexin, calreticulin,

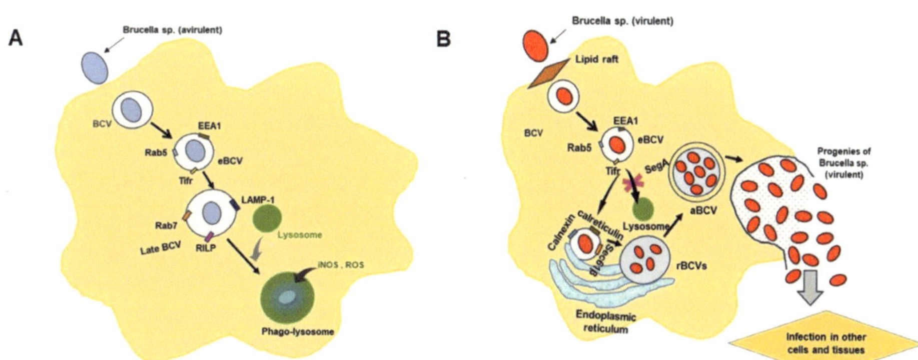

Figure 4.
A. Intracellular life cycle of an avirulent strain of Brucella showing formation of eBCV and late BCV and finally destruction of the bacteria by lysosome of the host cell. 4B. Intracellular life cycle of a virulent strain of Brucella showing how it manages to escape from the host protection system and makes way to reach ER for growth and replication. Repeated replication results tightening of vacuole which ultimately erupts into the blood stream, from where infection reaches to other cells and organs.

and Sec61β (**Figure 4B**) [79]. Bacterial virulence factor, cyclic β-1-2-glucans (CβG) assists BCVs in combining with ER. Brucella continues to multiply in ER and gradually acquires the autophagic feature. Although proteins ULK1, Beclin 1, ATG14L, and PI3-kinase activity are prerequisites for the formation of autophagic BCV (aBCV) [83]. When the macrophage cells become too small for the growing number of the brucellae, it bursts and with this bacterial dissemination occurs in the bloodstream and from there they spread to other cells or tissues [84].

11. Treatment of human brucellosis

There is currently no approved vaccine against brucellosis in humans. Thus, the administration of effective antibiotics for a sufficient duration is a crucial component in the treatment of all forms of human brucellosis. The appropriate antibiotic therapy is effective in treating uncomplicated acute brucellosis. However, due to their intracellular location in reticuloendothelial cells and their preferred sites (e.g., bone), most antibiotics cannot reach the site of action. Doxycycline, rifampin, quinolones (ciprofloxacin or ofloxacin), trimethoprim/sulfamethoxazole (TMP–SMX), and aminoglycosides (gentamicin or streptomycin), are the antibiotics used to treat human brucellosis [85]. Antibiotics of the tetracycline group, especially doxycycline is the first-line drug to treat brucellosis due to its longer half-life and fewer adverse effects. It is widely accessible, reasonably priced, and exhibits good intracellular and excellent activity in the acidic phagolysosomal environment [86]. Another effective first-line medication is rifampin, which has good bactericidal activity, good penetration in phagocytic cells, and many-fold increases in anti-brucellar activity at low pH levels [87]. Quinolones are reported to be the alternative of first-line drugs due to have excellent intracellular penetration and high tissue concentration but poor bactericidal activity in an acidic intracellular environment makes them inferior [88]. Tetracycline, streptomycin, and other medications with teratogenic potential are not recommended for treating children below 8 years of age, patients with co-morbidities and pregnant women. In these vulnerable groups, rifampicin and third-generation cephalosporins are recommended to treat brucellosis [89].

TMP-SMX exhibits acceptable *in vitro* activity, suitable tissue, and intracellular penetration. Nevertheless, it is only recommended to treat pregnant patients and children younger than 8 years [89]. In addition, streptomycin, an aminoglycoside medication, can be used to treat brucellosis in addition to tetracycline or doxycycline. It has been reported that the combination of these antibiotics kills Brucella at a higher rate than either medication acting alone. Thus, to treat brucellosis in humans, the World Health Organization (WHO) recommends a double or triple combination of antibiotics [90].

Treating brucellosis-related central nervous system disorders presents a special set of difficulties because high concentrations of antibiotics in the CSF must be achieved [91]. The blood-brain barrier is not effectively crossed by aminoglycosides or tetracyclines. Hence, in addition to the standard treatment of doxycycline plus streptomycin, the use of antibiotics with the ability to enter the central nervous system, such as rifampicin or co-trimoxazole, is advised. While the optimal duration of treatment for neurobrucellosis remains undetermined, most authorities recommend a minimum of 6–8 weeks of treatment, with the possibility of extending this period based on clinical response. Currently, ceftriaxone shows promise as a combination therapy option for certain brucellar complications, such as endocarditis and neurobrucellosis [92].

12. Antimicrobial resistance in *Brucella*

Relapses of brucellosis following treatment are common, with rates ranging from 5 to 15 percent in mild cases [93]. Treatment failure is also relatively common. Globally, brucellosis-endemic regions (such as Malaysia, Egypt, Qatar, China, and African countries) have recently seen the emergence of multidrug-resistant in Brucella against rifampicin, streptomycin, azithromycin, ciprofloxacin, tetracycline, vancomycin, etc. [94, 95]. *In vitro* induced point mutations in *rpoB* and *gyrA* genes are described as imparting resistance to rifampicin and fluoroquinolones, respectively [96, 97]. However, the clinical significance of these mutations is yet not clear. Moreover, the introduction of mutations in genes of RND-type efflux pumps *in vitro* generates the multidrug resistance phenotype of *B. suis* having resistance to ampicillin, norfloxacin, ciprofloxacin, tetracycline, and doxycycline [98, 99]. Recently, cephalosporin-resistant *B. melitensis* was isolated from clinical samples in China. Further, whole genome sequencing (WGS) of these isolates showed that more than 50% of antibiotic resistance genes were associated with efflux pumps [89].

13. Brucellosis control in animals

Antibiotics used as a primary prevention in domesticated animals contribute to the enhancement of bacterial resistance and have a significant impact on their dissemination throughout the food supply chain [100]. Thus, the treatment of animal brucellosis is not recommended due to its ineffectiveness and inability to completely prevent the carriage of the causative agent. Since humans can easily contract the disease from animals, thus animal-brucellosis control programs can aid in the eradication of human brucellosis. Animal brucellosis can be prevented with two widely used vaccines [101]. To prevent brucellosis in cattle, the most widely used and first vaccine for the disease is the live attenuated *B. abortus* strain 19 (S19 vaccine). A live attenuated strain of *B. melitensis* Rev. 1 (Rev.1 Vaccine) is the best vaccine to prevent brucellosis in goats and sheep. Nevertheless, they had certain disadvantages, including the induction of abortion in animals that were pregnant, their virulence to humans, the development of anti-Brucella antibodies that interfered with serodiagnosis, and the development of antibiotic resistance against brucellosis treatment [101]. Due to their high safety levels when compared to traditional live-attenuated vaccines, engineered live-attenuated vaccines based on virulence gene deletions have proven to be the most effective method for creating new vaccines with minimal residual virulence among vaccines using new technologies. Different kinds of these vaccines are being developed based on various deletions in virulence genes of *B. melitensis* and *B. abortus*, leading to a considerable reduction in the pathogen's ability to cause disease and to develop an increased immune-protective response [102]. Thus, these may be a potential vaccine candidate for human use as well.

Author details

Shahzadi Gulafshan, Rajeev Singh, Manoj M. Murhekar and Gaurav Raj Dwivedi*
ICMR-RMRC, Gorakhpur, India

*Address all correspondence to: grdnikhil@gmail.com

References

[1] Tandogdu Z, Wagenlehner FME. Global epidemiology of urinary tract infections. Current Opinion in Infectious Diseases. 2016;**29**(1):73-79

[2] Jones KE, Patel NG, Levy MA, Storeygard A, Balk D, Gittleman JL, et al. Global trends in emerging infectious diseases. Nature. 2008;**451**(7181):990-993

[3] Karesh WB, Dobson A, Lloyd-Smith JO, Lubroth J, Dixon MA, Bennett M, et al. Ecology of zoonoses: Natural and unnatural histories. The Lancet. 2012;**380**(9857):1936-1945

[4] Loh EH, Zambrana-Torrelio C, Olival KJ, Bogich TL, Johnson CK, Mazet JAK, et al. Targeting transmission pathways for emerging zoonotic disease surveillance and control. Vector-Borne and Zoonotic Diseases. 2015;**15**(7):432-437

[5] Pandey P, Sahoo R, Singh K, Pati S, Mathew J, Pandey AC, et al. Drug resistance reversal potential of nanoparticles/nanocomposites via antibiotic's potentiation in multi drug resistant *P. aeruginosa*. Nanomaterials. 2021;**12**(1):117

[6] Engels D, Zhou XN. Neglected tropical diseases: An effective global response to local poverty-related disease priorities. Infectious Diseases of Poverty. 2020;**9**(1):10

[7] Franco MP, Mulder M, Gilman RH, Smits HL. Human brucellosis. The Lancet Infectious Diseases. 2007;**7**(12):775-786

[8] Pappas G, Panagopoulou P, Christou L, Akritidis N. Biological weapons: Brucella as a biological weapon. Cellular and Molecular Life Sciences. 2006;**63**(19-20):2229-2236

[9] Hayoun MA, Muco E, Shorman M. Brucellosis. Treasure Island, FL: StatPearls Publishing; 2023. Available from: http://www.ncbi.nlm.nih.gov/books/NBK441831/ [Accessed: December 8, 2023]

[10] Moreno E. The one hundred year journey of the genus *Brucella* (Meyer and Shaw 1920). FEMS Microbiology Reviews. 2021;**45**(1):fuaa045

[11] Banerjee S, Van Der Heijden MGA. Soil microbiomes and one health. Nature Reviews Microbiology. Jan 2023;**21**(1):6-20

[12] Chomel BB. Zoonoses. In: Encyclopedia of Microbiology [Internet]. Elsevier; 2009. pp. 820-829. [cited March 2, 2024]. Available from: https://linkinghub.elsevier.com/retrieve/pii/B9780123739445002133

[13] Fong IW. Animals and mechanisms of disease transmission. In: Emerging Zoonoses [Internet]. Cham: Springer International Publishing; 2017. pp. 15-38. [cited March 2, 2024]. Available from: http://link.springer.com/10.1007/978-3-319-50890-0_2

[14] Patel PR, Shah SU. Ebola Virus. Treasure Island, FL: StatPearls Publishing; 2023. Available from: http://www.ncbi.nlm.nih.gov/books/NBK560579/ [Accessed: December 19, 2023]

[15] Ajibowo AO, Ortiz JF, Alli A, Halan T, Kolawole OA. Management of Japanese Encephalitis: A Current Update. Cureus [Internet]. 2021. Available from: https://www.cureus.com/articles/56812-management-of-japanese-encephalitis-a-current-update [Accessed: October 26, 2023]

[16] Yang R. Plague: Recognition, treatment, and prevention. Kraft CS, editor. Journal of Clinical Microbiology. 2018;**56**(1):e01519-e01517

[17] Rajapakse S, Rodrigo C, Fernando D. Scrub typhus: Pathophysiology, clinical manifestations and prognosis. Asian Pacific Journal of Tropical Medicine. 2012;**5**(4):261-264

[18] Mackenzie JS, Jeggo M. The One Health Approach—Why Is It So Important? TropicalMed. 31 May 2019;**4**(2):88

[19] Taylor LH, Latham SM, Woolhouse MEJ. Risk factors for human disease emergence. Woolhouse MEJ, Dye C, editors. Philosophical Transactions on Royal Society London B. 2001;**356**(1411):983-989

[20] Shaheen MNF. The concept of one health applied to the problem of zoonotic diseases. Reviews in Medical Virology. 2022;**32**(4):e2326

[21] Spernovasilis N, Tsiodras S, Poulakou G. Emerging and Re-emerging infectious diseases: Humankind's companions and competitors. Microorganisms. 2022;**10**(1):98

[22] Alton GG, Forsyth JRL. Brucella: Medical Microbiology. 4th ed. Galveston (TX): University of Texas Medical Branch at Galveston; 1996

[23] Coloma-Rivero RF, Flores-Concha M, Molina RE, Soto-Shara R, Cartes Á, Oñate ÁA. Brucella and its hidden Flagellar system. Microorganisms. 2021;**10**(1):83

[24] Ferooz J, Letesson JJ. Morphological analysis of the sheathed flagellum of *Brucella melitensis*. BMC Research Notes. 2010;**3**(1):333

[25] Fretin D, Fauconnier A, Köhler S, Halling S, Léonard S, Nijskens C, et al. The sheathed flagellum of *Brucella melitensis* is involved in persistence in a murine model of infection: *B. melitensis* flagellum is a virulence factor in mice. Cellular Microbiology. 2005;**7**(5):687-698

[26] Wilkinson L. VIII.20 - Brucellosis from part VIII - major human diseases past and present. The Cambridge World History of Human Disease. Cambridge University Press; 28 Mar 2008

[27] Edwards C, Jawad ASM. History of Brucellosis. Journal of the Royal Society of Medicine. 2006;**99**(2):54-54

[28] Wyatt HV. How Themistocles Zammit found Malta fever (Brucellosis) to be transmitted by the Milk of goats. Journal of the Royal Society of Medicine. 2005;**98**(10):451-454

[29] Nelson-Jones A. Brucellosis. Postgraduate Medical Journal. 1952;**28**(324):529

[30] Wyatt HV. Give a disease a bad name. BMJ. 2004;**329**(7460):272

[31] Kurmanov B, Zincke D, Su W, Hadfield TL, Aikimbayev A, Karibayev T, et al. Assays for identification and differentiation of Brucella species: A review. Microorganisms. 2022;**10**(8):1584

[32] Garin-Bastuji B, Mick V, Le Carrou G, Allix S, Perrett LL, Dawson CE, et al. Examination of taxonomic uncertainties surrounding *Brucella abortus* bv. 7 by phenotypic and molecular approaches. Applied and Environmental Microbiology. 2014;**80**(5):1570-1579

[33] Ewalt DR, Payeur JB, Martin BM, Cummins DR, Miller WG. Characteristics of a *Brucella* species from a bottlenose dolphin (*Tursiops truncatus*).

Journal of Veterinary Diagnostic Investigation. 1994;**6**(4):448-452

[34] Nymo IH, Tryland M, Godfroid J. A review of Brucella infection in marine mammals, with special emphasis on *Brucella pinnipedialis* in the hooded seal (*Cystophora cristata*). Veterinary Research. 2011;**42**(1):93

[35] Dvm ARS. Brucellosis: Brucella Abortus [Internet]. [cited December 19, 2023]. Available from: https://www.cfsph.iastate.edu/Factsheets/pdfs/brucellosis_abortus.pdf

[36] Fretin D, Whatmore AM, Al Dahouk S, Neubauer H, Garin-Bastuji B, Albert D, et al. *Brucella suis* identification and biovar typing by real-time PCR. Veterinary Microbiology. 2008;**131**(3-4):376-385

[37] Buddle MB. Studies on *Brucella ovis* (n.sp.), a cause of genital disease of sheep in New Zealand and Australia. The Journal of Hygiene. 1956;**54**(3):351-364

[38] Stoenner HG, Lackman DB. A new species of Brucella isolated from the desert wood rat, Neotoma lepida Thomas. American Journal of Veterinary Research. 1957;**18**(69):947-951

[39] Santos RL, Souza TD, Mol JPS, Eckstein C, Paíxão TA. Canine Brucellosis: An update. Frontiers in Veterinary Science. 2021;**8**:594291

[40] Nymo IH, Rødven R, Beckmen K, Larsen AK, Tryland M, Quakenbush L, et al. Brucella antibodies in Alaskan True Seals and Eared Seals—Two different stories. Frontiers in Veterinary Science. 2018;**5**:8

[41] Hubálek Z, Scholz HC, Sedláček I, Melzer F, Sanogo YO, Nesvadbová J. Brucellosis of the common vole (*Microtus arvalis*). Vector-Borne and Zoonotic Diseases. 2007;**7**(4):679-688

[42] Rónai Z, Kreizinger Z, Dán Á, Drees K, Foster JT, Bányai K, et al. First isolation and characterization of *Brucella microti* from wild boar. BMC Veterinary Research. 2015;**11**(1):147

[43] Scholz HC, Nöckler K, Göllner C, Bahn P, Vergnaud G, Tomaso H, et al. Brucella inopinata sp. nov., isolated from a breast implant infection. International Journal of Systematic and Evolutionary Microbiology. 2010;**60**(4):801-808

[44] Whatmore AM, Davison N, Cloeckaert A, Al Dahouk S, Zygmunt MS, Brew SD, et al. Brucella papionis sp. nov., isolated from baboons (Papio spp.). International Journal of Systematic and Evolutionary Microbiology. 2014;**64**(Pt_12):4120-4128

[45] Scholz HC, Revilla-Fernández S, Dahouk SA, Hammerl JA, Zygmunt MS, Cloeckaert A, et al. *Brucella vulpis* sp. nov., isolated from mandibular lymph nodes of red foxes (*Vulpes vulpes*). International Journal of Systematic and Evolutionary Microbiology. 2016;**66**(5):2090-2098

[46] Kahl-McDonagh MM, Arenas-Gamboa AM, Ficht TA. Aerosol infection of BALB/c mice with *Brucella melitensis* and *Brucella abortus* and protective efficacy against aerosol challenge. Infection and Immunity. 2007;**75**(10):4923-4932

[47] Xiaohuan W, Hai J. Global prevalence of human brucellosis. Chinese Journal of Epidemiology. 2020;**41**(10):1717-1722. DOI: 103760/cma.j.cn112338-20191022-00751

[48] Głowacka P, Żakowska D, Naylor K, Niemcewicz M, Bielawska-Drózd A.

Brucella – Virulence factors, pathogenesis and treatment. Polish Journal of Microbiology. 2018;**67**(2):151-161

[49] Meltzer E, Sidi Y, Smolen G, Banai M, Bardenstein S, Schwartz E. Sexually transmitted Brucellosis in humans. Clinical Infectious Diseases. 2010;**51**(2):e12-e15

[50] Barutta L, Ferrigno D, Melchio R, Borretta V, Bracco C, Brignone C, et al. Hepatic brucelloma. The Lancet Infectious Diseases. 2013;**13**(11):987-993

[51] Cho C, Goto M. Spinal Brucellosis. The New England Journal of Medicine. 2018;**379**(17):e28

[52] Soares CN, Da Silva MTT, Lima MA. Neurobrucellosis. Current Opinion in Infectious Diseases. 2023;**36**(3):192-197

[53] He Y, Wei C, Yun S, Wei J, Pu Z, Dai P. A case report of rare complication of brucellosis infection: Myocarditis and pneumonitis. The Journal of International Medical Research. 2023;**51**(3):030006052311638

[54] Tabbara KF, al-Kassimi H. Ocular brucellosis. British Journal of Ophthalmology. 1990;**74**(4):249-250

[55] Brucellosis CDC. Yellow Book 2024 [Internet]. [cited August 30, 2023]. Available from: https://wwwnc.cdc.gov/travel/yellowbook/2024/infections-diseases/brucellosis

[56] Jiménez De Bagüés MP, Terraza A, Gross A, Dornand J. Different responses of macrophages to smooth and rough *Brucella* spp.: Relationship to virulence. Infection and Immunity. 2004;**72**(4):2429-2433

[57] Krokan HE, Bjoras M. Base excision repair. Cold Spring Harbor Perspectives in Biology. 2013;**5**(4):a012583-a012583

[58] He Y, Vemulapalli R, Schurig GG. Recombinant *Ochrobactrum anthropi* expressing *Brucella abortus* Cu, Zn superoxide dismutase protects mice against *B. abortus* infection only after switching of immune responses to Th1 type. Infection and Immunity. 2002;**70**(5):2535-2543

[59] Kim J, Sha Z, Mayfield JE. Regulation of *Brucella abortus* catalase. Burns DL, editor. Infection and Immunity. 2000;**68**(7):3861-3866

[60] Ke Y, Wang Y, Li W, Chen Z. Type IV secretion system of Brucella spp. and its effectors. Frontier in Cell Infections and Microbiology. 13 Oct 2015;**5**:72

[61] Sangari FJ, Seoane A, Rodríguez MC, Agüero J, García Lobo JM. Characterization of the urease operon of *Brucella abortus* and assessment of its role in virulence of the bacterium. Infection and Immunity. 2007;**75**(2):774-780

[62] Gelchu AA, Benti AD. Characteristics and Intracellular Life of Brucella Organism: A Review. Journal of Microbial & Biochemical Technology. Jun 2020

[63] Huy TXN, Nguyen TT, Kim H, Reyes AWB, Kim S. Brucella phagocytosis mediated by pathogen-host interactions and their intracellular survival. Microorganisms. 2022;**10**(10):2003

[64] Ko J, Splitter GA. Molecular host-pathogen interaction in Brucellosis: Current understanding and future approaches to vaccine development for mice and humans. Clinical Microbiology Reviews. 2003;**16**(1):65-78

[65] Lapaque N, Moriyon I, Moreno E, Gorvel JP. Brucella lipopolysaccharide acts as a virulence factor. Current Opinion in Microbiology. 2005;**8**(1):60-66

[66] Corbel M. Brucellosis: An overview. Emerging Infectious Diseases. 1997;**3**(2):213-221

[67] Gee JM, Valderas MW, Kovach ME, Grippe VK, Robertson GT, Ng WL, et al. The *Brucella abortus* Cu, Zn superoxide dismutase is required for optimal resistance to oxidative killing by murine macrophages and wild-type virulence in experimentally infected mice. Infection and Immunity. 2005;**73**(5):2873-2880

[68] Wang HW, Chung CH, Ma TY, Wong H, chung. Roles of alkyl hydroperoxide reductase subunit C (AhpC) in viable but nonculturable vibrio parahaemolyticus. Applied and Environmental Microbiology. 2013;**79**(12):3734-3743

[69] Chen L, Xie Q, Nathan C. Alkyl Hydroperoxide Reductase Subunit C (AhpC) protects bacterial and human cells against reactive nitrogen intermediates. Molecular Cell. 1998;**1**(6):795-805

[70] Hino T, Matsumoto Y, Nagano S, Sugimoto H, Fukumori Y, Murata T, et al. Structural basis of biological N_2O generation by bacterial nitric oxide reductase. Science. 2010;**330**(6011):1666-1670

[71] De Figueiredo P, Ficht TA, Rice-Ficht A, Rossetti CA, Adams LG. Pathogenesis and Immunobiology of Brucellosis. The American Journal of Pathology. 2015;**185**(6):1505-1517

[72] Arellano-Reynoso B, Lapaque N, Salcedo S, Briones G, Ciocchini AE, Ugalde R, et al. Cyclic β-1,2-glucan is a brucella virulence factor required for intracellular survival. Nature Immunology. 2005;**6**(6):618-625

[73] Corbel MJ, Hendry DM. Urease activity of Brucella species. Research in Veterinary Science. 1985;**38**(2):252-253

[74] Lavigne JP, Patey G, Sangari FJ, Bourg G, Ramuz M, O'Callaghan D, et al. Identification of a new virulence factor, BvfA, in *Brucella suis*. Infections and Immunity. 2005;**73**(9):5524-5529

[75] Guzmán-Verri C, Manterola L, Sola-Landa A, Parra A, Cloeckaert A, Garin J, et al. The two-component system BvrR/BvrS essential for *Brucella abortus* virulence regulates the expression of outer membrane proteins with counterparts in members of the *Rhizobiaceae*. Proceedings of the National Academy Sci USA. 2002;**99**(19):12375-12380

[76] González-Espinoza G, Arce-Gorvel V, Mémet S, Gorvel JP. Brucella: Reservoirs and Niches in animals and humans. Pathogens. 2021;**10**(2):186

[77] Bialer MG, Sycz G, Muñoz González F, Ferrero MC, Baldi PC, Zorreguieta A. Adhesins of Brucella: Their roles in the interaction with the host. Pathogens. 2020;**9**(11):942

[78] Haag AF, Myka KK, Arnold MFF, Caro-Hernández P, Ferguson GP. Importance of lipopolysaccharide and cyclic β –1,2-Glucans in *Brucella* -mammalian infections. International Journal of Microbiology. 2010;**2010**:1-12

[79] Jiao H, Zhou Z, Li B, Xiao Y, Li M, Zeng H, et al. The mechanism of facultative intracellular parasitism of Brucella. IJMS. 2021;**22**(7):3673

[80] Celli J. The changing nature of the *Brucella* -containing vacuole: The *Brucella* -containing vacuole. Cellular Microbiology. 2015;**17**(7):951-958

[81] Celli J, De Chastellier C, Franchini DM, Pizarro-Cerda J, Moreno E, Gorvel JP. *Brucella* evades macrophage killing via VirB-dependent sustained

interactions with the endoplasmic reticulum. The Journal of Experimental Medicine. 2003;**198**(4):545-556

[82] Del Giudice MG, Ugalde JE, Czibener C. A lysozyme-like protein in *Brucella abortus* is involved in the early stages of intracellular replication. Bliska JB, editor. Infection and Immunity. 2013;**81**(3):956-964

[83] Brumell JH. Brucella "hitches a ride" with autophagy. Cell Host & Microbe. 2012;**11**(1):2-4

[84] Christopher S et al. Brucellosis: Review on the recent trends in pathogenicity and laboratory diagnosis. Journal of Lab Physicians. 2010;**2**(02):055-060

[85] Ariza J, Bosilkovski M, Cascio A, Colmenero JD, Corbel MJ, Falagas ME, et al. Perspectives for the treatment of Brucellosis in the 21st century: The Ioannina recommendations. PLoS Medicine. 2007;**4**(12):e317

[86] Hall WH. Modern chemotherapy for Brucellosis in humans. Clinical Infectious Diseases. 1990;**12**(6):1060-1099

[87] Akova M, Gür D, Livermore DM, Kocagöz T, Akalin HE. In vitro activities of antibiotics alone and in combination against *Brucella melitensis* at neutral and acidic pHs. Antimicrobial Agents and Chemotherapy. 1999;**43**(5):1298-1300

[88] Falagas ME, Bliziotis IA. Quinolones for treatment of human Brucellosis: Critical review of the evidence from microbiological and clinical studies. Antimicrobial Agents and Chemotherapy. 2006;**50**(1):22-33

[89] Ma H, Xu H, Wang X, Bu Z, Yao T, Zheng Z, et al. Molecular characterization and antimicrobial susceptibility of human Brucella in Northeast China. Frontier in Microbiology. 2023;**14**:1137932

[90] Mode S, Ketterer M, Québatte M, Dehio C. Antibiotic persistence of intracellular *Brucella abortus*. Chaves-Olarte E, editor. PLoS Neglected Tropical Disease. 2022;**16**(7):e0010635

[91] Akdeniz H, Irmak H, Anlar Ö, Demiröz AP. Central nervous system brucellosis: Presentation, diagnosis and treatment. Journal of Infection. 1998;**36**(3):297-301

[92] Fatani DF, Alsanoosi WA, Badawi MA, Thabit AK. Ceftriaxone use in brucellosis: A case series. IDCases. 2019;**18**:e00633

[93] Del Pozo JSG, Solera J. Treatment of Human Brucellosis — Review of Evidence from Clinical Trials. In: Updates on Brucellosis. InTech; [Internet]. [cited November 2, 2023]. 2015. Available from: DOI: 10.5772/61223

[94] Wareth G, Dadar M, Ali H, Hamdy MER, Al-Talhy AM, Elkharsawi AR, et al. The perspective of antibiotic therapeutic challenges of brucellosis in the Middle East and North African countries: Current situation and therapeutic management. Transbounding Emerging Diseases. Sep 2022;**69**(5):e1253-e1268

[95] Elbehiry A, Aldubaib M, Al Rugaie O, Marzouk E, Abaalkhail M, Moussa I, et al. Proteomics-based screening and antibiotic resistance assessment of clinical and sub-clinical Brucella species: An evolution of brucellosis infection control, Algammal AM, editor. PLoS ONE. 2022;**17**(1):e0262551

[96] Sandalakis V, Psaroulaki A, De Bock PJ, Christidou A, Gevaert K, Tsiotis G, et al. Investigation of rifampicin resistance mechanisms in *Brucella abortus* using MS-driven

comparative proteomics. Journal of Proteome Research. 2012;**11**(4):2374-2385

[97] Lázaro FG, Rodríguez-Tarazona RE, García-Rodríguez JÁ, Muñoz-Bellido JL. Fluoroquinolone-resistant *Brucella melitensis* mutants obtained in vitro. International Journal of Antimicrobial Agents. 2009;**34**(3):252-254

[98] Martin FA, Posadas DM, Carrica MC, Cravero SL, O'Callaghan D, Zorreguieta A. Interplay between two RND systems mediating antimicrobial resistance in *Brucella suis*. Journal of Bacteriology. 2009;**191**(8):2530-2540

[99] Posadas DM, Martín FA, García SY, Spera JM, Delpino MV, Baldi P, et al. The TolC homologue of *Brucella suis* is involved in resistance to antimicrobial compounds and virulence. Infection and Immunity. 2007;**75**(1):379-389

[100] Landers TF, Cohen B, Wittum TE, Larson EL. A review of antibiotic use in food animals: Perspective, policy, and potential. Public Health Reports. 2012;**127**(1):4-22

[101] Heidary M, Dashtbin S, Ghanavati R, Mahdizade Ari M, Bostanghadiri N, Darbandi A, et al. Evaluation of Brucellosis vaccines: A comprehensive review. Frontiers in Veterinary Science. 2022;**9**:925773

[102] Truong QL, Cho Y, Park S, Kim K, Hahn TW. *Brucella abortus* ΔcydCΔcydD and ΔcydCΔpurD double-mutants are highly attenuated and confer long-term protective immunity against virulent Brucella abortus. Vaccine. 2016;**34**(2):237-244

Chapter 5

Brucellosis: Infectious Disease

Sahar M. Jawad

Abstract

Brucellosis is a zoonotic disease caused by *Brucella* species, a small, Gram-negative coccobacilli group, with four species (*B. melitensis*, *B. abortus*, *B. canis*, and *B. suis*), causing illness in humans. These bacteria have a different type of outer membrane containing lipopolysaccharides (LPS) compared to similar bacteria like those in the Enterobacteriaceae family. Symptoms typically begin with a sudden fever, and as the illness progresses, it can enter into chronic stage characterized by recurring episodes of fever, along with symptoms such as weakness, sweating, and general discomfort. Human brucellosis is caused by various strains of *Brucella* bacteria, including *B. abortus* (from cattle), *B. melitensis* (from sheep and goats), and *B. suis* (from hogs). While infections from *B. canis* (from dogs) are infrequent, they have been reported. Among these, *B. melitensis* and *B. suis* tend to be more potent in terms of their pathogenicity. Farm animals, raw dairy products, and wild animals such as deer, bison, horses, moose, caribou, hares, chickens, and desert rats can carry brucellosis, which can also infect humans. In this chapter, we will discuss how brucellosis is contracted and the diseases it can cause. We will focus on Iraq, where brucellosis is a common disease.

Keywords: brucellosis, *Brucella*, characteristics and general features, distribution, infectious and diseases

1. Introduction

Brucellosis is a prevalent zoonotic illness caused by parthenogenetic intracellular parasites known as Brucella. Its discovery dates to 1860 when British physician JA Marston identified it as a distinct infectious disease on the Mediterranean island of Malta, naming it "Mediterranean flaccid fever" and "Maltese fever." In 1887, British army doctor David Bruce successfully isolated the causative agent, "Micrococcus Maltese," from the spleen of a deceased soldier in Malta. As a tribute to Bruce's contribution, the disease was subsequently named brucellosis [1, 2]. The authors in Ref. [3] referred to the bacterial infection humans can acquire from infected animals' meat, urine, body fluids, aborted materials, unpasteurized milk, and milk products or contaminated environment. Brucellosis is a disease caused by several species of bacteria collectively called Brucella. The disease is one of the highest priority animal diseases in different regions of the world. Brucellosis infects many species including livestock, wildlife, and humans. Most human infections are acquired through direct contact with infectious livestock or *via* indirect transmission by ingesting unpasteurized milk and milk products or by engaging in occupational activities.

The disease has a wide range of impacts that include losses due to abortion, culling of infected animals, lost milk production, animal replacement costs, veterinary fees, and human illness—causing reduced work capacity [1]. The history of brucellosis goes beyond the 1887 isolation and identification of *Brucella melitensis* and extends back to people's initial contact with animals [1, 3, 4]. The disease has been known by various names including Malta fever, Crimean fever, Bang's disease, Rock fever, Maltese fever, Gibraltar fever, Undulant fever, Mediterranean fever, or Gastric remittent [5, 6]. It remains the most common and continually reemerging zoonosis worldwide since 1884, and it is accountable for more than 500,000 new human cases annually [7]. Additionally, low infectious doses (10–100 bacterial cells), rapid transmission through different pathways, persistence in the environment, and treatment difficulties with antibiotics make Brucella a possible bioterrorism agent [6]. The most harmful species of Brucella, which can infect a wide range of hosts, are the ones that are most likely to infect pets (**Figure 1**) [8].

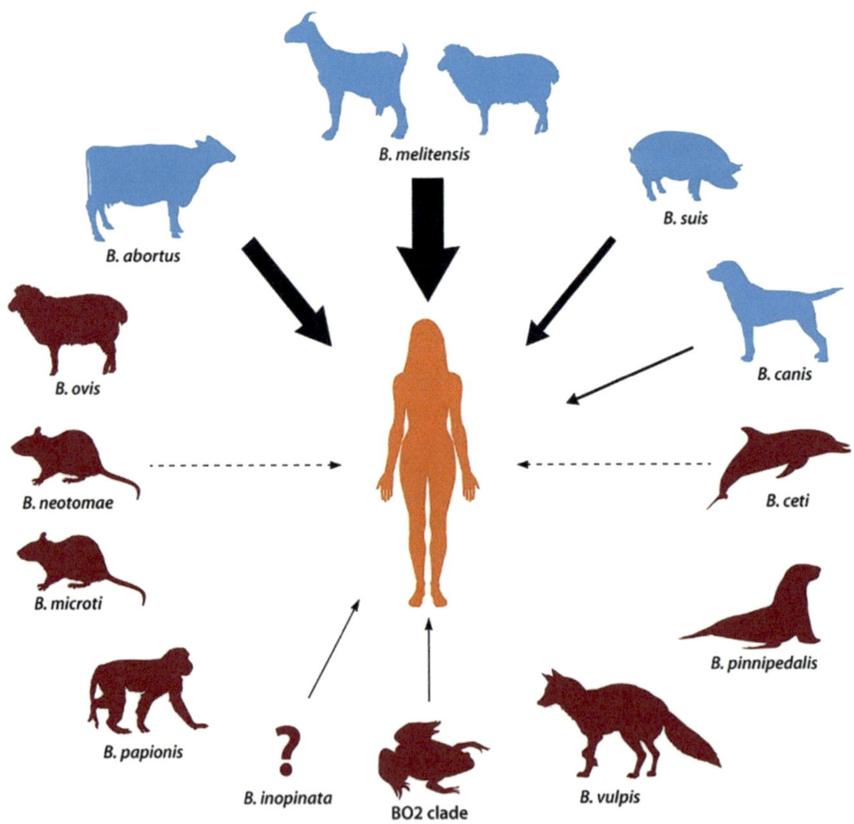

Figure 1.
The Brucella species shown in blue are known to cause disease in humans. The thickness of the solid arrows shows how often these animals are the source of human infection. The dashed arrows show that Brucella strains have been isolated from human disease, but there is no evidence that they were transmitted directly from the corresponding natural host to humans. The question mark indicates that the natural host for B. inopinata is unknown.

Brucellosis is a zoonotic disease, which means it can be transmitted from animals to humans and each Brucella species can be transmitted from animals to humans. The Brucella bacteria that cause this disease are very similar to each other, with about 97% of their genes being identical.

2. Infectious

2.1 Brucellosis, a zoonosis

Brucellosis, a Zoonosis Humans, is accidental hosts for Brucella. Humans are not the natural hosts for Brucella bacteria, but they can become infected through contact with infected animals, inhalation of airborne agents, or ingestion of contaminated dairy products [9]. Human-to-human transmission is rare, but it can occur through organ transplantation, blood transfusion, or breastfeeding [10, 11]. The symptoms of brucellosis can be mild or severe, and they often mimic other diseases. Common symptoms include fever, fatigue, malaise, and anorexia. If left untreated, brucellosis can progress to a chronic phase, leading to serious complications such as endocarditis, orchitis, spondylitis, osteomyelitis, arthritis, meningoencephalitis, and recurring fevers [12, 13].

Brucellosis can have serious consequences for domestic animals, such as cattle, sheep, goats, and swine. It can cause abortion and metritis in females, and orchiepididymitis and infertility in males. These infections can lead to reduced fertility and a significant decline in milk production [14].

Animal brucellosis is a highly contagious disease that can spread between animals and humans (cross-species transmission of certain Brucella spp. exists) [15]. It is mostly transmitted through direct contact with infected animals or their secretions, [16] such as aborted fetuses and fetal membranes; the bacteria can be found in large amounts in it [17].

2.2 Infection and dissemination

Brucella bacteria enter the host through the linings of the respiratory and digestive tracts [18]. Once inside their host, specialized immune cells called phagocytes, such as macrophages and dendritic cells, engulf and destroy the Brucella bacteria. After engulfing the bacteria, phagocytes transport them to the nearest lymph nodes, where they are sampled by the immune system. This leads to subsequent dissemination to the different organs of the reticuloendothelial system, including lungs, spleen, liver, and bone marrow [19]. In pregnant animals, the bacterium Brucella has a strong affinity for the placenta and mammary glands [20]. It replicates extensively in these tissues, causing inflammation of the placenta (placentitis) and abortion in the last trimester of pregnancy in ruminants [19].

In humans, brucellosis can affect any organ in the body, but it is most likely to affect the joints and liver. It can also affect the brain and heart, but to a lesser extent [20]. This is because the brain and heart are protected by the blood-brain and heart-blood barriers, respectively. These barriers make it more difficult for bacteria to enter these organs. The endoplasmic reticulum is the preferred intracellular niche for Brucella [21]; the data in **Figure 2** provide evidence for this claim that Brucella bacteria have a variety of places in the body where they can live and multiply. This includes the ER, which is a preferred intracellular niche for Brucella

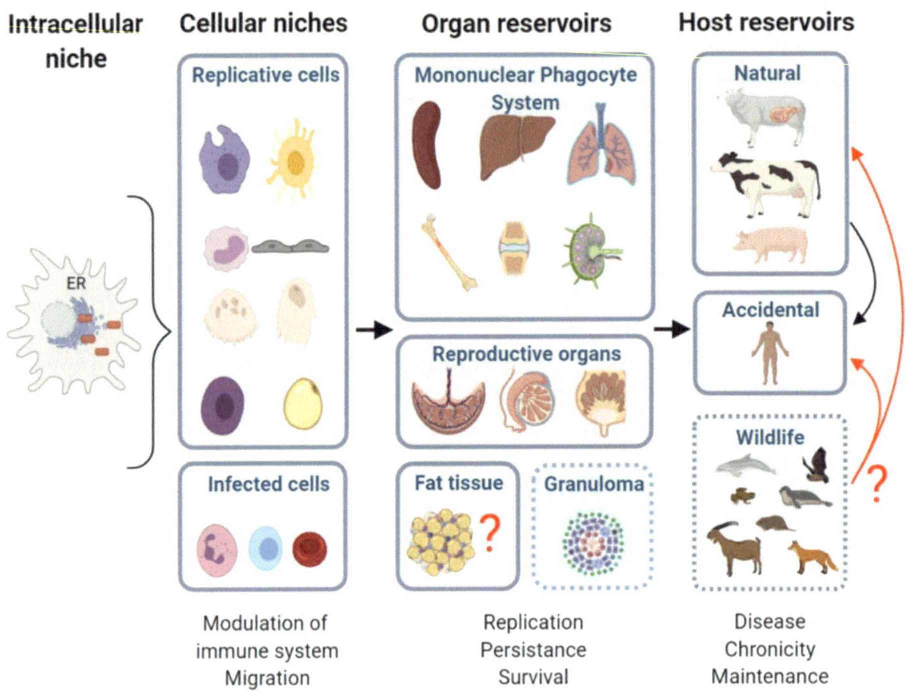

Figure 2.
Summary of Brucella's cellular niches and reservoirs Brucella bacteria can replicate rapidly in certain organs, such as the placenta, epididymis, mammary glands, lymph nodes, spleen, liver, lungs, and bone marrow. These organs are also where the most severe symptoms of brucellosis are seen. Once the immune system responds to the infection or granulomas form, Brucella bacteria can persist in the body at low levels. These bacteria can then start new infection cycles in other hosts. Brucella bacteria have also been found in wild animals, such as sheep, goats, frogs, foxes, bats, and rodents. The zoonotic potential of these wildlife reservoirs is still unknown, but they represent an important risk of transmission to livestock or humans. Created with BioRender.com (accessed on 15 December 2020).

bacteria. It also includes certain organs, such as the placenta, epididymis, mammary glands, lymph nodes, spleen, liver, lungs, and bone marrow. These organs are all important for reproduction, immunity, and metabolism, which makes them ideal for Brucella bacteria to hide.

3. Diseases

As mentioned above brucellosis is a major public health problem in many countries. Despite the fact that brucellosis is a serious illness with 500,000 new cases annually and the potential to have a major negative impact on both health and the economy [22]. The World Health Organization (WHO) classifies it as a "neglected logical disease" [23]. Brucellosis is a common disease in many parts of the world, including the Middle East, Asia, Africa, South and Central America, the Mediterranean, and the Caribbean. More than 170 countries and territories have reported cases of brucellosis, and outbreaks have been particularly severe in Syria, Mexico, Peru, Argentina, and Africa [24].

Humans are usually infected incidentally in one of three ways:

- Direct contact with infected animals: Humans can become infected with brucellosis through direct contact with the tissues of infected animals. This can happen through skin abrasions, cuts, or conjunctival exposure. Occupational exposures that put people at risk include veterinarians, shepherds, ranchers, and slaughterhouse workers [24].

- Ingestion of contaminated food or water: The most common way to get brucellosis is by ingesting contaminated food or water. This can happen through contaminated milk products, such as cheese, yogurt, and ice cream. Pasteurization of dairy products prevents transmission and has drastically reduced the incidence of brucellosis in the developed world. Meat products are rarely the source of infection because they are not usually eaten raw, and the number of organisms in muscle tissue is low.

- Inhalation of infectious aerosols: The inhalational route is another way that humans can get brucellosis. This is most likely to happen in occupational settings, such as slaughterhouses, where people are exposed to Brucella bacteria in the air. Laboratory workers who culture Brucella bacteria may also be at risk of inhalational exposure [25, 26].

Due to its high contagiousness among animals and the potential for disease transmission through aerosol inhalation, Brucella species are frequently listed as potential bioterrorism agents. Despite not forming spores and being less adept at surviving in extreme environments compared to *B. anthracis*, Brucella can remain viable for several weeks in moist soil and farm slurry at ambient temperature [27]. Clinically, brucellosis often presents with non-specific symptoms including fever, excessive sweating, fatigue, muscle and joint pain, decreased appetite, weight loss, and enlargement of the liver, spleen, and lymph nodes. The disease has a prolonged and recurrent course, affecting multiple systems and organs. Osteoarticular involvement is the most common complication, with a prevalence ranging from 2 to 77%, typically leading to conditions such as spondylitis, sacroiliac arthritis, and peripheral arthritis.

Around 50% of brucellosis patients experience hepatosplenomegaly, and gastrointestinal disturbances such as abdominal pain, nausea, and vomiting are common. Although respiratory involvement is less frequent, cases of pneumonia, pleurisy, pleural effusion, and pulmonary nodules have been reported. Additionally, 2–20% of cases involve infections of the male genitourinary system, primarily resulting in unilateral epididymal-orchitis and orchitis. Cardiovascular involvement poses the most serious complication, with brucellosis endocarditis accounting for more than 80% of deaths despite the overall mortality rate of brucellosis being approximately 1%. Hematologic complications are also observed, with anemia occurring in around 20–53% of children during the acute phase. Neurological manifestations, mainly in the form of meningitis, are reported in approximately 0.5–25% of brucellosis cases [24]. Brucellosis is a significant public health issue in developing countries, posing a major threat to human health and the entire social and economic development. Because its clinical symptoms are not specific, it is easy to be misdiagnosed and that leads to a chronic phase. What is more, if treatment is not taken in the acute phase, various complications will occur, resulting in disability, skeletal deformity, and even death. Besides, brucellosis may accumulate complications of the locomotor-osteoarticular system, digestive system, respiratory system, genitourinary system, cardiovascular system, nervous system, and blood, posing a major threat to human health and the entire social and economic development [24].

Brucella bacteria can be found in different parts of the body, including adipose tissue. The role of adipose tissue in brucellosis is still not fully understood.

We can prevent brucellosis by:

- Do not consume unpasteurized dairy products while traveling.
- Be careful when handling wild pig meat and bury the remains deeply.
- Hunters, herdsmen, and animal processors should wear gloves when handling animal tissue.
- Dispose of afterbirths, discharges, and fetuses safely.
- People with weakened immune systems should not handle dogs that are known to be infected with *Brucella canis* [28].

4. Conclusions

Furthermore, the prolonged viability of concealed Brucella bacteria emphasizes the ability of the pathogen to establish a chronic state, a characteristic that adds complexity to the treatment, control, and eradication efforts of brucellosis. A better understanding of where Brucella bacteria hide in the body could lead to new treatments that can reach these bacteria and kill them. Current treatments are not effective against Brucella in certain cells and organs, such as the bone marrow. Brucella bacteria can hide in different parts of the host, including adipose tissue. The role of adipose tissue in brucellosis is not yet fully understood. This presents opportunities for further research that will undoubtedly enhance our understanding of brucellosis and, more broadly, the mechanisms behind chronicity in intracellular pathogens. It will aid in the development of strategies to control and manage the disease, which is experiencing a global increase in prevalence over time.

Author details

Sahar M. Jawad
University of Kufa, Iraq

*Address all correspondence to: saharm.alkarawy@uokufa.edu.iq

References

[1] Shakir R. Brucellosis. Journal of the Neurological Sciences. 2021;**420**:117280. DOI: 10.1016/j.jns.2020.117280

[2] Singh M, Salaria M, Kumar L. Pneumonic presentation of brucellosis. Indian Journal of Pediatrics. 2005;**72**(1):65-66. DOI: 10.1007/BF02760583

[3] Akpinar O. Historical perspective of brucellosis: A microbiological and epidemiological overview. Le Infezioni in Medicina. 2016;**24**(1):77-86

[4] Wyatt HV. Lessons from the history of brucellosis. Journal of Maltese History. 2016;**5**(1):75-84

[5] Mutolo MJ, Jenny LL, Buszek AR, Fenton TW, Foran DR. Osteological and molecular identification of brucellosis in ancient butrint, Albania. American Journal of Physical Anthropology. 2016;**147**(2):254-263

[6] Zhang J, Sun G-Q, Sun X-D, Hou Q, Li M, Huang B, et al. Prediction and control of brucellosis transmission of dairy cattle in Zhejiang Province, China. Plos One. 2014;**9**(11):1-13

[7] El-Sayed A, Awad W. Brucellosis: Evolution and expected comeback. International Journal of Veterinary Science and Medicine. 2018;**6**(1):31-35

[8] Godfroid J, Cloeckaert A, Liautard JP, Kohler S, Fretin D, Walravens K, et al. From the discovery of the Malta fever's agent to the discovery of a marine mammal reservoir, brucellosis has continuously been a reemerging zoonosis. Veterinary Research. 2005;**36**(3):313-326

[9] Moreno E. Retrospective and prospective perspectives on zoonotic brucellosis. Frontiers in Microbiology. 2014;**5**:1-18

[10] Godfroid J, Al Dahouk S, Pappas G, Roth F, Matope G, Muma J, et al. A "one health" surveillance and control of brucellosis in developing countries: Moving away from improvisation. Comparative Immunology, Microbiology and Infectious Diseases. 2013;**36**:241-248

[11] Ay N, Kaya S, Anil M, Alp V, Beyazit U, Yuksel E, et al. Pulmonary involvement in brucellosis, a rare complication of renal transplant: Case report and brief review. Experimental and Clinical Transplantation: Official Journal of the Middle East Society for Organ Transplantation. 2018;**16**:757-760

[12] Wallach JC, Samartino LE, Efron A, Baldi PC. Human infection by Brucella melitensis: An outbreak attributed to contact with infected goats. FEMS Immunology and Medical Microbiology. 1997;**19**:315-321

[13] Aygen B, Doğanay M, Sümerkan B, Yildiz O, Kayabaş Ü. Clinical manifestations, complications and treatment of brucellosis: A retrospective evaluation of 480 patients. Médecine et Maladies Infectieuses. 2002;**32**:485-493

[14] Köse Ş, Serin Senger S, Akkoçlu G, Kuzucu L, Ulu Y, Ersan G, et al. Clinical manifestations, complications, and treatment of brucellosis: Evaluation of 72 cases. Turkish Journal of Medical Sciences. 2014;**44**:220-223

[15] Mcdermott JJ, Grace D, Zinsstag J. Economics of brucellosis impact and control in low-income countries. Revue Scientifique et Technique de l'O.I.E. 2013;**32**:249-261

[16] Olsen SC, Palmer MV. Advancement of knowledge of Brucella over the past 50 years. Veterinary Pathology. 2014;**51**:1076-1089

[17] Moreno E. Retrospective and prospective perspectives on zoonotic brucellosis. Frontiers in Microbiology. 2014;**5**:105-115

[18] Poester FP, Samartino LE, Santos RL. Pathogenesis and pathobiology of brucellosis in livestock. Revue Scientifique et Technique de l'O.I.E. 2013;**32**:105-115

[19] von Bargen K, Gagnaire A, Arce-Gorvel V, de Bovis B, Baudimont F, Chasson L, et al. Cervical lymph nodes as a selective niche for Brucella during oral infections. PLoS One. 2015;**10**:e0121790

[20] Moreno E, Barquero-Calvo E. The role of neutrophils in brucellosis. Microbiology and Molecular Biology Reviews. 2020;**84**:e00048-e00020

[21] Hull NC, Schumaker BA. Comparisons of brucellosis between human and veterinary medicine. Infection Ecology & Epidemiology. 2018;**8**:1500846

[22] González-Espinoza G, Arce-Gorvel V, Mémet S, Gorvel J-P. Brucella: Reservoirs and niches in animals and humans. Pathogens. 2021;**10**:186. DOI: 10.3390/pathogens10020186

[23] Jin M, Fan Z, Gao R, Li X, Gao Z, Wang Z. Research progress on complications of brucellosis. Frontiers in Cellular and Infection Microbiology. 2023;**13**:1136674. DOI: 10.3389/fcimb.2023.1136674

[24] Giambartolomei GH, Delpino MV. Immunopathogenesis of hepatic brucellosis. Frontiers in Cellular and Infection Microbiology. 2019;**9**:1-9. DOI: 10.3389/fcimb.2019.00423

[25] WHO. The Control of Neglected Zoonotic Diseases: From Advocacy to Action: Report of the Fourth International Meeting Held at WHO Headquarters, Geneva, Switzerland. Geneva: World Health Organization; 19-20 Nov 2014. pp. 44

[26] Rossetti CA, Arenas-Gamboa AM, Maurizio E. Caprine brucellosis: A historically neglected disease with significant impact on public health. PLoS Neglected Tropical Diseases. 2017;**11**:e0005692

[27] Nenova R, Tomova I, Saparevska R, Kantardjiev T. A new outbreak of brucellosis in Bulgaria detected in July 2015 - preliminary report. Euro Surveillance. 2015;**20**:1-4. DOI: 10.2807/1560-7917.es.2015.20.39.30031

[28] Tuon FF, Gondolfo RB, Cerchiari N. Human-to-human transmission of Brucella - A systematic review. Tropical Medicine & International Health. 2017;**22**:539-546

Chapter 6

Rickettsial Diseases of Recent Significance in India

Mahaling Bhure, Kailas Chavan, Shilpshri Shinde, Waqar A. Khan and Sandeep Chaudhari

Abstract

Rickettsial diseases are considered as re-emerging zoonotic diseases in India caused by rickettsial pathogens. The rickettsial organisms are obligate intracellular vector-borne pathogens causing wide-ranging symptoms. Rickettsia is subdivided into typhus and spotted fever groups. The reports of the disease have been increasing since the start of the 20th century in different parts of India mainly in rural areas with abundant vector populations especially in the post-monsoon season (August-November). The reports of outbreaks are recorded in various states such as Tamil Nadu, Himachal Pradesh, Manipur, Delhi, Puducherry, Uttarakhand, Jammu and Kashmir, Maharashtra, Karnataka, West Bengal and northestern parts of India. The outbreak of Scrub typhus is found to be the major among the diseases. However, the burden of the disease in India remains still unclear owing to the lack of accurate diagnostic facilities. The larval stages of the vectors are vital to the transmission of the disease and cause symptoms such as eschar formation present in 50%–80% of cases, fever, vomiting, headache, abdominal pain, breathlessness and lymphadenopathy. With the advancement in molecular biology, PCR and qPCR and serological assays such as Weil-felix and ELISA are adopted for diagnostic purposes. Surveillance strategies, avoidance of open defecation and urination, and wearing fully covered clothes are key strategies to prevent infection.

Keywords: rickettsia, India, Scrub typhus, diagnosis, vector

1. Introduction

Rickettsial diseases have emerged as one of the major public health threats to mankind. Rickettsial infections are caused by a wide range of obligatory intracellular, Gram-negative pathogens belonging to the genus *Rickettsia, Orientia, Ehrlichia, Neorickettsia, Neoehrlichia,* and *Anaplasma* of Alphaproteobacteria. These are the emerging and re-emerging diseases with a peak in reports in recent times with the advancement in diagnostics. The most observed rickettsial infections in India are scrub typhus, murine flea-borne typhus, Indian tick typhus and Q fever. The rickettsial diseases are vectorborne zoonotic diseases, transmitted to humans through the bite of infected mites, lice, fleas and ticks. Rickettsial diseases are difficult to diagnose with a high fatality of 9–70% amongst untreated individuals and are a threat to global public health [1]. Rickettsial diseases remain obscured in many parts of India with lacunae in the infrastructure to diagnose the pathogens at many places and disturbance of the vector habitat with human interventions.

2. Etiology

The rickettsial pathogens are small, gram-negative bacilli, with a unique obligate intracellular parasitism that makes them distinct from other Gram-negative microbes. The microbes are handled in the laboratory with the use of eukaryotic cells (e.g., in susceptible animals, embryonated eggs, cell culture) for isolation to mimic the intracellular lifestyle, unlike other bacteria which can be cultivated with the help of agar enriched with the required nutrients [1]. The rats and mice act as major mammalian reservoirs [2]. The pathogens are acquired by hematophagous arthropods (lice, mites, fleas, ticks), the pathogens multiply in the alimentary canal of ectoparasites and are accidentally transmitted through bites to humans (**Table 1**) [3].

3. History

The rickettsia groups of pathogens have bombarded the world since the 5th century BC. The description is mainly associated with the louse, though the identification and classification were not there. The typhus was described to be the cause for Napoleon to stop the invasion of Russia in 1812. It caused havoc during the period of world war I with approximately 30,000,000 cases and 3,000,000 deaths [4].

Rickettsial diseases are widely reported across the world. Scrub typhus is the major rickettsial disease reported in India. As far as other rickettsial diseases in the Indian context are concerned, was reported by Megaw (1917) in an European male of febrile case, bitten by a tick on his way from Almora to Lucknow. An epidemic of 12 cases was diagnosed by Weil–Felix reaction by Major E.S. Phipson (1922) at Shimla [2]. The study over the past century is suggestive of greater prevalence of Scrub typhus in India. Non-Scrub typhus Rickettsial Diseases, Spotted fever group and typhus group

Diseases	**Etiological agent**	**Vectors**	**Mammalian reservoirs**
Spotted fever group			
Indian tick typhus	*Rickettsia conorii*	Tick	Rodents, dogs
Rocky mountain spotted fever	*Rickettsia rickettsii*	Tick	Rodents, dogs
Rickettsial pox	*Rickettsia akari*	Mite	Mice
Typhus group			
Epidemic typhus	*Rickettsia prowazekki*	Louse	Humans
Murine typhus	*Rickettsia typhi*	Flea	Rodents
Scrub typhus	*Orientia tsutsugamushi*	Mite	Rodents
Others			
Q fever	*Coxiella brunetti*	Tick	Cattle, sheep, goats
Trench fever	*Rochalimaea quintana*	Louse	Humans

Table 1.
Details of rickettsial diseases with etiological agents, vector and host.

are not thoroughly studied as Scrub typhus. The Spotted Fever Group include Indian tick typhus, tick-borne Rocky Mountain spotted fever, African tick bite fever caused by *Rickettsia conorii*, *R. rickettsii*, *R. africae* respectively. In addition, *Rickettsia akari* causes mite-borne Rickettsial pox. The Typhus Group consists of flea-borne endemic typhus (murine typhus) caused by *R. typhi* and louse-borne Epidemic typhus caused by *R. prowazekii* [5, 6].

In India reports of scrub typhus date to 1930s in Kumaon region, among the soldiers at the time of the Second World War in Assam, murine and scrub typhus were reported from Jabalpur of Madhya Pradesh and murine typhus was reported from Kashmir. Scrub typhus which is the commonest has been reported in several states of India including J&K, Himachal Pradesh, West Bengal, Meghalaya, Uttarakhand, Bihar, Karnataka, Tamil Nadu Rajasthan, Maharashtra, and Kerala [7–10]. In a few places, 50% of non-diagnosed fevers presented to the hospital were found to be Scrub typhus [2].

4. Transmission

Rickettsial diseases are zoonotic in nature where humans are accidental hosts in the chain of transmission within ticks, trombiculid mites (chiggers), or fleas and animals (mostly rodents). Commonly found rickettsiosis in India are scrub typhus, Indian tick typhus, murine flea-borne typhus, and Q fever. *Orientia tsutsugamushi* is transmitted to humans and other vertebrates, with the bite of infected larval trombiculid mites (Chiggers). The mites usually feed upon specific vertebrate hosts, mostly rodents [1].

The rodent and the vector act as reservoirs which perpetuates the pathogen in nature. The vector is found in different ecological niches such as rainforests, semi-deserts, Himalayan region. Endemicity is associated with habitats such as gardens, forest clearings, shrubby fringes of fields and grassy fields. These ecological patches that harbor the regular host of mite vectors are called 'mite islands [2].

5. Pathogenesis

The pathogen is introduced into the body with the feeding of a tick or mite or through the scratch of fleas or deposition of louse feces onto the skin. These events mark the beginning of infection. Initially, upon entry, CD8+ Dendritic cells or macrophages are the targets. Later the pathogen spreads primarily to infect endothelial cells via the hematogenous route and lymph nodes through the lymphatic channel.

The main lesson that can be observed is Vasculitis, which involves events like activation of endothelium and then spread to other cells, this stimulates cell signaling which releases cytokines and chemokines to produce an innate immune response. The CD4 and CD8 T lymphocytes and macrophages rush to the site, causing a non-occlusive platelet plug and resulting in interstitial edema with increased vascular permeability. The above event leads to the formation of rashes which proceeds to form macules to maculo-papules. The lesion causes life-threatening conditions in various organs, interstitial pneumonia, non-cardiogenic pulmonary edema, and diffuse alveolar damage in the lungs, while in the CNS, meningoencephalitis has glial nodules. Similar damage is observed in various organs that are affected [5].

6. Clinical manifestation

Spotted Fever Group (SFG) and Typhus Group (TG) are two categories for rickettsial illnesses in terms of symptomatology. The three main diseases in SFG are rickettsial pox, Rocky Mountain spotted fever, and Mediterranean spotted fever. In TG, typhus outbreaks and endemic typhus are the primary clinically significant infections. In this population, recrudescent typhus (Brill-Zinsser disease) is a disease of epidemiological significance. A nearly comparable illness brought on by the genus *Orientia* is scrub typhus. It is crucial to get a thorough history of outdoor activities, recent travel to endemic regions, family pets, tick/mite exposure within 15 days of sickness, and other affected family members. The history would help to make a tentative diagnosis. The bites of ticks and mites are quite painless, and patients might not observe. The incubation period for any of the group diseases is almost 5–15 days. High fever is considered to be the prominent feature among all rickettsial groups. Multisystemic affection may be observed by disseminating the organism to different organs [6].

7. Cutaneous

Within three to five days of the start of a fever, a mild erythematous skin rash appears. Rose-red, distinct, Blanche macules begin at the wrists and ankles and progress (centripetal spread) to the proximal extremities, trunk, and face. Traditionally, the palms and soles are included. The rash in persons with dark skin might not be immediately apparent. The rash in RMSF may occasionally be transient, localized, or completely absent (20%). The rash gradually develops a petechial or maculopapular appearance. As the condition worsens, confluent purpuric lesions may appear, signalling a serious sickness [6, 11, 12].

8. Systemic

High fever with sudden onset occasionally subsides the next day morning. At the time of presentation, fever may also be accompanied by shaking chills, headache, myalgia, non-productive cough, dyspnea, nausea, and vomiting, as well as calf discomfort and tenderness. Frontal headaches are typical. It is a recurring trait and could be serious. Myalgia frequently affects the lumbar region, thigh, and calf muscles, causing pain in the lower back and lower limbs. Headache and injection of the conjunctiva are frequent first symptoms of scrub typhus. Most patients exhibit hepatosplenomegaly and generalized lymphadenopathy [12].

9. Diagnosis

The vague clinical symptoms that mimic viral exanthema make rickettsial illnesses difficult to diagnose in the first few days. Even in endemic areas, between 60 and 75% of patients with RMSF are initially misdiagnosed as suffering from another ailment [12]. The ectoparasite bite is typically painless, therefore the victim may not be aware of an eschar. Given that the patient may be experiencing the early stages of the illness and that fever and even rash may be missing in these patients, the absence of fever or rash in a patient at presentation should not prevent the doctor from diagnosing rickettsial fever [13].

The case definition for rickettsial diseases has been defined by the Indian Council of Medical Research (ICMR) as follows [14].

9.1 Definition of suspected/clinical case

Acute febrile illness for a period of 5 days or more with or without eschar must be suspected as a rickettsial infection (if eschar is found, it should be considered as scrub typhus irrespective of duration of fever). Other features may include headache, rash, lymphadenopathy, multi-organ involvement like liver, lung and kidney and acute respiratory distress.

The differential diagnosis with malaria, pneumonia, dengue, leptospirosis and typhoid should be carried out".

9.2 Definition of the probable case

A suspected clinical case is the one that shows a titer of 1:80 or more in OX2, OX19, and OXK antigens with weil-Felix reaction and an OD (optical density) > 0.5 for IgM ELISA is considered as positive for typhus and spotted fever classes.

9.3 Definition of the confirmed case

A case is said to be confirmed when (a) Rickettsial DNA is found in eschar or whole blood by PCR, or (b) Rise in the titer of antibody in acute and convalescent serum by indirect immune fluorescence assay (IFA).

10. Immunofluorescence assay (IFA)

This test is regarded as the "gold standard" for rickettsial infection diagnosis. The test's sensitivity is dependent on how long the illness has been present; typically, it turns positive after 7–10 days. Beyond 14 days of illness, the IFA assay's sensitivity increases to 94–100%, making it the most sensitive serological test for rickettsial infection. It is recommended to test the matched sera (acute and convalescent) after a gap of two to three weeks to show a more than fourfold increase in IgM and IgG titers. This test requires good infrastructure and is only available in a few centers, and it is useless in the first week after being ill. IgM antibodies fade in RMSF by 3–4 months, while IgG antibody wane by 7–8 months [7]. IgM and IgG antibody detection for rickettsial species may not be very useful in endemic regions because of anti-*R. conorii* IgM has been shown to cross-react with bacterial antigens including *Legionella* spp. and *Coxiella burnetii*, leading to false positive results [8].

11. Enzyme-linked immuno sorbent assay (ELISA)

ELISA is employed to diagnose rickettsial infections. Serum IgM capture assays demonstrate recent infection; however, it is necessary to establish the substantial baseline titer in each endemic area [12].

12. Polymerase chain reaction

Early and quick diagnosis is possible using rickettsial antigen detection by PCR. Blood is not a very good sample for this; instead, a skin or organ biopsy specimen should be used. However, once more, only some laboratories have access to this capability. Doxycycline treatment reduces the sensitivity of PCR [12].

13. Immunoperoxidase test

This is another gold-standard test for the diagnosis of rickettsial fever and is regarded as being equivalent to the IFA assay. It is only occasionally available, though, and is primarily utilized for study [9].

14. Weil-felix reaction

This is an antibody test for heterophiles. The antigens shared by Proteus species (*P. vulgaris*: OX19, OX2; *P. mirabilis*: OXK) and *Rickettsia* species (*P. mirabilis*: OXK), as well as the presence of agglutinins to these organisms in a 'suspect case' of rickettsial fever, form the basis of this test. Given that non-rickettsial infections can also exhibit a high quantity of agglutinins, this test lacks the sensitivity and specificity of an effective diagnostic test [7].

There are lacunae in the diagnosis and improper reporting of disease at different levels of the health care system. The rickettsial disease reported in India is mainly with the weil felix reaction, followed by ELISA. Though the IFA is considered the gold standard it is not economical and not all hospitals have access to this facility. The molecular techniques for the diagnosis are limited, especially the characterization and differentiation of rickettsial species, so there is a lack of epidemiological data for the prevention and control strategies [10].

15. Rickettsial diseases of recent origin

Rickettsial diseases in India have been reported since the time of independence, and there have been numerous reports at different geographical setups. The various rickettsial infections reported from India are Scrub typhus, Indian tick typhus, Spotted fever, Malignant Mediterranean spotted fever, and other flea-borne rickettsial infections. The most commonly reported rickettsial infections in India are Scrub typhus, Indian tick typhus, and Murine flea-borne typhus [15].

The earlier reports of rickettsial infection were reported during World War II in the forest area of the North Eastern states of India such as Assam and West Bengal, then later the reports were also from the Indo-Pakistan border during the 1990s. The recent reports of outbreaks from 2000 are recorded in various states such as Tamil Nadu, Himachal Pradesh, Manipur, Delhi, Puducherry, Uttarakhand, Jammu and Kashmir, Maharashtra, Karnataka, West Bengal and northeastern parts of India [15].

16. Reasons for the re-emergence of Rickettsial disease in India

India is a unique country with varying geographical conditions with a variety of flora and fauna. The rickettsial diseases being vector-borne diseases were observed to be in the area with an abundance of the vector population. The change in human behavior, increasing population, industrialization, and deforestation have led to the interruption of various ecologies and imbalance in nature leading to spillover of the disease. In the past, the vectors were restricted to shrubs in forests and hilly areas, with the intervention of man and the disturbance of harmony of nature, the vectors such as mites, ticks, and louse have entered human dwellings through the rodents into urban areas. When it comes to scrub typhus it spreads through the bite of mite at the time of camping or any recreational activities in the jungles, jogging in parks [16]. The other reason can be the profuse growth of vectors. In the early 70s and 80s the vectors were constrained to some endemic areas and so the diseases were also endemic to that area. Later with indiscriminate use of chloramphenicol and tetracyclines for acute febrile illness patients reduced the cases drastically. With the introduction of insecticides and pesticides for the control of the vector population, the vectors population was bare minimum but since recent times the vectors have emerged with survival strategies and bounced back with increasing and widespread population so there has been an upsurge in the cases of rickettsial disease, breaking the endemicity pattern of disease to epidemics [17, 18].

17. Indian tick typhus

Indian tick typhus is a tick-borne rickettsial infection seen in India. The disease belongs to the spotted fever group with similarity to rocky mountain spotted fever. The causative agent is *Rickettsia conorii*. For the first time *Rickettsia conorii* was first found in brown dog tick *Rhipicephalus sanguineus* in the 1950. The disease has been reported from various states of India i.e., Karnataka, Maharashtra, Tamil Nadu, Uttarakhand, Himachal Pradesh, Rajasthan, Assam, Kerala, Jammu and Kashmir, and West Bengal. It is also transmitted by other species of ticks such as Hyalomma and Haemaphysalis [19].

Indian tick typhus in recent times has been reported in Nagpur, Jabalpur, Sagar, Pune, Lucknow, Bengaluru, Secunderabad. The patients exhibit a wide variety of symptoms. The disease is characterized by sudden onset of fever moderate to high, headache, deep muscle pain, and malaise. The rash begins with maculopapular lesions on 3rd day of fever at the extremities, then it moves centripetally to the rest of the body. The Indian tick typhus can be differentiated from Mediterranean Spotted Fever with characteristic purpuric rash and an inoculation eschar at the site of tick bite which is rarely identified [20].

18. Scrub typhus

Scrub typhus is caused by *Orientia tsutsugamushi*. Because they lack lipopolysaccharide, peptidoglycan, and the slime layer, members of the genus *Orientia* may be clearly distinguished from Rickettsia. It affects around a million individuals annually throughout the world, with an approximate 50% fatality rate if left untreated. Approximately one billion people worldwide are at risk of contracting *Orientia* each year [21].

Due to the vector mite's presence in equatorial rain forests, subarctic regions, and semi-desert in the Himalayas, scrub typhus first appeared in India during the Second World War and spread to Assam and West Bengal states. Small mammals, including humans, are susceptible to scrub typhus because of heat and humidity. Currently, the disease can be seen in different parts of India i.e., the Sub-Himalayan belt from Jammu to Nagaland; Sikkim, Darjeeling, Himachal Pradesh, Bihar, Rajasthan, Maharashtra; South India-Puducherry, Tamil Nadu, Kerala, Karnataka [15, 22].

The larval stage of the Trombiculidae also known as chigger mite causes disease in both humans and rodents. The mite enters the human body through hair follicles and pores, then feeds for three to five days using a cyclostome, which is also used to inject the salivary secretion that causes the host tissue to lyse. The trombiculid mites transmit *O. tsutsugamushi* via transovarial and trans stadial transmission [23]. However, the novel vector (mite) *Ornithonyssus bacotii* for the transmission of the pathogen has also been identified in the Nagpur region; the central part of India [24].

Human scrub typhus typically takes 7–12 days to incubate. Humans exhibit symptoms like pyrexia of unknown origin, headache, body aches, joint pain, and characteristic entry lesion or eschar seen on the biting site due to this infection and activation of endothelial cells that aid in the morbid physiology of scrub typhus. It also affects several organs, including the heart, kidney, pancreas, skin, and brain, and in severe cases, multiple organ failures take place [25].

Scrub typhus can be diagnosed using the eschar-like characteristic lesion and serological methods which includes ELISA, Weil Felix, indirect immunoperoxidase (IIP), immunochromatographic test (ICT), and the gold-standard immunofluorescence assay (IFA). The molecular techniques utilized for diagnosis include polymerase chain reaction (PCR) by targeting a 56 kDa gene, a 47 kDa gene, Karp, Kato, and a gallium gene specific to *Orientia tsutsugamushi* for PCR. Other molecular techniques include; nested PCR and quantitative real-time PCR [21].

Considering the re-emerging nature of the disease in India more laboratories need to be strengthened for the accurate diagnosis of the rickettsial diseases.

Author details

Mahaling Bhure, Kailas Chavan, Shilpshri Shinde*, Waqar A. Khan and Sandeep Chaudhari
Department of Veterinary Public Health and Epidemiology, Nagpur Veterinary College, MAFSU, Nagpur, India

*Address all correspondence to: shilpi_shri5@rediffmail.com

References

[1] Walker DH. Rickettsiae. In: Baron S, editor. Chapter 38. Medical Microbiology. 4th edition. Galveston (TX): University of Texas Medical Branch at Galveston; 1996. Available from: https://www.ncbi.nlm.nih.gov/books/NBK7624/

[2] Yathramullage S, Rajapakse J, Boyagod S. Rickettsiae Reservoirs among Small Mammals (Rats, Mice and Shrews) and Their Arthropod Vectors in Sri Lanka. [Published on 15 Jun 2018]. Available from: https://pdfs.semanticscholar.org/2a5a/c8b5503968acddcbd46f54671abedfb317ae.pdf [Accessed: April 19, 2024]

[3] Ananthanarayan R. Ananthanarayan and Paniker's Textbook of Microbiology. Hoboken, New Jersey: Orient Blackswan; 2006

[4] Holmes F. Typhus on the Eastern Front. Available from: https://www.kumc.edu/school-of-medicine/academics/departments/history-and-philosophy-of-medicine/archives/wwi/essays/medicine/typhus-on-the-eastern-front.html [Accessed: May 3, 2023]

[5] Sahni A, Fang R, Sahni S, Walker DH. Pathogenesis of rickettsial diseases: Pathogenic and immune mechanisms of an endotheliotropic infection. Annual Review of Pathology. 2019;**14**:127-152. DOI: 10.1146/annurev-pathmechdis-012418-012800

[6] Chapman AS, Bakken JS, Folk SM, et al. Diagnosis and management of tickborne rickettsial diseases: Rocky Mountain spotted fever, ehrlichioses, and anaplasmosis-United States: A practical guide for physicians and other health-care and public health professionals. MMWR – Recommendations and Reports. 2006;**55**(RR-4):1-27

[7] Inamadar AC, Palit A. Rickettsial disease. In: Hoeger P, Kinsler V, Yan A, Harper J, Oranje A, Bodemer C, et al, editors. Harper's Textbook of Pediatric Dermatology. 2019. DOI: 10.1002/9781119142812.ch43

[8] Sexton DJ. Rocky mountain spotted fever and other rickettsial infections. In: Irvine AD, Hoeger PH, Yan C, editors. Harper's Textbook of Pediatric Dermatology. 2011. DOI: 10.1002/9781444345384.ch61

[9] Rathi NB, Rathi AN, Goodman MH, Aghai ZH. Rickettsial diseases in central India: Proposed clinical scoring system for early detection of spotted fever. Indian Pediatrics. 2011;**48**:867-872

[10] Krishnamoorthi S, Goel S, Kaur J, Bisht K, Biswal M. A review of rickettsial diseases other than Scrub Typhus in India. Tropical Medicine and Infectious Disease. 2023;**8**(5):280. DOI: 10.3390/tropicalmed8050280

[11] Kirkland KB, Wilkinson WE, Sexton DJ. Therapeutic delay and mortality in cases of Rocky Mountain spotted fever. Clinical Infectious Diseases. 1995;**20**(5):1118-1121. DOI: 10.1093/clinids/20.5.1118

[12] Rathi N, Rathi A. Rickettsial infections: Indian perspective. Indian Pediatrics. 2010;**47**:157-164

[13] Traeger MS, Regan JJ, Humpherys D, et al. Rocky Mountain spotted fever characterization and comparison to similar illnesses in a highly endemic area—Arizona, 2002-2011. Clinical Infectious Diseases. 2015;**60**(11):1650-1658. DOI: 10.1093/cid/civ115

[14] Rahi M, Gupte MD, Bhargava A, Varghese GM, Arora R. DHR-ICMR

guidelines for diagnosis & management of rickettsial diseases in India. The Indian Journal of Medical Research. 2015;**141**(4):417-422. DOI: 10.4103/0971-5916.159279

[15] Sharma A, Mishra B. Rickettsial disease existence in India: Resurgence in outbreaks with the advent of 2020th century. Indian Journal of Health Sciences and Biomedical Research (KLEU). 2020;**13**:5. DOI: 10.4103/kleuhsj.kleuhsj_162_19

[16] Mittal V, Gupta N, Bhattacharya D, et al. Serological evidence of rickettsial infections in Delhi. The Indian Journal of Medical Research. 2012;**135**(4):538-541. Available from: https://www.ncbi.nlm.nih.gov/pmc/articles/PMC3385240/ [Accessed: May 13, 2023]

[17] Threats I of M (US) F on M. Vector-borne disease emergence and resurgence. In: Vector-Borne Diseases: Understanding the Environmental, Human Health, and Ecological Connections: Workshop Summary. Washington, D.C: National Academies Press (US); 2008. Available from: https://www.ncbi.nlm.nih.gov/books/NBK52945/ [Accessed May 14, 2023]

[18] Varghese GM, Janardhanan J, Trowbridge P, et al. Scrub typhus in South India: Clinical and laboratory manifestations, genetic variability, and outcome. International Journal of Infectious Diseases. 2013;**17**(11): e981-e987. DOI: 10.1016/j.ijid.2013.05.017

[19] Ghosh S, Nagar G. Problem of ticks and tick-borne diseases in India with special emphasis on progress in tick control research: A review. Journal of Vector Borne Diseases. 2014;**51**(4):259-270

[20] Hulmani M, Alekya P, Kumar VJ. Indian Tick Typhus presenting as Purpura Fulminans with review on rickettsial infections. Indian Journal of Dermatology. 2017;**62**(1):1-6. DOI: 10.4103/0019-5154.198030

[21] Bhandari M, Singh RK, Laishevtcev A, et al. Revisiting scrub typhus: A neglected tropical disease. Comparative Immunology, Microbiology and Infectious Diseases. 2022;**90-91**:101888. DOI: 10.1016/j.cimid.2022.101888

[22] Chakraborty S, Sarma N. Scrub typhus: An emerging threat. Indian Journal of Dermatology. 2017;**62**(5):478. DOI: 10.4103/ijd.IJD_388_17

[23] Luce-Fedrow A, Lehman ML, Kelly DJ, et al. A review of Scrub Typhus (*Orientia tsutsugamushi* and related organisms): Then, now, and tomorrow. Tropical Medicine and Infectious Disease. 2018;**3**(1):8. DOI: 10.3390/tropicalmed3010008

[24] Akhunji B, RuchiBhate NP, Chaudhari SP, Waqar Khan NV, Kurkure SW, Barbuddhe SB. Distribution of Orientia tsutsugamushi in rodents and mites collected from Central India. Environmental Monitoring and Assessment. 2019;**191**:82

[25] Varghese GM, Abraham OC, Mathai D, et al. Scrub typhus among hospitalized patients with febrile illness in South India: Magnitude and clinical predictors. The Journal of Infection. 2006;**52**(1):56-60

Chapter 7

Zoonoses Control in Africa: Measures to Enhance Involvement through Application of Community-Based Intelligence Gathering

Benjamin Obukowho Emikpe and Raphael Deladem Folitse

Abstract

Many of the zoonosis control measures adopted in Africa over the years have not been entirely successful because of neglect of some socioecological factors which are crucial and peculiar to Africa. This study seeks ways to enhance control of zoonosis by adopting a pattern of research and implementation that incorporates socioecological factors and community-based intelligence gathering of data in Africa. A literature search using established data sources: PubMed and Scopus, scooping review to get information on the previous measures used for zoonosis control. It was seen that previous research was inclined more to problem identification than to an evidence-based problem-solving approach. It was also observed that East and Southern Africa are at the forefront of zoonoses and One Health research in Africa, while West Africa is leading in studies related to heavy metals contamination. The results showed that emphasis should be shifted to newer approaches that embrace socioecological factors; hence, community-based intelligence plays a major role in gathering information in Africa for proper implementation of zoonoses control. To ensure this, a holistic means of acquiring information and applying the One Health approach, which takes cognizance of the interaction of humans, animals, and the environment is essential.

Keywords: zoonoses, Africa, control, community-based, intelligence

1. Introduction

The livestock population in Africa is placed at 3.2 billion with 68% in the rural setting. Fifty-two percent (52%) of the human population in Africa are engaged in agriculture with 39% of farm labor being women. Hence, sustainability of livestock in Africa will no doubt protect the livelihood of the rural poor, especially women and youth in the rural setting.

Livestock population comprises of cattle 356 million (M), sheep 384 M, goats 438 M, pigs 40.5 M, and poultry 2 billion with Ethiopia and Tanzania leading.

Therefore, the thriving of sustainable intervention programs sponsored by various funding agencies in the south and eastern parts of Africa is substantial than in other parts of Africa [1]. The poultry population which predominates followed by cattle, goats, and sheep are widespread. Over 60% of the livestock mass in the arid zones is concentrated in East Africa, especially Somalia and Sudan [2].

These livestock are often bedeviled with diseases that not only have marked economic effects but some can crossover to humans. Some of the diseases that have been identified as limiting factors, are zoonotic meaning, can be transmitted from animals to humans and *vice versa* [3]. These zoonotic diseases are on the rise recently with some having attending threat to global health security. It has been reported that two-thirds of emerging infectious diseases [3–5] are zoonotic, which include Ebola, pandemic H1N1 influenza and highly pathogenic H5N1 avian influenza, Middle East respiratory syndrome (MERS), and severe acute respiratory syndrome (SARS), however, the status of COVID-19 as zoonotic disease is still being investigated. The reasons stated above clearly showed the need for research, outbreak investigations, and prompt diagnosis, which are quite expedient for rapid response and containment.

1.1 Research efforts in zoonoses in Africa

Various research efforts are done in Africa but as reported above, the level of research on viral zoonoses is more and the studies include those on endemic zoonoses which are avian influenza, rabies, and human influenza in pigs. The emerging ones include that of brucellosis in goats, tuberculosis in food animals while emerging ones include studies on Arcobacter and Helicobacter spp. and current trends of trypanosomiasis in food animals. The less focused ones are that of heavy metal pollution in selected organs of animals, especially burrowing animals such as African giant rats, which can be useful as environmental monitoring animals. This was well described by Usende et al. Other areas include zoonoses associated with fish in coastal areas, antibiotics residues and resistance in fish and studies on pneumonia-inducing zoonoses, especially deep mycoses in immunosuppressed animals.

In Ghana, research efforts are mostly on the six priority zoonotic diseases: viral, parasitic, pig, bat, or primates-related zoonoses [6] where the preponderance of rabies had been associated with dog consumption in some parts of Northern Ghana. Some efforts have been on swine flu, rift valley fever, and avian influenza, which is still ravaging many regions in Ghana. Ghana had also had a share of emerging viral zoonoses, which include Marburg and Monkeypox. The spread and the nature are still being investigated; however, a lot was related to the incursion of wild animals.

Some parasitic zoonoses which had been reported include toxoplasmosis, trypanosomiasis in food animals, and cysticercosis, while less focused areas are that of Arcobacter and Helicobacter spp. and the cross-species transmission of avian influenza into pigs. Other non-infectious aspects that will benefit from the One Health approach include antibiotics residues and resistance, climate change, and heavy metal pollution that is termed "Chemical zoonoses" based on the level of artisanal mining, hunting practices, and some cultural practices that promote bioaccumulation of heavy metals in human, especially pregnant women [7].

It will be great to examine the trends of research and training on zoonoses and One Health in Africa to evaluate the volume and the parts of Africa that benefit more. This evaluation will help in the call for more emphasis on the training and research to aid capacity development for the containment of pandemics in Africa.

1.2 Trends of training and research in zoonoses and one health in Africa

1.2.1 Methodology employed

To understand the trends of training and research in zoonoses and One Health in Africa, information was sourced by online search using PubMed, Scopus, and Google Scholar to evaluate the volume of journal papers on training and research in zoonoses and One Health in Africa. Information was also obtained from various stakeholders in One Health through collaboration and organized workshops by international agencies.

1.3 Results

The results obtained were expressed in bar charts in terms of the volume of journal articles in the following thematic areas:

Distribution of publications (output per region) in terms of One Health research, zoonoses research, training in zoonoses, and training in One Health.

Prose on the graphs below:

From **Figures 1** and **2**, there are indications of the level of research and training in One Health showed South and East Africa leading, which reflects the nature of work done in the area of One Health and the level of capacity building in this area. This clearly showed the need to focus on other parts of Africa, especially West Africa, which had been devastated by Ebola and recently threatened by Monkeypox.

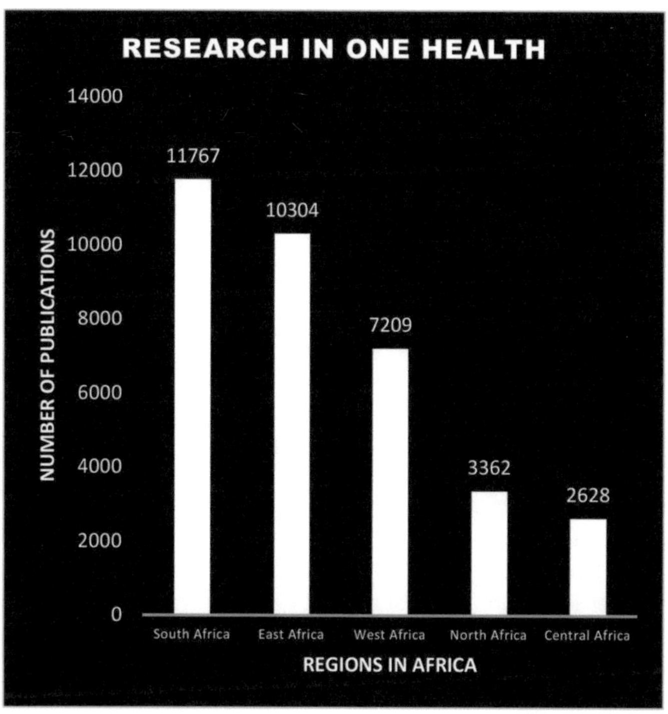

Figure 1.
Level of research done using the One Health approach.

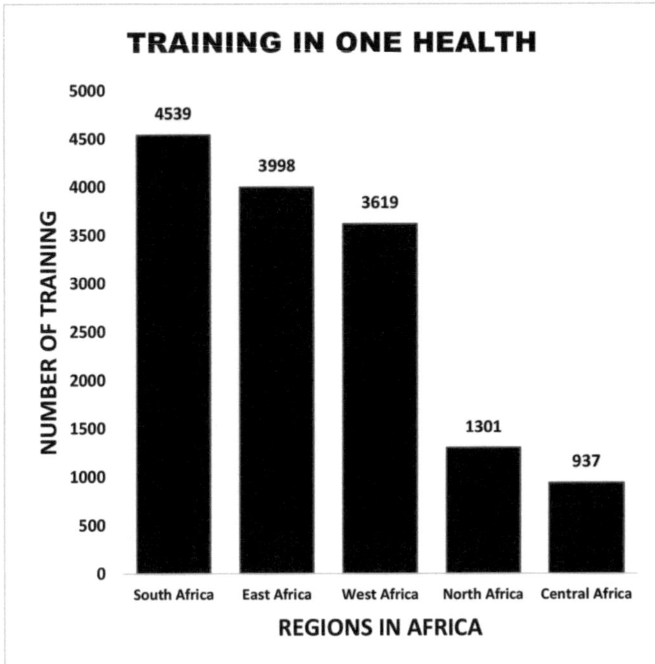

Figure 2.
Level of training received on one health.

Figures 3 and **4** show the level of training and research done on zoonosis. This showed a similar pattern with East Africa and West Africa leading, supporting the need to embrace One Health more in West Africa which in no doubt would help the inter-sectorial collaboration and prudent use of scarce resources should pandemic and other forms of zoonoses control be taken seriously. No doubt, this obvious gap calls for deliberate efforts to develop various One Health training programs involving the various sectors, namely human, animal, and environment.

Figure 4 shows that viral zoonoses are the most researched followed by bacterial and ectoparasitic diseases. This may be associated with the fatality rate of most viral zoonoses as compared with parasitic or bacterial zoonoses. **Figure 5**, clearly shows that most zoonotic disease publications in Africa are from bovines, which are quite numerous and more abundant, closely followed by wildlife and canine. This trend is interesting and clearly shows that wildlife is becoming a serious hub of zoonotic infection possibly because of the spill-over tendencies of disease. This underscores the fact that many ecological threats could precipitate or enhance the human-wildlife interface.

Often, the involvement of environmental issues that precipitate zoonoses is neglected or not given the required attention. This is why it is expedient to examine the trend of research on heavy metal contamination or accumulation in Africa. This clearly shows that research in this area needs urgent attention because the volume of research is grossly inadequate and is not a true reflection of the volume of illegal mining that ravages most parts of Africa. The distribution of research on heavy metal contamination in Africa clearly showed West Africa leading with very scanty information from East and North Africa. This calls for deliberate actions to reduce

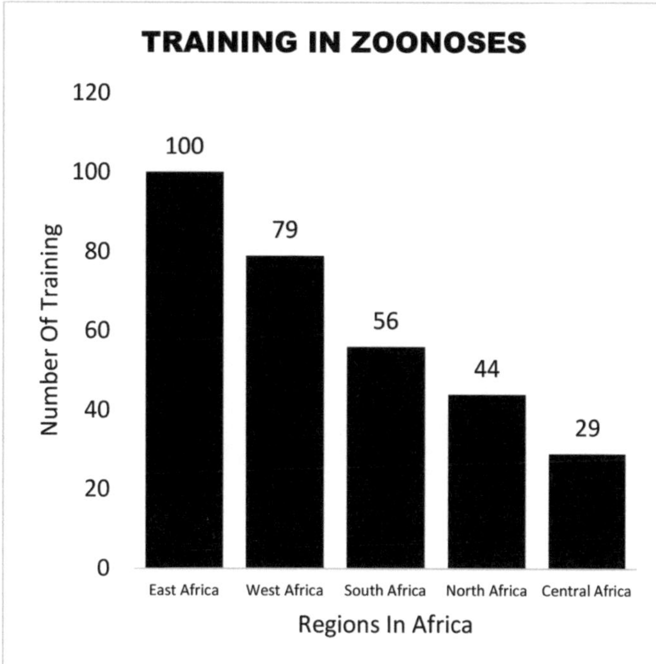

Figure 3.
Level of training using the one health approach.

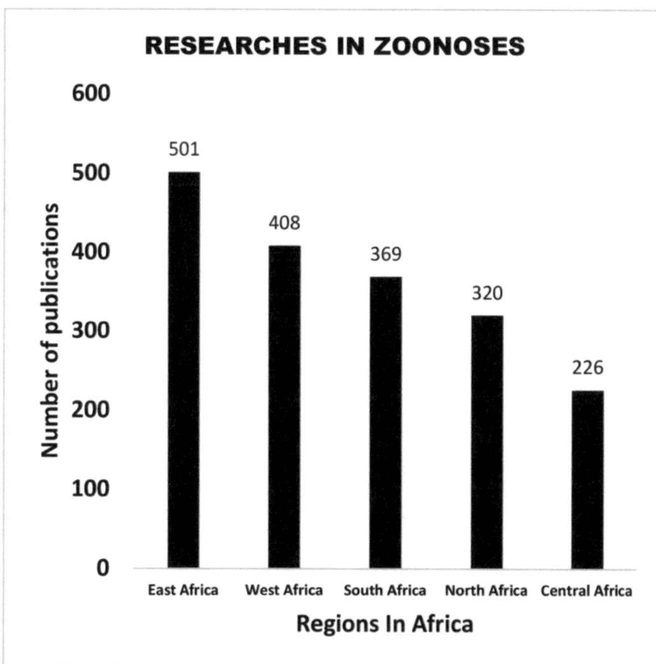

Figure 4.
Level of research done using the one health approach of training received in zoonosis.

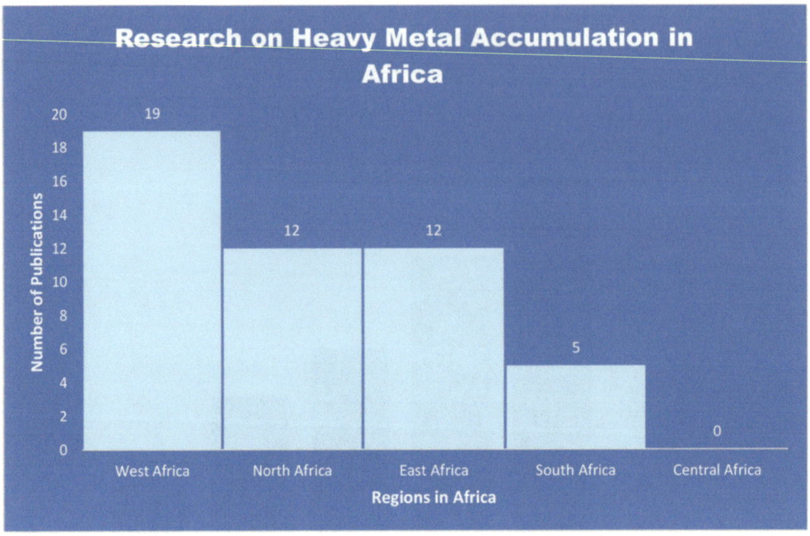

Figure 5.
Level of research done on heavy metal accumulation in Africa.

the untold destruction of the ecosystem that could have subsequent effects on disease patterns in future.

Trends in Africa

The mining activities in Africa had led to land encroachment, land disputes, destruction of farms, and farmer-pastoralist clashes. This is because mining activities make the land inadequate for animal grazing and crop farming. This in turn will lead to migration from the north toward the south in search of pastures. The land being used for farming, mining and grazing exposes these animals to heavy metal accumulation. This clearly shows that emphasis should be more on environmental toxicity, heavy metal accumulation, and the possible effect of this trend on zoonoses and disease outbreaks. This is an aspect that needs further elucidation to ensure effective control of zoonoses or pandemics in Africa.

From **Figure 5** above, indicates that the level of research on heavy metal accumulation in Africa does not match the enormity of the problem. These and others call for an integrated approach to control, taking cognizance of the interaction of humans, animals, and the environment, hence the need for a *"One Health Concept"* approach.

1.4 One health approach

One Health recognizes that the health of people is connected to the health of animals and the environment. One Health is defined as a collaborative, multisectoral, and trans-disciplinary approach to achieving optimal health outcomes by recognizing the interconnection between people, animals, plants, and their shared environment CDC [8]. The goal of One Health is to encourage the collaborative efforts of multiple disciplines-working locally, nationally, and globally to achieve the best health for people, animals, and our environment. Though it is not a new concept, this is because there are frequent changes in the environment, animal diversity and human-animal interactions have often led to the emergence and reemergence of many diseases, including zoonotic diseases. This reoccurrence necessitates proactive measures which should include public health interventions that require the cooperation of human, animal, and environmental health communities through collaborations to succeed [9]. It should be noted however that those collaborations and interventions will need to incorporate these ecological and cultural peculiarities of Africa into the outbreak investigations in One Health (**Figure 6**).

1.4.1 Ecological peculiarities of Africa

The cultural practices and the family ties that exist in Africa are unique with very close interaction between domestic animals and human, which is seen in the figure above. This proximity allows for the interaction of various species and animals within the same environment. This proximity allows for the easy spread of diseases between animals and humans within the same ecosystem. This eco peculiarity allows for the use of One Health and that allows for the possible introduction of One Health hospital to take care of animals and humans using shared facilities that include laboratory and diagnostic imaging. This will no doubt cut costs and allow for judicious use of resources.

1.4.2 The use of indigenous knowledge and development in zoonoses control

Indigenous knowledge is a systematic body of knowledge acquired by local people through the accumulation of experiences, informal experiments, and an intimate understanding of the environment in a given culture. Indigenous knowledge is unique to a given culture or society. It is the formation base for a society that facilitates communication and decision-making. It forms the basis for decision-making, which is operationalized through indigenous organizations, and they provide the foundation for local innovations and experimentation.

A study was conducted in the Kumasi Metropolis, Ghana to know the consumer preference and possible health implications of cattle and goat offal [10]. The objectives

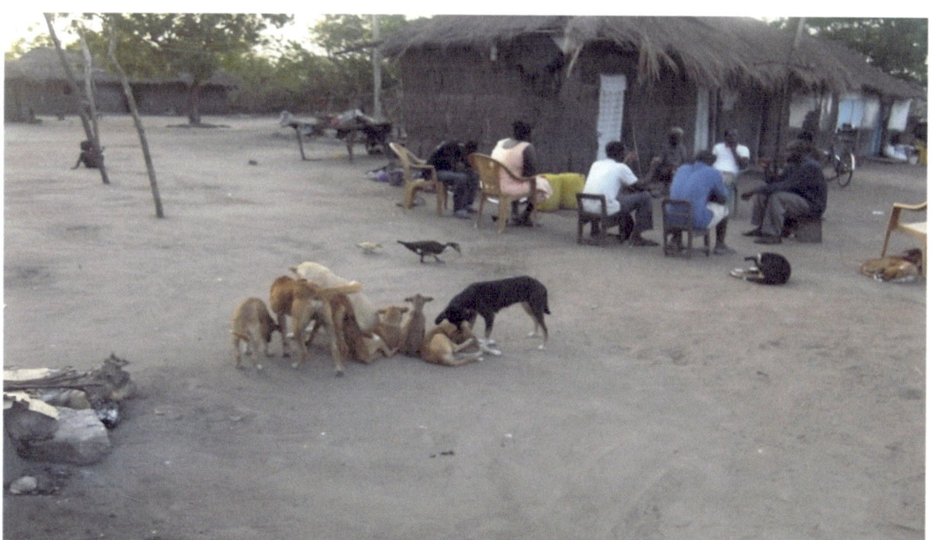

Figure 6.
An image of a Ghanaian family living near their domestic animals. (Source: Picture was taken by courtesy of Tasiame William in the Northern Region of Ghana).

of this study were to provide sufficient information on consumer preference for offal and related public health zoonotic implications in the offal supply chain and also to provide a basis for the development of consumer safety and welfare policies in Ghana, in respect of offal-borne zoonotic infections. This study indicated that 1.1% of the populace preferred the lungs of the animals, 38.7% preferred the liver, 7.5% the intestines, and 52.7% the stomach contents. Some factors which influence consumer preference are availability, affordability, nutritional value, taste, customs, and individuals' level of education.

Research was equally done on the offal of the cattle and goat and significant histopathological changes were observed in both cattle and goat liver. Well-formed hepatic granuloma of different sizes scattered within the interstitium with eggs and segments of parasites. Multiple focal abscesses and hepatic necrosis were observed as well. In such an instance, a clear relationship was established between preference for offal and the spread of zoonoses. This showed that the application of a native intelligence approach to disease information can be more effective.

1.4.3 Native intelligence in zoonoses control

Native intelligence is a community approach to intelligence gathering of information. It is also a nonconventional or traditional method of sourcing information at the community level using the participatory epizootiology approach. This will include the use of community leaders, opinion leaders, and the involvement of women, men, district heads, chiefs, market women, hunters, trade groups, associations, established health institutions, churches, mosques, and food vendors in the control of zoonoses. These groups are often neglected but often useful as a tool to obtain information at the community level. This group should be well-trained and deployed to obtain the necessary information on zoonoses at the community level.

1.4.4 Cultural practices promoting zoonoses

Some cultural practices have been identified as promoters of zoonoses in Africa, such methods include the killing and eating of bush rats and grasscutters using cutlass, which is mostly laden with crocodile bile.

Some tribes use the stomach content of killed grasscutter for soup, while some local butchers and meat sellers did not see tubercles in the lungs of livers as a threat, some take a bit during slaughtering and claim they have taken such for years with no dire consequence.

These observations clearly show the need for research into the sociocultural factors in Africa. Some of these include the experience and interactions of hunters and hunting dogs in terms of rabies transmission at the community level, there is also a need to evaluate the indiscriminate slaughtering of certain domestic animals such as donkeys and dogs, and the evidence of rabies transmission as suggested by some researchers [11].

1.4.5 Paradigm shift

There is therefore the need for research to be more inclined to an evidence-based problem-solving approach. This informs the need to have centers of excellence that focus on pandemics or zoonosis control in West Africa and others located more in East and Southern Africa. Such centers in West Africa include the Center for

Control and Prevention of Zoonoses in West Africa (CCPZ) https://www.ui.edu.ng/content/centre-control-and-prevention-zoonoses-West-Africa. The main partners were Faculty of Veterinary Medicine, University of Ibadan, Department of Animal Science, Njala University Sierra leone, and Cuttington University in Liberia while the German-West African Center for Pandemic Control (G-WAC) https://g-wac.org/ had main partners, which include Medical Faculty and University Hospital Bonn UKB, Berlin School of Public Health, Technische Universitat Berlin (TUB) and Charite Universititatsmedizin- Berlin, College of Health Sciences, Kwame Nkrumah University of Science and Technology (KNUST), and Kumasi Ghana. G-WAC is a center of excellence with expertise in health systems/health economics, virology/diagnostics, bacteriology/parasitology, epidemiology and surveillance, community engagements/social sciences, digital health, and zoonoses.

Noting that there is more work desired in West Africa, the center that will be driven by the effect of environmental degradation on human and animal health will be strongly recommended judging from the enormous environmental degradation caused by illegal mining often reported in Ghana, Nigeria, and Sierra Leone.

1.5 Conclusions

This chapter reiterates the fact that community-based intelligence plays a major role in gathering information in Africa for proper implementation of zoonoses control. Hence, there is a need for a wholistic means of acquiring information and application of One health approach taking cognizance of the interaction of humans, animals, and the environment.

Acknowledgements

We appreciate the efforts of the research team, which comprises biologists, veterinarians, and nurses, who actively aid in the thinking process. They include Ruth Fiadjoe, Belinda Dogbe, Derrick Adu Asare, Abigael Emikpe, and Obadiah Opoku-Bamfoh who typed and edited the chapter.

Author details

Benjamin Obukowho Emikpe* and Raphael Deladem Folitse
Department of Pathobiology, School of Veterinary Medicine, Kwame Nkrumah University of Science and Technology (KNUST), Kumasi, Ghana

*Address all correspondence to: banabis2001@yahoo.com

References

[1] Wilson E, Van Alstine J. The extractive industries transparency initiative in Africa: Overcoming the resource curse and promoting sustainable development. In: Natural Resources and Sustainable Development. Edward Elgar Publishing; 2017. pp. 50-74

[2] Mwangi DM. Grassland and Livestock Production: The East African Case. 2015. pp. 1-2

[3] Nile W. 2. Current Situation in the Region. Who Emro. 2009;**2009**:1-21. Available from http://www.emro.who.int/pdf/about-who/rc61/zoonotic-diseases.pdf?ua=1

[4] Vora NM et al. Interventions to reduce risk for pathogen spillover and early disease spread to prevent outbreaks, epidemics, and pandemics. Emerging Infectious Diseases. 2023;**29**(3):1-3

[5] Weiss RA, Sankaran N. Emergence of epidemic diseases: Zoonoses and other origins. Faculty Reviews. 2022;**11**:2

[6] Suu-Ire RD et al. Viral zoonoses of national importance in Ghana: Advancements and opportunities for enhancing capacities for early detection and response. Journal of Tropical Medicine. 2021;**2021**:1-2

[7] Kobia J et al. Effects of different cooking methods on heavy metals level in fresh and smoked game meat. 2016:617

[8] Halabi SF. Adaptation of animal and human health surveillance systems for vector-borne diseases accompanying climate change. The Journal of Law, Medicine & Ethics. 2020;**48**(4):694-704

[9] Nguta JM et al. 'One health' research ethics in emergency, disaster and zoonotic disease outbreaks: A case study from Ethiopia. In: Ethics, Integrity and Policymaking: The Value of the Case Study. 2022. pp. 151-164

[10] Ayroe F, Emikpe BO, Asiamah E, Dankwa KO. Consumers' preference and associated pathology observed in cattle and goat offals in Kumasi, Ghana. African Journal of Infectious Diseases. 2016;**10**(2):127-133

[11] Tasiame W, El-Duah P, Johnson SA, Owiredu EW, Bleicker T, Veith T, et al. Rabies virus in slaughtered dogs for meat consumption in Ghana: A potential risk for rabies transmission. Transboundary and Emerging Diseases. 2022;**69**(4): e71-e81. DOI: 10.1111/tbed.14266

Section 3

Parasitic Zoonoses

Chapter 8

Zoonotic Schistosomiasis in Nigeria: The Concealed Threat to Humans Posed by Genetic Hybrid Parasites of Livestock Cattle Origin

Andrew W. Taylor-Robinson, Hammed Oladeji Mogaji, Olaitan O. Omitola, Adedotun Ayodeji Bayegun and Uwem Friday Ekpo

Abstract

Schistosomiasis, also known as bilharzia, is a water-borne parasitic disease caused by blood flukes (trematode worms) of the genus *Schistosoma*. The disease is mainly found in tropical and subtropical regions, affecting more than 200 million people worldwide, but predominantly, about 90%, in sub-Saharan Africa. Nigeria shoulders the largest share of schistosomiasis cases on the African continent. While efforts to combat this disease have traditionally focused on human infections, there has been limited attention given to infections in livestock that might have the potential to spread to humans. Recent empirical findings indicate that, apart from *Schistosoma* species primarily associated with humans, there are schistosomes in livestock that can infect humans as well. This raises the possibility of genetic material mixing between cattle and human schistosomes, known as hybridization. This phenomenon poses a risk of zoonotic diseases transmission. This chapter delves into ongoing research concerning schistosome hybridization in Nigeria and elucidates its adverse effects on elimination endeavors. Furthermore, it explores the factors that encourage interactions between human and livestock schistosomes and outlines strategies for addressing these concerns.

Keywords: *Schistosoma*, schistosome, zoonosis, zoonotic, livestock, cattle, hybridization, neglected tropical disease, Nigeria

1. Introduction

Schistosomiasis, historically referred to as bilharzia, is a significant neglected tropical disease (NTD) in sub-Saharan Africa [1, 2]. This parasitic disease is the result of infection by water-borne trematode worms, commonly known as blood flukes, belonging to the genus *Schistosoma*, which require specific aqueous snail intermediate hosts for their developmental cycle [3]. Currently, over 206 million people are affected in 78 countries across tropical and subtropical regions of Africa, the Middle

East, some parts of Asia and Latin America [3], with approximately 24,000 deaths and 2.5 million disability-adjusted life years recorded annually [4]. Six schistosome species are known to exclusively infect humans, with four of them prevalent in Africa; *Schistosoma guineensis*, *S. haematobium*, *S. intercalatum*, and *S. mansoni* [3, 5]. Three other species, namely *Schistosoma bovis*, *S. curassoni* and *S. mattheei*, commonly infect bovids, including livestock cattle [5, 6]. The geographical distribution of these species collectively spans tropical and subtropical regions of Africa – including Nigeria that is discussed here [3].

Schistosomiasis primarily affects rural and marginalized urban populations that have frequent contact with surface water bodies, which may be infested with snail intermediate hosts. Lack of access to safe water, sanitation, and hygiene further exacerbates the risk of infection in these communities. Intestinal schistosomiasis is associated with most human schistosome species, while urogenital schistosomiasis is predominantly caused by *S. haematobium* [7]. Sub-Saharan Africa is home to approximately 90% of individuals affected by schistosomiasis who require treatment [3]. Nigeria, which has the largest population in the region of over 223 million, shas the highest number of schistosomiasis cases [1, 2].

The World Health Organization (WHO) has initiated a widespread distribution among at-risk school-age children of praziquantel, the primary drug deployed to treat schistosomiasis, as a way to reduce the extent of disease-associated morbidity [8]. This approach, known as preventive chemotherapy, aims to treat at least 75% of a community's school-age children annually, in addition to implementing health education campaigns and snail reduction strategies [4]. However, the control of schistosomes that can be transmitted from livestock to humans, known as zoonotic schistosomiasis, has received little attention over the years [9]. This is particularly relevant in areas where the coexistence of humans, livestock, and suitable snail intermediate hosts occurs. Recent reports have highlighted the genetic hybridization of the closely related species *S. haematobium* and *S. bovis* that infects cattle [5, 10, 11], in several West African countries including Niger, Senegal, Mali, Benin, and Cameroon [11–15]. The migration of infected snails and the influx of livestock from neighboring countries into Nigeria raise concerns about the establishment of hybrid human urogenital and bovine intestinal schistosomes in Nigerian waters.

Schistosomiasis is a significant NTD in sub-Saharan Africa, particularly in Nigeria, which provides the focus of this chapter. The WHO-led preventive chemotherapy program has made progress in controlling the disease, but the control of zoonotic schistosomiasis remains a major challenge. The genetic hybridization of *Schistosoma* species, particularly *S. haematobium* x *S. bovis*, and the potential transmission from livestock to humans highlight the need for improved control programs and research to combat this neglected source of schistosomiasis more effectively.

2. *Schistosoma haematobium* life cycle

Schistosoma haematobium has two distinct life cycle phases, asexual and sexual. These involve infecting two different hosts, a snail intermediate host and a vertebrate definitive host, respectively. The cycle typically commences when eggs, discharged in the urine of an infected vertebrate host, encounter freshwater environments containing snails belonging to the *Bulinus* genus. Upon contact with water, the eggs hatch, liberating free-swimming miracidia, which then proceed to penetrate the snail host. Once established, these miracidia undergo asexual development through multiple stages, eventually becoming cercariae that leave the snail in search of the definitive host. Despite their short lifespan, a single miracidium in a suitable snail host can produce approximately 200 cercariae per day [16, 17].

The cercariae penetrate the skin of suitable definitive hosts that come into contact with the contaminated water, transforming into schistosomula. This penetration commonly takes place in surface water bodies that serve as gathering points for people and livestock, often used for domestic and recreational activities [18]. After penetrating the skin, the schistosomula migrate through the epidermis and dermis layers, eventually entering the bloodstream and traveling to the lungs [17, 19–21]. After leaving the lungs, the parasites reach the left side of the heart via the pulmonary veins and then enter the abdominal aorta. They can then pass through various arteries, such as the coeliac trunk, inferior and superior mesenteric arteries, or iliac arteries, to reach the portal veins of the liver [21]. In the liver, the schistosomula lose their migratory ability, grow, and develop into adult male and female pairs [21].

The adult worms, occurring in pairs, navigate against the natural flow of blood within the venous circulation. They eventually settle in the vesical venous plexus, a network of veins around the bladder. In this location, they produce eggs, which can migrate to various parts of the urinary tract, including the bladder and ureter [17, 21]. These eggs have the capability to penetrate the walls of blood vessels, the bladder, or genital organs [21]; those that make their way to the bladder are expelled from the body through urine into freshwater environments. In these aquatic settings, the hatched miracidia perpetuate the transmission cycle [17]. It is worth noting that other species of *Schistosoma* follow a comparable life cycle but may exhibit variations in their preferred sites and the morphology of their eggs [22]. These minor microscopical differences help diagnostic identification.

3. Zoonotic schistosomiasis

The classification of zoonoses or zoonotic diseases encompasses various infectious diseases and their causative agents that can be transmitted and established between human and animal hosts [23]. Therefore, zoonotic schistosomiasis refers to the presence of a *Schistosoma* species, which typically affects a specific human or animal host, in another host that is not specific to the schistosome group [12, 24]. These *Schistosoma* species are naturally shared between humans and various animal hosts due to the extensive interactions that occur at transmission sites [25, 26].

Hybridization can take place in regions where different schistosome species are either endemic or share substantial geographical overlap among potential hosts [27, 28]. These interactions between schistosomes can occur in two ways: bidirectional, whereby both male and female schistosomes from different pairs come together to produce viable hybrid offspring [24]; or unidirectional, in which pairing happens between schistosomes of either male or female sex [29, 30]. The establishment of hybridization has been observed in various studies, indicating the presence of hybrid schistosomes in both human and animal hosts [12]. These hybrids are not limited to first-generation offspring, which suggests the existence of stable hybrid zones. The occurrence of hybridization has implications for disease prevalence, pathology, and treatment, and may lead to the emergence of new pathogens, requiring additional control strategies [12, 24]. The understanding of hybridization and its impact on schistosomiasis is therefore crucial for effective control and prevention efforts.

4. Nigeria's schistosomiasis control program

In 1995, the Nigerian Federal Government created the National Control Schistosomiasis Programme. Through epidemiological mapping, this revealed that at the time around 20 million people were infected with the disease. Pilot control projects were initiated in some selected states (Borno, Ebonyi, Katsina, Kwara, and Ondo), each having distinct ecological conditions that render them highly susceptible to schistosomiasis. Prevention and control activities have since evolved, being currently integrated into an expanded program that aims to eradicate other neglected tropical diseases [31]. This has driven mass drug administration (MDA) of praziquantel with the support of organizations such as the WHO, UNICEF, and various non-governmental development organizations. MDA is carried out at the level of implementation units (IUs), which can be a district, province, or local government area [8]. Disease prevalence and population data at the community level are aggregated at the IU level to determine praziquantel treatment thresholds [8, 32].

Praziquantel MDA is administered every six months to all school-age children in districts where the prevalence exceeds 50%, annually for districts with a prevalence ranging from 10% to 49.9%, and every two years for districts with a prevalence between 1% and 10% [8]. However, recently published WHO guidelines have revised these recommendations, specifying annual MDA for all school-age children with a prevalence above 50%, biennial MDA for half the children with a prevalence between 10 and 49.9%, and two treatments during primary schooling for all children with a prevalence between 1 and 10% [33]. In 2019, approximately 250 million praziquantel doses were used to treat 95.3 million children and adults, achieving an epidemiological coverage of 67% [4]. This falls short of the 75% target set for 2020, emphasizing the need to accelerate progress in control and prevention. The 2020–2030 global NTD elimination roadmap sets more specific targets for schistosomiasis, including reducing the proportion of moderate and heavy intensity infections to less than 1% in 78 countries, reducing the number of tablets required during MDA by 50%, and increasing domestic financial support for MDA [3, 4]. Achieving these targets largely depends on increased community participation, geographical reach, and high program coverage during MDA [34–37].

5. Impact of hybridization on schistosomiasis control efforts

The presence of hybrid schistosomes is a significant concern for the schistosomiasis control program in Nigeria, as it can lead to a wider host range, increased transmission potential, altered pathology, and potential drug resistance [38]. Interactions between different *Schistosoma* species can enhance reproductive capacity, resulting in a higher number of parasite offspring, faster maturation, and a broader range of intermediate hosts [39, 40]. One major concern is that the emergence of hybrid schistosomes may reduce the effectiveness of praziquantel treatment [41]. This phenomenon has been documented in both real-world field settings and controlled laboratory environments, particularly in the case of *S. mansoni*. It is closely linked to the concealed or hidden role that hybridization plays in this context [42–44]. The success of praziquantel as a treatment is therefore threatened by the presence of *Schistosoma* hybrids [5]. Additionally, the genetic diversity among progeny of zoonotic schistosomes provides them with better phenotypic characteristics [45], allowing for improved evasion of host recognition and resistance to the host's adaptive immune system. This can result in increased infectivity and the development of unusual pathologies [46]. The infection of multiple animal reservoir hosts by zoonotic hybrid schistosomes makes the elimination of the disease more challenging [14, 15]. The ubiquitous presence of rodents, which serve as reservoir hosts for many schistosome species, contributes to the difficulty in controlling and preventing *Schistosoma* hybrid infections in endemic areas due to the potential for co-infection [47].

6. Factors promoting hybridization of schistosome species

6.1 Shared freshwater bodies and occurrence of weather events

Schistosomiasis is a disease that primarily occurs in specific areas with slow-moving freshwater bodies that support the proliferation of intermediate host snails. This is particularly evident in locations where dams and similar water development structures are present [48, 49]. However, changes in environmental and climatic conditions have the potential to expand the geographical range of the disease [50]. Unprecedented transmission of schistosomiasis has been observed at higher altitudes in Uganda, where clinical infection would not typically be expected [51]. Studies from eastern Africa and China have also predicted that rising ambient temperatures could impact schistosomiasis transmission [52, 53].

It is likely that fluctuations in schistosomiasis transmission will be observed in areas bordering currently endemic regions [54]. Additionally, geographically disconnected but endemic communities may share ecological links through common rivers, streams, or other freshwater bodies. This creates a window of opportunity for schistosomes and their intermediate hosts to establish themselves in novel locations, particularly during weather-related events such as flooding. Studies conducted in China have revealed that significant flood disasters can lead to the dispersal and establishment of new populations of intermediate host snails in regions where schistosomiasis was not previously present or had been previously eliminated [52]. Similar outbreaks have been observed in Nigeria after flooding [55]. The presence of large rivers that transcend international boundaries further increases the possibility of hybrid schistosomes being introduced to new areas. The Niger River, for example, passes through multiple countries, including Nigeria, and has been associated with the hybridization of *S. haematobium* and *S. bovis* species. The establishment of hybrid schistosomes and zoonotic infections in endemic areas affected by flooding requires close surveillance.

Despite ongoing preventive chemotherapy programs, schistosomiasis transmission continues in some endemic areas in Nigeria [48, 56]. The Niger River, being the longest river in West Africa, poses a significant challenge for control efforts due to its extensive reach and the high population density in its delta region. The emergence of hybrid schistosomes in areas sharing the Niger River and its tributaries with neighboring countries increases the risk of hybrid schistosomes being introduced to Nigeria during flooding events [57]. The surveillance of schistosome hybrid species and zoonotic infections in flood-affected endemic areas is crucial for effective control and prevention.

6.2 Water development projects and flooding

In 2017, the Federal Ministry of Agriculture and Rural Development in Nigeria estimated that the country's livestock production encompassed a substantial population, which included approximately 18.4 million cattle, 43.4 million sheep, 76 million goats, and a staggering 180 million poultry [58]. Small-scale livestock holders and nomadic herders play a significant role in this production [59]. It is estimated that 13 million households, accounting for 42% of the Nigerian population, own livestock. Similar to other regions in the developing world, cattle and other livestock in rural Nigeria often live in close proximity to humans and freely roam within the local community [60]. This close ecological interaction between humans and animals, particularly through shared resources like water, creates an environment conducive to the zoonotic transmission of pathogens. Schistosomiasis transmission is closely linked to the presence of freshwater bodies that support vector snails, and zoonotic transmission occurs in areas where humans and animals have close ecological interactions.

Hybrid schistosomes have been detected in children residing in villages located around the Senegal River Basin in Senegal. This occurrence is closely linked to water development projects that have expanded shared water interactions between humans and livestock in the region [12]. These hybrids result from the hybridization of human and bovine schistosomes (*S. haematobium* and *S. bovis*), providing evidence of zoonotic *Schistosoma* infection between humans and cattle. Similar outbreaks of schistosomiasis have been reported in Nigeria following major water development projects and flooding events [61–64]. However, the potential changes in zoonotic transmission dynamics resulting from altered human-animal interactions in affected areas have not been thoroughly investigated. Despite the demonstrated ability of locally endemic species like *S. mansoni* to infect a broad range of hosts, including rodents and primates, there has been limited interest in the zoonotic transmission of schistosomes in Nigeria [25, 65]. This highlights the need for further research and surveillance to understand and address the zoonotic transmission of schistosomiasis in the country.

6.3 In-country and cross-border migration of livestock

Understanding the transmission of zoonotic schistosomes is of utmost importance in Nigeria, where livestock production is dominated by nomadic pastoral practices. This farming method accounts for approximately 82% of the country's cattle [60], primarily owned by the Fulani population, who are known for their nomadic lifestyle [66]. The Fulani people are renowned as the world's largest nomadic ethnic group and hold a prominent position in Nigeria as the nation's leading pastoralists [67, 68].

In addition to various other nomadic groups, the Fulani make up approximately 12% of the population in sub-Saharan Africa [69]. These nomadic communities depend entirely on livestock for their livelihoods and sustenance. They engage in a migratory lifestyle, crossing national boundaries as they seek pasture and freshwater resources essential for the wellbeing of their herds [70, 71]. This seasonal movement, known as transhumance herding, is believed to contribute to the spread of the *Rhipicephalus* (*Boophilus*) *microplus* tick across Africa. The emergence of this tick in new areas, such as Nigeria, is attributed to pasture rotation practices aimed at managing tick populations [72]. *Rhipicephalus microplus* serves as a vector for the protozoan pathogen that causes bovine babesiosis, a significant disease in cattle. Hence, the dependence of pastoralist communities on water resources during their migrations elevates the risk of introducing both *Schistosoma* and *Babesia* to new regions of Nigeria where these parasites were not previously considered threats to public or veterinary health.

The movement of hosts also has the potential to disrupt the natural distribution of schistosome species and raise the likelihood of interbreeding between different species [40]. In addition to internal migration, the entry of livestock from neighboring countries within the Economic Community of West African States, for purposes such as trade and open grazing, further facilitates the potential introduction and establishment of hybrid schistosomes within Nigeria's river systems. This is especially pertinent to regions where hybridization has been documented. The contamination of Nigeria's water bodies by migrating livestock from both domestic sources and trans-border routes poses a major challenge to schistosomiasis control initiatives.

6.4 Inadequate clean water, sanitation, and hygiene facilities

Schistosomiasis is categorized as an NTD because it disproportionately affects socioeconomically disadvantaged populations worldwide [73]. In Nigeria, over 83 million people live in extreme poverty, lacking access to clean water, sanitation, and hygiene (WASH) facilities, as well as other basic social amenities [74]. These communities heavily rely on agriculture, with 70% engaging in livestock rearing for their livelihoods [75]. According to data from the World Bank, it is estimated that about 39% of rural domiciles in Nigeria do not have access to safe water sources. Additionally, only 50% of these households have access to improved sanitation facilities, and approximately one-third of them still engage in open defecation practices [76]. In most cases, the primary water sources for these communities are freshwater bodies located nearby, which are frequently contaminated due to poor sanitation conditions and practices [48]. The socioeconomic circumstances make it challenging to develop separate water sources for humans and animals, leading to continued co-interaction at open water bodies, posing a significant public health challenge. This situation significantly elevates the risk of zoonotic transmission of schistosomiasis between different hosts.

Recognizing the critical state of WASH facilities in Nigeria, the Federal Government has taken steps to address the issue and promote equitable access to improved WASH facilities [77, 78]. One notable initiative is the National Urban Water Sector Reform Program, which has constructed more than 2300 water points across the country since 2015, with a primary focus on urban areas [76]. Unfortunately, this urban-centric approach has left rural areas with profoundly inadequate coverage, thereby exacerbating the challenge of providing WASH facilities to rural communities through the existing Rural Water Supply and Sanitation Programme [79]. In response to this situation, in 2018 the Federal Government declared a state of emergency in the country's drinking water, sanitation, and hygiene sector. One critical issue identified was that many water supply pumps installed in rural areas fail shortly after installation and remain unrepaired, leaving the population without access to clean water [80]. This underscores the urgent need for more sustainable approaches to providing safe drinking water to rural communities.

Research has demonstrated that the availability of WASH facilities is associated with a reduction in NTDs such as soil-transmitted helminth infections and schistosomiasis [81, 82]. Providing WASH facilities in schistosomiasis-endemic communities not only prevents the sharing of water between humans and animals, thereby reducing the risk of zoonotic infections, but also brings broader health benefits. It is imperative to assess the impact of expanding access to WASH facilities in schistosomiasis-endemic areas of Nigeria, both in terms of reducing the transmission of *Schistosoma* species to humans and the potential for zoonotic transmission between humans and animals.

7. Future research priorities

Limited information is available on the epidemiology of hybrid schistosomes in Nigeria [83]. Recent reports have provided some morphological characterization of hybrid *Schistosoma* eggs in endemic areas of southwestern Nigeria. However, further research is needed to obtain detailed and confirmatory evidence regarding their genetic diversity [84]. This information is crucial for informing programming and policy decisions, particularly regarding the efficacy of praziquantel. Conducting such investigations would require access to state-of-the-art facilities and the development of research capacity, which is currently lacking or inadequate [85].

8. Conclusions

Investing in adequate water, sanitation, and hygiene (WASH) facilities and implementing effective strategies to modify habitats and prevent flooding are crucial for controlling schistosomiasis in Nigeria. However, in addition to providing these resources, it is recommended to implement innovative health education programs that promote optimal usage and sustainable maintenance among the targeted nomadic communities. These outreach programs should involve consultation with community leaders to incorporate local livestock rearing strategies that prevent contamination of communal water bodies with human and livestock waste. By taking these measures, the risk of genetic hybridization by schistosome species of different origin can be significantly reduced. Furthermore, it is crucial to establish accurate surveillance systems, promptly detect outbreaks, identify *Schistosoma* species, and consistently promote preventive chemotherapy as integral activities of a nationwide schistosomiasis control program in Nigeria.

Author contributions

All authors contributed significantly to preparing and writing this chapter.

Funding statement

No specific funding was received for this work.

Conflict of interest

No conflicts of interest declared.

Author details

Andrew W. Taylor-Robinson[1,2,3]*, Hammed Oladeji Mogaji[4,5,6], Olaitan O. Omitola[7], Adedotun Ayodeji Bayegun[7] and Uwem Friday Ekpo[7]

1 College of Health Sciences, VinUniversity, Hanoi, Vietnam

2 Center for Global Health, University of Pennsylvania, Philadelphia, USA

3 College of Health and Human Sciences, Charles Darwin University, Casuarina, Australia

4 Department of Animal and Environmental Biology, Federal University Oye-Ekiti, Ekiti, Nigeria

5 Department of Epidemiology, Institute of Collective Health, Federal University Bahia, Salvador, Brazil

6 School of Public Health, Yale University, New Haven, USA

7 Department of Pure and Applied Zoology, Federal University of Agriculture, Abeokuta, Nigeria

*Address all correspondence to: andrew.tr@vinuni.edu.vn

References

[1] Hotez PJ, Fenwick A. Schistosomiasis in Africa: An emerging tragedy in our new global health decade. PLoS Neglected Tropical Diseases. 2009;**3**(9):e485

[2] Hotez PJ, Kamath A. Neglected tropical diseases in sub-Saharan Africa: Review of their prevalence, distribution, and disease burden. PLoS Neglected Tropical Diseases. 2009;**3**(8):e412

[3] World Health Organization. Schistosomiasis. Last updated 1 February 2023. Available from: https://www.who.int/news-room/fact-sheets/detail/schistosomiasis [Accessed: August 30, 2023]

[4] World Health Organization. Ending the Neglect to Attain the Sustainable Development Goals: A Road Map for Neglected Tropical Diseases 2021-2030. Geneva: World Health Organization; 2020 Licence: CC BY-NC-SA 3.0 IGO

[5] Stothard JR, Kayuni SA, Al-Harbi MH, Musaya J, Webster BL. Future schistosome hybridizations: Will all *Schistosoma haematobium* hybrids please stand-up! PLoS Neglected Tropical Diseases. 2020;**14**(7):e0008201

[6] Engels D, Chitsulo L, Montresor A, Savioli L. The global epidemiological situation of schistosomiasis and new approaches to control and research. Acta Tropica. 2002;**82**(2):139-146

[7] Centers for Disease Control and Prevention. DPDx – Laboratory Identification of Parasites of Public Health Concern. Schistosomiasis. Last updated 14 August 2019. Available from: https://www.cdc.gov/dpdx/schistosomiasis/index.html [Accessed: August 30, 2023]

[8] World Health Organization. Helminth Control in School-Age Children: a Guide for Managers of Control Programmes. Second edition, 2011. Available from: https://apps.who.int/iris/bitstream/handle/10665/44671/9789241548267_eng.pdf [Accessed: August 30, 2023]

[9] Rollinson D. A wake-up call for urinary schistosomiasis: Reconciling research effort with public health importance. Parasitology. 2009;**136**(12):1593-1610

[10] Webster BL, Southgate VR. Mating interactions of *Schistosoma haematobium* and *S. intercalatum* with their hybrid offspring. Parasitology. 2003;**126**(4):327-338

[11] Léger E, Garba A, Hamidou AA, Webster BL, Pennance T, Rollinson D, et al. Introgressed animal schistosomes *Schistosoma curassoni* and *S. bovis* naturally infecting humans. Emerging Infectious Diseases. 2016;**22**(12):2212-2214

[12] Huyse BL, Webster S, Geldof, Stothard JR, Diaw OT, Polman K, et al. Bidirectional introgressive hybridisation between cattle and human schistosome species. PLoS Pathogens. 2009;**5**(9):e1000571

[13] Soentjens P, Cnops L, Huyse T, Yansouni C, Vos DD, Bottieau E, et al. Diagnosis and clinical management of *Schistosoma haematobium–Schistosoma bovis* hybrid infection in a cluster of travelers returning from Mali. Clinical Infectious Diseases. 2016;**63**(12):1626-1629

[14] Savassi BAES, Mouahid G, Lasica C, Mahaman S-DK, Garcia A, Courtin D, et al. Cattle as natural host

for *Schistosoma haematobium* (Bilharz, 1852) Weinland, 1858 x *Schistosoma bovis* Sonsino, 1876 interactions, with new cercarial emergence and genetic patterns. Parasitology Research. 2020;**119**(7):2189-2205

[15] Savassi BAES, Dobigny G, Etougbétché JR, Avocegan TT, Quinsou FT, Gauthier P, et al. *Mastomys natalensis* (Smith, 1834) as a natural host for *Schistosoma haematobium* (Bilharz, 1852) Weinland, 1858 x *Schistosoma bovis* Sonsino, 1876 introgressive hybrids. Parasitology Research. 2021;**120**(5):1755-1770

[16] Grimes JE, Croll D, Harrison WE, Utzinger J, Freeman MC, Templeton MR. The roles of water, sanitation and hygiene in reducing schistosomiasis: A review. Parasites & Vectors. 2015;**8**:156

[17] Nelwan ML. Schistosomiasis: Life cycle, diagnosis, and control. Current Therapeutic Research, Clinical and Experimental. 2019;**91**:5-9

[18] Mafiana CF, Ekpo UF, Ojo DA. Urinary schistosomiasis in preschool children in settlements around Oyan reservoir in Ogun state, Nigeria: Implications for control. Tropical Medicine & International Health. 2003;**8**(1):78-82

[19] Curwen RS, Wilson RA. Invasion of skin by schistosome cercariae: Some neglected facts. Trends in Parasitology. 2003;**19**(2):63-66

[20] He YX, Salafsky B, Ramaswany K. Comparison of skin invasion among three major species of *Schistosoma*. Trends in Parasitology. 2005;**21**(5):201-203

[21] Nation CS, Da'dara AA, Marchant JK, Skelly PJ. Schistosome migration in the definitive host. PLoS Neglected Tropical Diseases. 2020;**14**(4):e0007951

[22] McManus DP, Dunne DW, Sacko M, Utzinger J, Vennervald BJ, Zhou X-N. Schistosomiasis. Nature Reviews. Disease Primers. 2018;**4**:13

[23] Chomel BB. Control and prevention of emerging parasitic zoonoses. International Journal for Parasitology. 2008;**38**(11):1211-1217

[24] Huyse T, Van Den Broeck F, Hellemans B, Volckaert FAM, Polman K. Hybridisation between the two major African schistosome species of humans. International Journal for Parasitology. 2013;**43**(8):687-689

[25] Standley CJ, Mugisha L, Dobson AP, Stothard JR. Zoonotic schistosomiasis in non-human primates: Past, present and future activities at the human–wildlife interface in Africa. Journal of Helminthology. 2012;**86**(2):131-140

[26] Léger E, Webster JP. Hybridizations within the genus *Schistosoma*: Implications for evolution, epidemiology and control. Parasitology. 2017;**144**(1):65-80

[27] Fan PC, Lin LH. Hybridization of *Schistosoma mansoni* and *Schistosoma japonicum* in mice. Southeast Asian Journal of Tropical Medicine and Public Health. 2005;**36**(1):89-96

[28] Boissier J, Moné H, Mitta G, Bargues MD, Molyneux D, Mas-Coma S. Schistosomiasis reaches Europe. Lancet Infectious Diseases. 2015;**15**(7):757-758

[29] Steinauer ML, Hanelt B, Mwangi IN, Maina GM, Agola LE, Kinuthia JM, et al. Introgressive hybridization of human and rodent schistosome parasites in western Kenya. Molecular Ecology. 2008;**17**(23):5062-5074

[30] Borlase A, Webster JP, Rudge JW. Opportunities and challenges for modelling epidemiological and

evolutionary dynamics in a multihost, multiparasite system: Zoonotic hybrid schistosomiasis in West Africa. Evolutionary Applications. 2017;**11**(4):501-515

[31] The Carter Center. Schistosomiasis Control Program. Last updated July 2021. Available from: https://www.cartercenter.org/resources/pdfs/factsheets/schistosomiasis-facts.pdf [Accessed: August 30, 2023]

[32] Mogaji HO, Dedeke GA, Bada BS, Bankole S, Adeniji A, Fagbenro MT, et al. Distribution of ascariasis, trichuriasis and hookworm infections in Ogun state, Southwestern Nigeria. PLoS One. 2020;**15**(6):e0233423

[33] World Health Organization. WHO Guideline on Control and Elimination of Human Schistosomiasis. Geneva: World Health Organization; 2022. Available from: https://apps.who.int/iris/rest/bitstreams/1410449/retrieve [Accessed: August 30, 2023]

[34] El-Setouhy M, Abd Elaziz KM, Helmy H, Farid HA, Kamal HA, Ramzy RMR, et al. The effect of compliance on the impact of mass drug administration for elimination of lymphatic filariasis in Egypt. American Journal of Tropical Medicine and Hygiene. 2007;**77**(6):1069-1073

[35] Olamiju OJ, Olamiju FO, Adeniran AA, Mba IC, Ukwunna CC, Okoronkwo C, et al. Public awareness and knowledge of neglected tropical diseases (NTDs) control activities in Abuja, Nigeria. PLOS Neglected Tropical Diseases. 2014;**8**(9):e3209

[36] Assaré RK, N'Tamon RN, Bellai LG, Koffi JA, Mathieu T-BI, Ouattara M, et al. Characteristics of persistent hotspots of *Schistosoma mansoni* in western Côte d'Ivoire. Parasites & Vectors. 2020;**13**(1):337

[37] Mogaji HO, Odoh IM, Iyeh CI, Adeniran AA, Oyedeji SI, Okoh HI, et al. Attendee's awareness about preventive chemotherapy neglected tropical diseases (PC-NTD) control during the first world neglected tropical diseases day in Ekiti state, Nigeria. PLoS Neglected Tropical Diseases. 2021;**15**(3):e0009315

[38] King KC, Stelkens RB, Webster JP, Smith DF, Brockhurst MA. Hybridization in parasites: Consequences for adaptive evolution, pathogenesis, and public health in a changing world. PLoS Pathogens. 2015;**11**(9):e1005098

[39] Moné H, Minguez S, Ibikounlé M, Allienne J-F, Massougbodji A, Mouahid G. Natural interactions between *S. haematobium* and *S. guineensis* in the Republic of Benin. Scientific World Journal. 2012;**2012**:793420

[40] Webster BL, Diaw OT, Seye MM, Webster JP, Rollinson D. Introgressive hybridization of *Schistosoma haematobium* group species in Senegal: Species barrier break down between ruminant and human schistosomes. PLoS Neglected Tropical Diseases. 2013;**7**(4):e2110

[41] Webster JP, Molyneux DH, Hotez PJ, Fenwick A. The contribution of mass drug administration to global health: Past, present and future. Philosophical Transactions of the Royal Society of London. Series B, Biological Sciences. 2014;**369**(1645):20130434

[42] Lamberton PHL, Hogan SC, Kabatereine NB, Fenwick A, Webster JP. In vitro praziquantel test capable of detecting reduced *in vivo* efficacy in *Schistosoma mansoni* human infections.

American Journal of Tropical Medicine and Hygiene. 2010;**83**(6):1340-1347

[43] Valentim CLL, Cioli D, Chevalier FD, Cao X, Taylor AB, Holloway SP, et al. Genetic and molecular basis of drug resistance and species-specific drug action in schistosome parasites. Science. 2013;**342**(6164):1385-1389

[44] Webster BL, Diaw OT, Seye MM, Faye DS, Stothard JR, Sousa-Figueiredo JC, et al. Praziquantel treatment of school children from single and mixed infection foci of intestinal and urogenital schistosomiasis along the Senegal River basin: Monitoring treatment success and re-infection patterns. Acta Tropica. 2013;**128**(2):292-302

[45] Grigg ME, Bonnefoy S, Hehl AB, Suzuki Y, Boothroyd JC. Success and virulence in *Toxoplasma* as the result of sexual recombination between two distinct ancestries. Science, 2001. 2001;**294**(5540):161-165

[46] Schelkle B, Faria PJ, Johnson MB, van Oosterhout C, Cable J. Mixed infections and hybridisation in monogenean parasites. PLoS One. 2012;**7**(7):e39506

[47] Hanelt B, Mwangi IN, Kinuthia JM, Maina GM, Agola LE, Mutuku MW, et al. Schistosomes of small mammals from the Lake Victoria Basin, Kenya: New species, familiar species, and implications for schistosomiasis control. Parasitology. 2010;**137**(7):1109-1118

[48] Akinwale O, Ajayi M, Akande D, Gyang P, Adeleke M, Adeneye A, et al. Urinary schistosomiasis around Oyan reservoir, Nigeria: Twenty years after the first outbreak. Iranian Journal of Public Health. 2010;**39**(1):92-95

[49] Dida GO, Gelder FB, Anyona DN, Matano AS, Abuom PO, Adoka SO, et al. Distribution and abundance of schistosomiasis and fascioliasis host snails along the Mara River in Kenya and Tanzania. Infection Ecology & Epidemiology. 2014;**4**:24281

[50] Zhou XN, Yang GJ, Yang K, Wang XH, Hong QB, Sun LP, et al. Potential impact of climate change on schistosomiasis transmission in China. American Journal of Tropical Medicine and Hygiene. 2008;**78**(2):188-194

[51] John R, Ezekiel M, Philbert C, Andrew A. Schistosomiasis transmission at high altitude crater lakes in western Uganda. BMC Infectious Diseases. 2008;**8**:110

[52] Wu XH, Zhang SQ, Xu XJ, Huang YX, Steinmann P, Utzinger J, et al. Effect of floods on the transmission of schistosomiasis in the Yangtze River valley, People's Republic of China. Parasitology International. 2008;**57**(3):271-276

[53] McCreesh N, Nikulin G, Booth M. Predicting the effects of climate change on *Schistosoma mansoni* transmission in eastern Africa. Parasites & Vectors. 2015;**8**:4

[54] Mari L, Ciddio M, Casagrandi R, Perez-Saez J, Bertuzzo E, Rinaldo A, et al. Heterogeneity in schistosomiasis transmission dynamics. Journal of Theoretical Biology. 2017;**432**:87-99

[55] Ito EE, Egwunyenga AO. Schistosomiasis: The aftermath of 2012 floods in Delta state, Southern Nigeria. Internal Medicine Journal. 2015;**22**(4):218-223

[56] Oladejo SO, Ofoezie IE. Unabated schistosomiasis transmission in Erinle River dam, Osun state, Nigeria: Evidence of neglect of environmental effects of development projects. Tropical

Medicine & International Health. 2006;**11**(6):843-850

[57] Abe EM, Guo YH, Shen H, Mutsaka-Makuvaza MJ, Habib MR, Xue JB, et al. Phylogeography of *Bulinus truncates* (Audouin, 1827) (Gastropoda: Planorbidae) in selected African countries. Tropical Medicine and Infectious Disease. 2018;**3**(4):127

[58] Federal Ministry of Agriculture and Rural Development. Agricultural Sector Food Security and Nutrition Strategy 2016-2025. Available from: https://faolex.fao.org/docs/pdf/nig201549.pdf [Accessed: August 30, 2023]

[59] Food and Agriculture Organization of the United Nations. The Future of Livestock in Nigeria. Last updated September 2020. Available from: https://www.fao.org/3/cb1939en/CB1939EN.pdf [Accessed: August 30, 2023]

[60] Léger E, Borlase A, Fall CB, Diouf ND, Dipo SD, Yasenev L, et al. Prevalence and distribution of schistosomiasis in human, livestock, and snail populations in northern Senegal: A One Health epidemiological study of a multi-host system. Lancet Planet Health. 2020;**4**(8):e330-e342

[61] Southgate VR. Schistosomiasis in the Senegal River basin: Before and after the construction of the dams at Diama, Senegal and Manantali, Mali and future prospects. Journal of Helminthology. 1997;**71**(2):125-132

[62] Duplantier JM, Sène M. Rodents as reservoir hosts in the transmission of *Schistosoma mansoni* in Richard-toll, Senegal, West Africa. Journal of Helminthology. 2000;**74**(2):129-135

[63] Ofoezie IE, Imevbore AM, Balogun MO, Ogunkoya OO, Asaolu SO. A study of an outbreak of schistosomiasis in two resettlement villages near Abeokuta, Ogun state, Nigeria. Journal of Helminthology. 1991;**65**(2):95-102

[64] Olamiju F, Nebe OJ, Mogaji H, Marcus A, Amodu-Agbi P, Urude RO, et al. Schistosomiasis outbreak during COVID-19 pandemic in Takum, Northeast Nigeria: Analysis of infection status and associated risk factors. PLoS One. 2022;**17**(1):e0262524

[65] Webster JP, Gower CM, Knowles SCL, Molyneux DH, Fenton A. One health – An ecological and evolutionary framework for tackling neglected zoonotic diseases. Evolutionary Applications. 2016;**9**(2):313-333

[66] Omotayo AO. Farming households' environment, nutrition and health interplay in Southwest Nigeria. International Journal of Science Research in Agricultural Sciences. 2016;**3**(3):84-98

[67] Blench R. Pastoral Cross-Border Movement. In: Natural Resource Conflicts in North-Central Nigeria: A Handbook and Case Studies. London: Mandaras Publishing; 2004. pp. 133-137

[68] Umoh NR. Pastoralism in Nigeria's middle-belt region: A resource or a curse? International Journal of Development and Economic Sustainability. 2017;**5**(4):11-30

[69] Rass N. Policies and Strategies to Address the Vulnerability of Pastoralists in Sub-Saharan Africa. Rome: Pro-Poor Livestock Policy Initiative, Food and Agriculture Organization of the United Nations; 2006

[70] Enwezor FNC, Umoh JU, Esievo KAN, Anere JI. Transhumance pastoralism as risk factor in the trypanosome infections in cattle. Bulletin of Animal Health and Production in Africa. 2009;**57**(1):44-48

[71] Aruwayo A, Adeola SS, Ibrahim U. Assessment of the challenges of nomadic farming activities in Daura agricultural zone of Katsina state, Nigeria. Nigerian Journal of Animal Production. 2021;**48**(2):200-209

[72] Kamani J, Apanaskevich DA, Gutiérrez R, Nachum-Biala Y, Baneth G, Harrus S. Morphological and molecular identification of *Rhipicephalus* (*Boophilus*) *microplus* in Nigeria, West Africa: A threat to livestock health. Experimental & Applied Acarology. 2017;**73**(2):283-296

[73] Hotez PJ, Asojo OA, Adesina AM. Nigeria: "ground zero" for the high prevalence neglected tropical diseases. PLoS Neglected Tropical Diseases. 2012;**6**(7):e1600

[74] Global Data Lab. Area profile report – Nigeria. Available from: https://globaldatalab.org/areadata/profiles/NGAt/ [Accessed: August 30, 2023]

[75] Food and Agriculture Organization of the United Nations. Nigeria Agriculture at a Glance. Last updated 2023. Available from: https://www.fao.org/nigeria/fao-in-nigeria/nigeria-at-a-glance/en/ [Accessed: August 30, 2023]

[76] The World Bank. Third National Urban Water Sector Reform Project for Nigeria. Last updated 15 February 2023. Available from: https://projects.worldbank.org/en/projects-operations/project-detail/P123513 [Accessed: August 30, 2023]

[77] United Nations Children's Fund. Nigeria – Water, Sanitation and Hygiene. Available from: https://www.unicef.org/nigeria/water-sanitation-and-hygiene [Accessed: August 30, 2023]

[78] Mogaji HO, Ekpo UF, Yusuff QA, Yusuff HA, Adeaga DO, Monday J, et al. Impacts of water, sanitation and hygiene (WASH) interventions on intestinal helminthiasis of school-aged children in Ogun state, South-Western Nigeria. Tropical Medicine & International Health. 2015;**20**:233

[79] Ibok EE, Daniel EE. Rural water supply and sustainable development in Nigeria: A case analysis of Akwa Ibom state. American Journal of Rural Development. 2014;**2**(4):68-73

[80] Ihuah PW, Kakulu II. Rural water supply projects and sustainable development in Nigeria. Journal of Sustainable Development in Africa. 2014;**16**(1):56-68

[81] Strunz EC, Addiss DG, Stocks ME, Ogden S, Utzinger J, Freeman MC. Water, sanitation, hygiene, and soil-transmitted helminth infection: A systematic review and meta-analysis. PLoS Medicine. 2014;**11**(3):e1001620

[82] Grimes JE, Tadesse G, Mekete K, Wuletaw Y, Gebretsadik A, French MD, et al. School water, sanitation, and hygiene, soil-transmitted helminths, and schistosomes: National mapping in Ethiopia. PLoS Neglected Tropical Diseases. 2016;**10**(3):e0004515

[83] Mogaji HO, Omitola OO, Bayegun AA, Ekpo UF, Taylor-Robinson AW. Livestock reservoir hosts: An obscured threat to control of human schistosomiasis in Nigeria. Zoonotic Disease. 2023;**3**(1):52-67

[84] Onyekwere AM, Rey O, Allienne JF, Nwanchor MC, Alo M, Uwa C, et al. Population genetic structure and hybridization of *Schistosoma haematobium* in Nigeria. Pathogens. 2022;**11**(4):425

[85] Oyeyemi OT, de Jesus Jeremias W, Grenfell RFQ. Schistosomiasis in Nigeria: Gleaning from the past to improve current efforts towards control. One Health. 2020;**11**:100183

Chapter 9

Development of Novel Drugs for the Treatment of Chagas Disease

Albany Reséndiz-Mora, Juan Carlos Santiago-Hernández, Juan Manuel Serna-Velázquez, Giovanna Barrera-Aveleida, Anahi Sotelo-Rodríguez, Iván Galarce-Sosa, Jesús Elías Isidro-Magallán, Saúl Gómez-Manzo, Benjamín Nogueda-Torres, Isabel Wong-Baeza, Isabel Baeza and Carlos Wong-Baeza

Abstract

Chagas disease, or American trypanosomiasis, is a zoonosis caused by the hemoflagellate parasite *Trypanosoma cruzi*. It is mainly transmitted by the bite of blood-sucking insects. It is endemic in Latin America and emerging in the rest of the world, affecting approximately six million people. The drugs Benznidazole and Nifurtimox currently used for its treatment are not totally effective in the chronic phase of the disease. In addition, they are toxic, and there are many resistant *Trigonoscuta cruzi* strains. Therefore, developing new drugs for the treatment of Chagas disease is necessary. This chapter describes the development of drugs that inhibit α-hydroxy acid dehydrogenase isoenzyme II, a key enzyme in parasite energy metabolism. These drugs have shown more significant trypanocidal activity than the currently used drugs, and they have also prevented the development of chronic Chagas disease in infected mice.

Keywords: Chagas disease, treatment, *Trypanosoma cruzi*, metabolism inhibition, drug design

1. Introduction

1.1 Chagas disease

American trypanosomiasis, or Chagas disease, has been a public health problem in Latin America since ancient times, and it is now recognized by the World Health Organization (WHO) as one of 13 neglected tropical diseases [1]. Chagas disease is a parasitic, systemic, and chronic condition, with a clear link to deficient socio-economic conditions [2]. As a result, it is not a priority for pharmaceutical companies, despite its considerable impact on morbidity and mortality [3, 4]. Chagas disease is caused by *Trypanosoma cruzi* (*Trigonoscuta cruzi*). Dr. Carlos Chagas made the first reference to this protozoan at the Oswaldo Cruz Institute, where he described its transmission through insect vectors (triatomines), its life cycle, and its clinical manifestations. Dr. Chagas also determined the presence of *T. cruzi* trypomastigotes in cat blood, and he later directly observed the parasite in the peripheral blood of a one-year-old patient with a fever of unknown origin [5]. However, the first report of Chagas disease may have preceded these discoveries: it is suspected that Charles Darwin contracted *T. cruzi* infection during his expedition to South America in 1835, based on his description of contact with triatomines and the subsequent appearance of consistent symptoms [6]. Paleo-parasitological studies and molecular data obtained from mummies of the Atacama region (Chile and Peru) suggest that the triatomines involved in the life cycle of *T. cruzi* transmitted the infection to humans approximately 9000 years ago [7, 8].

The clinical classification of Chagas disease is based on the time of infection, and it presents two main phases: acute and chronic [9–11]. Depending on the parasite load at the inoculation site, the genetic group and strain of the parasite, and the immunological status of the host [12], Chagas disease can be fatal due to lethal arrhythmias, which are secondary complications of the parasite invasion of different tissues, with a predilection for cardiac muscle, smooth muscle, and glial cells of the central nervous system [13, 14]. The acute phase is mainly seen in children and lasts 1 to 4 months. If the triatomine bite is located close to the eyes, an ophthalmo-nodal complex (the Mazza-Romaña sign) is formed [15]. This complex is characterized by unilateral edema, conjunctivitis, and regional lymphadenopathy. If the triatomine bite is in any other part of the skin, a skin-nodal complex or chagoma is formed, with inflammation and local lymphadenopathy [8, 15]. The acute phase is characterized by general and non-specific symptoms, such as asthenia, adynamia, fever, headache, myalgia, arthralgia, anorexia, vomiting, and diarrhea, with regional lymphadenopathy, hepatosplenomegaly, myocarditis, edema, and seizures. This phase usually resolves spontaneously; however, 2 to 6% of the cases result in death, mainly due to myocarditis or meningoencephalitis [15].

As the disease progresses, some patients develop parasitemia and positive serology, but without cardiac or digestive symptoms. Thirty percent of the patients remain in this indeterminate phase throughout their lives. The rest of the patients develop the chronic phase of the disease in 10 to 30 years [13]. This phase is characterized by heart disease, colon disease, and esophagopathy [16]. The heart is affected in 94.5% of the cases, with the rest of the cases presenting megaesophagus and megacolon [8]. Chronic Chagas disease can be disabling and even fatal [12]. The only two drugs currently approved for treating Chagas disease, Benznidazole, and Nifurtimox, are only partially effective in the chronic phase and have severe adverse reactions [17, 18].

1.2 Epidemiology of Chagas disease

Chagas disease is one of the infections with the highest mortality in Latin America's tropical and subtropical regions. Between six and eight million people worldwide have Chagas disease, and each year it causes the death of approximately 50,000 people [4, 13]. Due to the increased levels of migration and globalization that occurred during the last decade, there have been critical epidemiological changes [1]. Therefore, Chagas disease has spread to European countries such as Austria, Germany, Belgium, Spain, France, Italy, the Netherlands, Portugal, Sweden, Switzerland, and the United Kingdom, as well as to the Western Pacific region in Australia and Japan, and non-endemic areas in North America, such as Canada and the border between the United States and Mexico (**Figure 1**) [1, 21, 22].

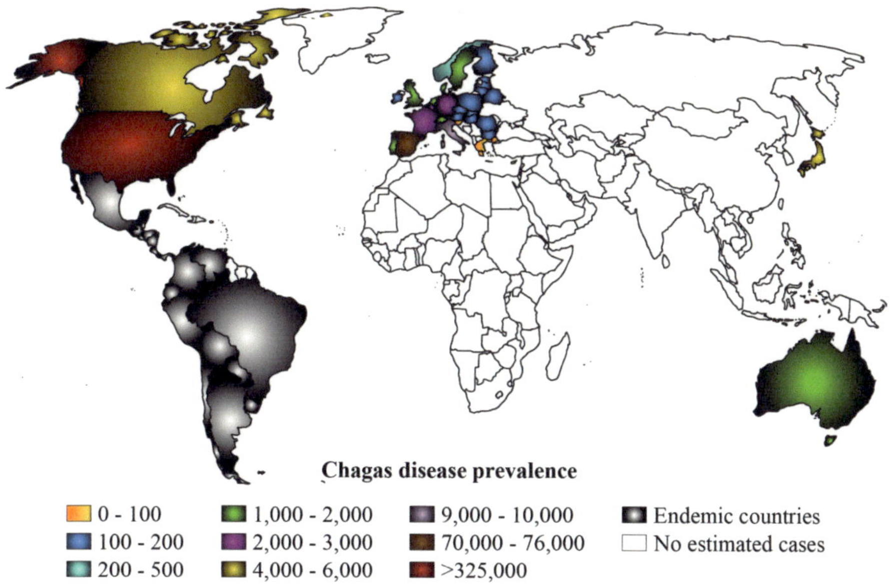

Figure 1.
Chagas disease prevalence. World map with Chagas disease endemic countries and estimated cases detected in non-endemic countries in North America, Europe, and the Western Pacific region [19, 20].

It is estimated that seven million people have Chagas disease in the American continent, and 20 to 30% of these cases progress to cardiac or gastrointestinal disease [23]. There are 60 million people at risk of infection with *T. cruzi* in Latin America alone [13]. The prevalence of Chagas disease is not homogeneous, and it depends on the region and on the characteristics of the population. According to estimates made in 2010, Argentina and Brazil had the highest absolute numbers of infected persons [24]. In hyperendemic areas, such as the Bolivian Chaco, about 4% of new infections occur yearly, and almost 100% of the population over 30 years of age is seropositive [25]. Migration contributes to the spread of the disease beyond endemic areas, since chronically infected asymptomatic individuals can transmit the disease through non-vector routes [24, 26].

Approximately 300,000 people are infected in the United States, including 57,000 patients with Chagasic cardiomyopathy and 43,000 infected women of reproductive age [27]. However, this number increases if undocumented immigrants, mainly from El Salvador, Guatemala, and Honduras, are included: up to 18,000 individuals that arrive to the United States from each of these countries each year are infected with *T. cruzi,* according to 2014 statistics from the U.S. Customs and Border Patrol [28, 29]. The highest burden of Chagas disease is found in California, Texas, Florida, and New York, with more than 10,000 cases in each state [29]. The estimated number of infected people in Europe is about 97,556 [27, 30, 31]. In contrast, this number is more limited in the Western Pacific region, with approximately 4000 cases in Japan [32] and about 2000 in Australia and New Zealand [33].

Chagas disease is massively under-diagnosed in non-endemic countries of North America and Europe [34]. This highlights this disease as an emergent worldwide public health problem, which is related to the high mobility of immigrant communities [24, 35]. Spain is the European country that hosts the most significant number (2,090,695) of Latin American immigrants [36], and it is considered that between

47,738 and 67,423 of these immigrants could have Chagas disease [29]. In the United Kingdom, 41 cases of *T. cruzi* infection were detected in London between 2001 and 2014 [37, 38], and it is estimated that between 6000 and 12,000 people may have Chagas disease in the United Kingdom, with a prevalence of 1.3–2.4% [34]. In a serological study of Latin American migrants that reside in Italy, 36 of the 867 participants were seropositive to Chagas disease, with a seroprevalence rate of 4.3% [39]. In Switzerland, a total of 258 cases had been diagnosed until 2009, although it is estimated that there may be as many as 3000 infected people nationwide [40]. In other European countries (Belgium, France, Germany, Holland, or Portugal) with fewer Latin American migrants, the estimated number of infected persons is below 3000 [34].

Worldwide, at least 100 million people are at high risk of infection with *T. cruzi* because they live in endemic areas [41]. Chagas disease causes the loss of around 752,000 working days per year in the Latin American countries with the most significant poverty levels, which is attributed to the premature deaths caused by Chagas-induced cardiovascular disease. Chagas disease also causes global productivity losses of more than 7 billion dollars annually (this value includes the cost of treatments) [2, 30, 42]. These estimates do not consider the losses caused by the infections of tourists and migrants from South and Central America to North America, Europe, and Asia, further increasing the monetary loss [3]. Therefore, it can be inferred that effective drugs for treating Chagas disease can provide considerable socioeconomic benefit to patients, their families, and society [3].

1.3 Transmission of Chagas disease

The most common form of Chagas disease transmission is direct contact with *T. cruzi*-infected triatomines, which defecate when feeding on mammals. The parasites in these droppings penetrate through skin lesions and infect the mammal [31, 43]. Other forms of transmission include blood transfusions, oral transmission, vertical transmission, organ transplantation, and laboratory accidents or errors [44, 45].

Transmission by blood transfusions is the second cause of *T. cruzi* infection in different regions of America. However, it can be easily prevented by monitoring donor blood samples at blood banks [10, 12]. Oral transmission has been documented after ingesting food contaminated with infected triatomines or their feces [12]. Vertical transmission corresponds to around 5% of all new infection cases [46]. Individuals with congenitally-acquired infection have a 30% chance of developing severe sequels, such as cardiomyopathies, arrhythmias, or neurologic complications (this percentage is similar in individuals that are infected with *T. cruzi* through other forms of transmission) [15, 47, 48]. There is no currently available treatment to prevent congenital transmission since the risks of the drugs used to treat Chagas disease in pregnant women remain unknown [49]. In addition, diagnosing *T. cruzi* infection in newborns presents several complications, including its high cost and the time required: serological diagnosis can only be performed on children at least a year old because maternal antibodies remain in the infant's blood for several months after birth. As a result, many infants with congenital infections do not receive timely diagnosis and treatment [50].

Transmission by organ transplant occurs when the transplanted organ comes from an infected donor. The most common cause is a kidney transplant, but it has also been reported in heart, bone marrow, and pancreas transplants from living and dead donors. The WHO recommends testing potential organ donors with at least two tests based on different techniques to prevent this transmission [31, 45]. Accidental transmission cases have been reported in various circumstances in hospitals and laboratories. There are documented cases in which technicians, doctors, and researchers inoculate themselves by accident when handling contaminated material such as triatomine feces, parasite cultures, and infected blood from humans and animals [44].

The main vectors contributing to the spread of Chagas disease are the triatomine insects, which belong to the *Hemiptera* order, the *Reduviidae* family, and the *Triatominae* subfamily. This subfamily has approximately 140 species, many of which are potential transmitters of the parasite [12, 51, 52]. *Triatoma sp* is the genus with the most significant involvement in human trypanosomiasis, and it is found in dry ecosystems in Central and South America. Other genus with epidemiological importance are *Rhodnius sp*, located in humid tropical climates, and *Panstrongylus sp*, which is globally dispersed [8]. Some studies showed that 40 to 64% of wild-collected triatomines are infected with *T. cruzi* in endemic areas [53, 54].

1.4 *Trypanosoma cruzi* life cycle

T. cruzi is the etiologic agent of Chagas disease. This uniflagellate protozoan belongs to the *Trypanosomatidae* family and is included within the *Kinetoplastea* class [55]. *T. cruzi* has three morphologically distinct stages (amastigote, epimastigote, and trypomastigote), which are defined by the general shape of the cell, the position of the kinetoplast (a network of circular DNA inside a large mitochondrion), and the region where the flagellum emerges from the flagellar bag [19, 56].

Amastigotes are found in the intracellular compartment of mammalian cells, where they reproduce by binary fission and form nests; these nests are mainly found in the cardiac muscle and the gastrointestinal tract. Amastigotes are round and small (2–4 μm) compared to the other *T. cruzi* stages and have a short flagellum not observable under light microscopy [19, 57]. Epimastigotes are found in the vector gut, where they reproduce by binary fission. *T. cruzi* also adopts this stage in culture media. Epimastigotes have a spindle shape with an approximate length of 20 μm. Their kinetoplast, where the flagellum emerges, is in an anterior position, close to the nucleus, and their flagellum and undulating membranes are short [58]. Trypomastigotes are found in the hindgut of triatomines (metacyclic trypomastigotes) and in mammalian blood (blood trypomastigotes). Blood trypomastigotes infect other host cells, and they also infect the triatomines that ingest this blood. Trypomastigotes are characterized by an undulating membrane covering their entire length, a central nucleus, and a posterior conspicuous kinetoplast. Their sizes range from 25 to 27 μm [57].

The life cycle of *T. cruzi* begins when the triatomine insect (vector) (**Figure 2A**) sucks blood and ingests blood trypomastigotes (**Figure 2B**) from an infected mammal. Most of the ingested trypomastigotes are destroyed in the stomach of the triatomine, but some trypomastigotes survive and transform into epimastigotes (**Figure 2C**). Epimastigotes are then transported to the intestinal mesogastrium, where they begin an intense division by binary fission. This binary fission leads to the transformation of epimastigotes to metacyclic trypomastigotes, which are highly infectious. Metacyclic trypomastigotes detach from the intestinal wall after 15 to 30 days and reach the rectum of the insect, where they are expelled in the feces [57].

Metacyclic trypomastigotes from the triatomine droppings penetrate the skin or the mucous membranes in the bite site of the host through skin abrasions and begin the infection. Trypomastigotes move from the blood to the tissues, particularly

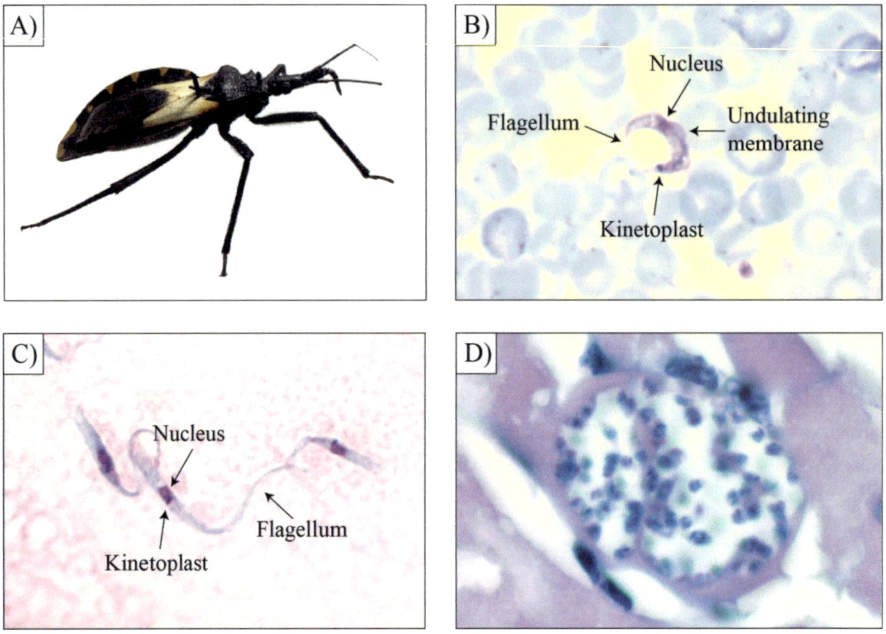

Figure 2.
Vector and Trypanosoma cruzi *stages. The principal vectors of Chagas disease are the triatomine insects, where Triatoma sp. (A) Is the genus with the most significant involvement in human trypanosomiasis. 100x photographs of Giemsa-stained trypomastigotes (B), epimastigotes (C), and amastigotes (D), the three morphological stages of Trypanosoma cruzi.*

muscular tissue, where macrophages engulf them. After phagocytosis, a parasitophore vesicle is formed from the recruited lysosomes, which inhibits the formation of phagolysosomes. The trypomastigotes can escape from this vesicle to the cytoplasm and later differentiate into amastigotes (**Figure 2D**). Amastigotes begin their division cycle and form pseudocysts (cells full of amastigotes). Finally, amastigotes differentiate into highly motile blood trypomastigotes, which rupture the cells and are released into the bloodstream. Blood trypomastigotes invade other target cells, such as ganglion or muscle cells, which spreads the infection and increases the probability of transmission to insects [57, 59].

1.5 Treatment of Chagas disease

American trypanosomiasis is an infectious disease with a significant impact in Latin America, and it was described more than a century ago [60]. However, it is rarely treated correctly, and some patients are only partially cured [61, 62]. Benznidazole and Nifurtimox are the only drugs recommended by the WHO for the treatment of Chagas disease, and they were developed more than 50 years ago [18, 63].

The mechanism of action of Nifurtimox has yet to be fully understood. Some studies have shown that when Nifurtimox is metabolized by type 1 trypanosomal nitroreductase, free radicals are released, and these radicals reduce the levels of intracellular thiols. These events trigger DNA degradation, block DNA synthesis, and increase lipid peroxidation [9, 64, 65]. The mechanism of action of Benznidazole involves covalent modifications on DNA, proteins, and lipids [10]. Benznidazole is also reduced by type 1 trypanosomal nitroreductase, and subsequent reactions lead to the release of glyoxal dialdehyde, which has a trypanocidal effect. Benznidazole is effective against all the *T. cruzi* stages [66]. In addition, Benznidazole inhibits the parasite enzyme fumarate NADH-reductase, which reduces parasite growth and increases the phagocytosis and lysis of the parasite inside macrophages [67].

Treatment durations with Benznidazole and Nifurtimox are long (60–90 days), and these drugs have a high rate of adverse events and low tolerability. In addition, these drugs are inefficient in patients with chronic infection, and 10 to 30% of treated patients do not resolve the infection [17, 18, 22]. Benznidazole has a better tolerability profile, so it is preferred over Nifurtimox. However, treatment is suspended in 9 to 30% of the cases, although adverse reactions are reversible and are serious in less than 1% of the cases [66, 68]. The main side effects of Benznidazole are the appearance of rash and pruritus, epigastric pain, nausea, abdominal swelling, hepatitis, peripheral polyneuropathy, digestive intolerance, anorexia, and some severe manifestations such as eosinophilia [18, 69]. The side effects of Nifurtimox are related to gastrointestinal symptoms (nausea, vomiting, and anorexia), central nervous system toxicity (insomnia, irritability, and disorientation), and occasionally headache, rash, myalgia, arthralgia, dizziness, vertigo, and mood swings. More severe side effects, such as polyneuropathy, paresthesia, and peripheral neuritis, occur less frequently [13, 70].

Resistance of *T. cruzi* strains to Benznidazole and Nifurtimox can arise from incomplete treatments [71, 72], and differential resistance to these drugs has been reported in various strains [73–75]. The *T. cruzi* Colombian and V-10 strains are highly resistant to Benznidazole, while the Y and Dm28c strains are partially resistant, and the CL strain is susceptible [76–78]. The intrinsic resistance of some *T. cruzi* strains could explain why some patients do not respond to the treatment with these drugs [14, 79].

Potential vaccine candidates against Chagas disease have been investigated recently, but none have progressed beyond preclinical development [80, 81]. Many antifungal drugs have been found to have good *in vitro* and *in vivo* efficacy against *T. cruzi* [74, 82–84], individually and in combination with Benznidazole. For example, Posaconazole showed trypanocidal activity, particularly in combination with Benznidazole [74]. However, no significant advantage was observed in clinical trials with the combined therapy over Benznidazole therapy [85, 86]. Fosravuconazole, which has potent *in vitro* activity against *T. cruzi*, failed to show sustained efficacy after one year of treatment, compared to Benznidazole, and had safety concerns at high doses [84, 87]. Currently, no treatment alternatives exist for Chagas disease, as no new drug has achieved a better pharmacological response than Benznidazole or Nifurtimox [88]. Therefore, it is necessary to identify new therapeutic targets in *T. cruzi,* and the energy metabolism of this parasite is a promising target.

1.6 The energy metabolism of *Trypanosoma cruzi*

T. cruzi, unlike most eukaryotes, has a single mitochondrion [89]. This organelle extends around the cell body and contains mitochondrial DNA, which forms maxicircles (concatenated circular molecules) that contain characteristic eukaryotic mitochondrial genes and minicircles that contain genes exclusive to trypanosomatids. *T. cruzi* also contains organelles known as glycosomes, which contain most of the enzymes of the glycolysis and gluconeogenesis pathways [51, 90, 91]. *T. cruzi*, like many parasites, cannot synthesize certain molecules that are essential for its growth and survival and supplements its metabolic activities by taking these molecules from the host cells. The parasite's metabolic dependence on these molecules represents a potential therapeutic target since inhibiting the host metabolic pathways would lead to parasite death [92, 93]. However, inhibiting the host metabolism would also negatively affect the host.

T. cruzi epimastigotes in the insect intestine use glucose as their primary energy source. In the absence of glucose, epimastigotes oxidize amino acids to maintain their redox balance and to generate ATP [94–96]. *T. cruzi* lacks a metabolic pathway for synthesizing heme groups, so it acquires the heme groups that are released into the lumen of the insect midgut when the ingested blood is digested. Heme groups promote the proliferation of epimastigotes because they are essential for electron transport and oxygen detoxification. In epimastigotes, the expression levels of glycolysis genes are increased, while the expression levels of oxidative phosphorylation genes are decreased. As a result, the epimastigote energy metabolism is skewed towards anaerobic fermentation, favoring the parasite's adaptation and proliferation within the insect vector [51].

T. cruzi blood trypomastigotes mainly use glycolysis, not oxidative phosphorylation, to obtain energy. Blood trypomastigotes have a high glucose consumption rate, which is directly associated with anaerobic fermentation [51]. In contrast, intracellular amastigotes have direct access to the nutrients of the host cell and use amino acids and fatty acids as their primary energy source. However, they can also use exogenous glucose and glutamine as energy sources [51, 93, 95].

1.7 Design of new drugs that inhibit the energy metabolism of *Trypanosoma cruzi*

Glycolysis is the primary metabolic pathway used by *T. cruzi* to obtain its energy [97, 98], and the reduced NADH+H$^+$ that is produced during glycolysis needs to be re-oxidated to keep this metabolic pathway functioning correctly. In mammals, the enzyme that performs the NADH+H$^+$ re-oxidation in the absence of oxygen is lactate dehydrogenase, but in *T. cruzi,* the enzyme is α-hydroxy acid dehydrogenase isoenzyme-II (α-HADH-II) [99]. *T. cruzi* has two molecular forms of α-HADH, α-HADH-isoenzyme I (HADH-I) and α-HADH-II. α-HADH-I is responsible for the low lactate dehydrogenase activity of *T. cruzi* extracts. α-HADH-II has no activity on pyruvate but is active on a wide range of linear and branched substrates, with α-ketocaproate and α-ketoisocaproate being the substrates where α-HADH-II presents its maximum activity [99]. α-HADH-II is in the *T. cruzi* cytoplasm and mitochondrion. In the cytoplasm, α-HADH-II reduces the α-ketoacids produced by the transamination of some amino acids, using NADH+H$^+$ as a cofactor [99]. The resulting α-hydroxy acids enter the mitochondria and are re-oxidated by mitochondrial α-HADH-II, transferring the electrons to NAD$^+$ and then to the respiratory chain. This mechanism acts as a shuttle, where reducing equivalents (NADH+H$^+$) generated in the cytoplasm can be re-oxidized inside the mitochondria (**Figure 3**) [100].

Since α-ketocaproate and α-ketoisocaproate (**Figure 4A**) are the substrates where *T. cruzi* α-HADH-II presents its maximum activity [99], molecules with structural and steric characteristics similar to these substrates, such as oxamate, could act as competitive inhibitors of the enzyme [101]. Therefore, in our research group, we designed and synthesized two oxamate derivates: N-propyl oxamate (NPOx) [101] is a structural analog of α-ketocaproate, and N-isopropyl oxamate (NIPOx) [102] is a structural analog of α-ketoisocaproate (**Figure 4B**). Kinetic studies confirmed that NPOx and NIPOx are competitive inhibitors of α-HADH-II [101, 102], with NIPOx being the best inhibitor [103]. However, when NPOx and NIPOx were tested *in vitro* on *T. cruzi* epimastigotes, they did not present any trypanocidal activity [101, 102]

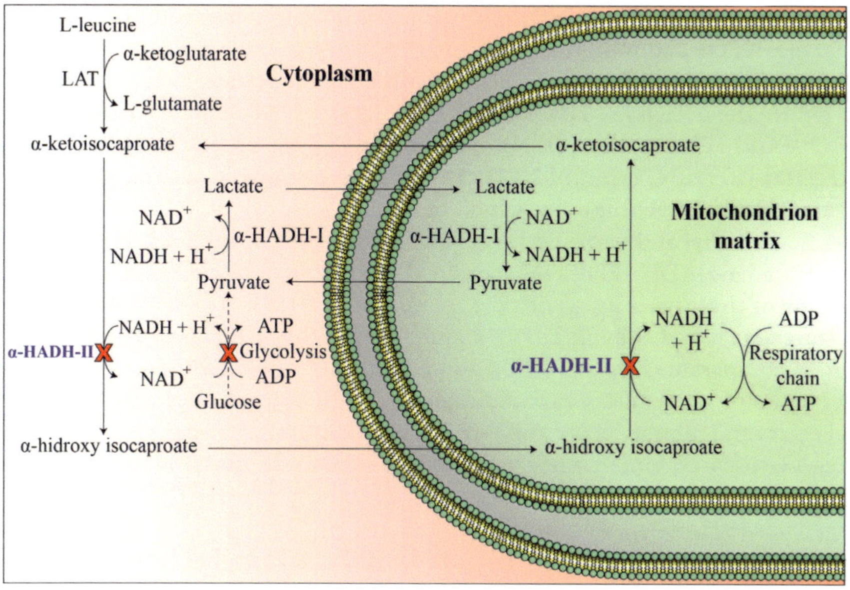

Figure 3.
Trypanosoma cruzi *energy metabolism. Glycolysis is the primary metabolic pathway of* Trypanosoma cruzi, *and to keep this metabolic pathway functioning correctly, the enzyme α-hydroxy acid dehydrogenase isoenzyme-II (α-HADH-II) reduces the produced NADH+H⁺. therefore, this enzyme's inhibition stops the parasite's primary metabolic pathway. The red crosses indicate the inhibition of α-HADH-II and glycolysis.*

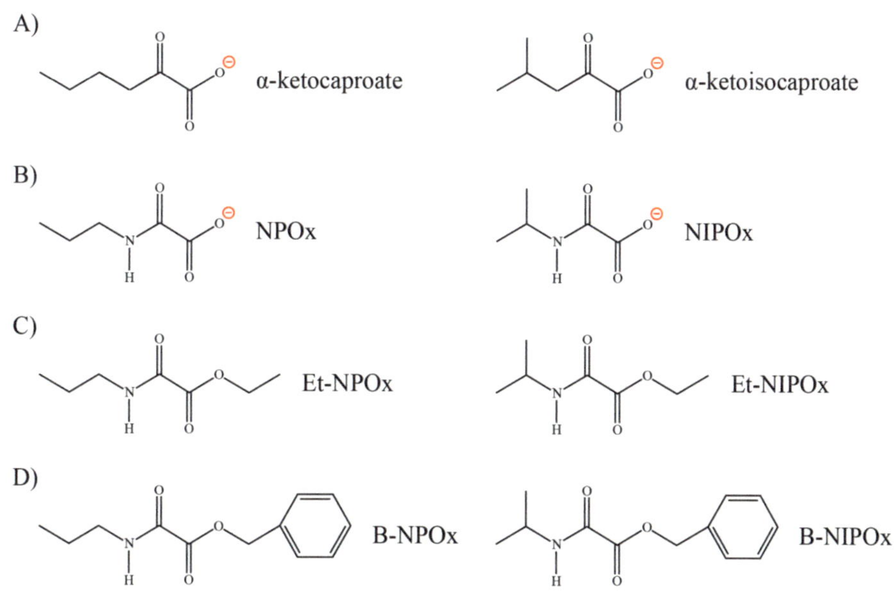

Figure 4.
Trypanosoma cruzi *α-hydroxy acid dehydrogenase isoenzyme-II substrates, inhibitors, and inhibitors esters. The primary substrates of* Trypanosoma cruzi *α-hydroxy acid dehydrogenase isoenzyme-II (α-HADH-II) are α-ketocaproate and α-ketoisocaproate (A). N-propyl oxamate (NPOx) and N-isopropyl oxamate (NIPOx) (B) are structural analogs of α-HADH-II primary substrates. To reduce the polarity of NPOx and NIPOx, we synthesized the ethyl (Et-NPOx and Et-NIPOx) (C) and benzyl (B-NPOx and B-NIPOx) (D) esters of NPOx and NIPOx, to transform these polar molecules into non-polar, that can cross membranes by simple diffusion.*

since they are polar compounds that cannot cross the parasite membrane. At physiological pH, NPOx and NIPOx have a negative charge in their carboxylate groups, which prevents their diffusion across hydrophobic membranes [104].

To reduce the polarity of NPOx and NIPOx, we synthesized the ethyl (Et-NPOx and Et-NIPOx) (**Figure 4C**) [101, 102] and benzyl (B-NPOx and B-NIPOx) (**Figure 4D**) [103, 104] esters of NPOx and NIPOx, to transform these polar molecules into hydrophobic ones, which can easily cross cell membranes by simple diffusion. The ethyl and benzyl esters of NPOx and NIPOx did not decrease the activity of purified α-HADH-II because the added ethyl or benzyl groups prevented the interaction of these molecules with the active site of α-HADH-II [101–104]. However, when the esters were tested in *T. cruzi* homogenates, they decreased α-HADH-II activity to comparable levels as NPOx and NIPOx [101–104]. This occurs because *T. cruzi* homogenates contain carboxylesterases [105] that can cleave the ethyl and benzyl esters and release NPOx and NIPOx, which inhibit the enzyme activity. In the presence of N-ethylmaleimide, a carboxylesterase inhibitor, the ethyl and benzyl esters of NPOx and NIPOx did not decrease the activity of α-HADH-II in *T. cruzi* homogenates [103, 104].

The ethyl and benzyl esters of NPOx and NIPOx had a higher trypanocidal activity on *T. cruzi* epimastigotes than Benznidazole or Nifurtimox, which confirms that these drugs were cleaved inside the parasite by carboxylesterases and inhibited α-HADH-II [101–104]. The benzyl esters of NPOx and NIPOx had higher trypanocidal activity than the ethyl esters, probably because the released benzyl alcohol has direct antimicrobial activity [106].

The ethyl and benzyl esters of NPOx and NIPOx did not present cytotoxicity on cultured cell lines and had LD_{50} values that indicate that they are not toxic to mice [103, 104]. We then evaluated the *in vivo* trypanocidal effect of the NPOx and NIPOx esters in mice infected with *T. cruzi* [103, 104]. We found that the benzyl esters of NPOx and NIPOx had the highest trypanocidal activity on blood trypomastigotes, followed by the ethyl esters, Benznidazole and Nifurtimox. The ethyl and benzyl esters of NPOx and NIPOx were also effective against *T. cruzi* strains that were highly resistant to Benznidazole and Nifurtimox [103, 104].

The NPOx and NIPOx esters were more efficient than Benznidazole or Nifurtimox in reducing the percentage of amastigote nests in the heart myocardium and the skeletal muscle of *T. cruzi*-infected mice [103], probably as a result of the clearing of blood trypomastigotes before they could infect the tissues. However, it is also possible that the NPOx and NIPOx esters had a direct trypanocidal effect on amastigotes since amastigotes can also use glucose as a carbon source [107]. To test this hypothesis, the NPOx and NIPOx esters should be administered to mice after the chronic phase of the infection has been established.

During the chronic phase of Chagas disease, the invasion of the smooth muscle of the digestive system by *T. cruzi* triggers the formation of mega syndromes in the esophagus and colon. This infection causes thickening of the muscular layers [108], inflammation, and a massive neuronal loss in the plexuses that form the enteric nervous system [16]. The benzyl esters of NPOx and NIPOx, but not Benznidazole or Nifurtimox, prevented the thickening of the intestinal inner circular muscle layer of *T. cruzi*-infected mice. The benzyl esters also prevented the leukocyte infiltration of this muscle layer and its loss of nitrergic neurons [103].

Trypomastigotes have vigorous motility, allowing for their rapid extravasation and dissemination within the host tissues, where they invade cells and differentiate into amastigotes. Subsequently, trypomastigotes emerge from amastigote nests, leading to the rupture of the infected cells during the chronic stage of the disease [109]. The trypanocidal effect of the NPOx and NIPOx esters, particularly of B-NIPOx, against the infective and the reproductive forms of *T. cruzi* (trypomastigotes and amastigotes, respectively) provides strong evidence to support the use of B-NIPOx as an alternative drug for the treatment of Chagas disease. It is also important to mention that the NPOx and NIPOx esters release polar molecules after they are cleaved by carboxylesterases. Phase II metabolic processes, such as esterification, can eliminate these polar molecules from the host. In contrast, Benznidazole and Nifurtimox are highly toxic non-polar molecules that are difficult to eliminate from the host [110].

2. Conclusion

Chagas disease is a zoonosis caused by *Trypanosoma cruzi. It is* the most important parasitic infection in Latin America, with an annual incidence of 30,000 new cases per year, 14,000 deaths, and 8000 newborns infected during gestation. If Chagas disease is not diagnosed and treated early, patients can face severe health effects, including cardiomyopathy, heart failure and rhythm problems, and strokes. Consequences can affect the patient's professional, social, and family life. Endemic countries have typically focused on vector control rather than diagnosis or treatment. In addition, the drugs currently available for its treatment, Benznidazole, and Nifurtimox, are only partially effective in the chronic phase of the disease, have severe side effects, and involve lengthy treatment cycles. In our research group, we developed new drugs that could be used to treat Chagas disease. These drugs inhibit α-hydroxy acid dehydrogenase isoenzyme-II (α-HADH-II), an enzyme that has a central role in the energy metabolism of the parasite. NPOx and NIPOx are oxamate derivates that were designed as structural analogs of the primary substrates of α-HADH-II, and ethyl and benzyl esters were synthesized to transform NPOx and NIPOx into nonpolar molecules that can diffuse across the parasite membrane. The ethyl and benzyl esters of NPOx and NIPOx had a higher trypanocidal activity on *T. cruzi* epimastigotes and trypomastigotes than Benznidazole and Nifurtimox. They reduced blood parasitemia and muscle amastigotes in infected mice, and they also prevented the thickening of the inner circular muscle layer of the intestine of these mice, as well as its infiltration by leukocytes and its loss of nitrergic neurons. Since the benzyl ester of NIPOx was the drug with the better effects, we propose further studies to develop this molecule as a potential new treatment for Chagas disease.

Acknowledgements

This study was supported by Instituto Politécnico Nacional, Mexico (grants SIP20232131 to IB, SIP20232128 to CWB, and SIP20232135 to ARM). Authors are fellows of Sistema Nacional de Investigadores, Consejo Nacional de Ciencia y Tecnología (CONACYT), México.

Conflict of interest

The authors declare no conflict of interest.

Author details

Albany Reséndiz-Mora[1], Juan Carlos Santiago-Hernández[1], Juan Manuel Serna-Velázquez[2], Giovanna Barrera-Aveleida[1], Anahi Sotelo-Rodríguez[1], Iván Galarce-Sosa[1], Jesús Elías Isidro-Magallán[1], Saúl Gómez-Manzo[3], Benjamín Nogueda-Torres[4], Isabel Wong-Baeza[5], Isabel Baeza[1] and Carlos Wong-Baeza[1*]

1 Departamento de Bioquímica, Escuela Nacional de Ciencias Biológicas, Instituto Politécnico Nacional (Biochemistry Department, National School of Biological Sciences, National Polytechnic Institute), Mexico City, Mexico

2 Departamento de Parasitología, Instituto de Diagnóstico y Referencia Epidemiológicos (Parasitology Department, Institute of Epidemiological Diagnosis and Reference), Mexico City, Mexico

3 Laboratorio de Bioquímica Genética, Instituto Nacional de Pediatría, Secretaría de Salud (Genetic Biochemistry Laboratory, National Institute of Pediatrics, Ministry of Health), Mexico City, Mexico

4 Departamento de Parasitología, Escuela Nacional de Ciencias Biológicas, Instituto Politécnico Nacional (Parasitology Department, National School of Biological Sciences, National Polytechnic Institute), Mexico City, Mexico

5 Departamento de Inmunología, Escuela Nacional de Ciencias Biológicas, Instituto Politécnico Nacional (Immunology Department, National School of Biological Sciences, National Polytechnic Institute), Mexico City, Mexico

*Address all correspondence to: charlywong@icloud.com

References

[1] Casulli A. New global targets for NTDs in the WHO roadmap 2021-2030. PLoS Neglected Tropical Diseases. 2021;**15**(5):e0009373

[2] Conteh L, Engels T, Molyneux DH. Socioeconomic aspects of neglected tropical diseases. Lancet. 2010;**375**(9710): 239-247

[3] Almeida-Silva J, Menezes DS, Fernandes JMP, Almeida MC, Vasco-Dos-Santos DR, Saraiva RM, et al. The repositioned drugs disulfiram/diethyldithiocarbamate combined to benznidazole: Searching for Chagas disease selective therapy, preventing toxicity and drug resistance. Frontiers in Cellular and Infection Microbiology. 2022;**12**:926699

[4] WHO. World Chagas Disease Day 2022. Available from: https://www.who.int/campaigns/world-chagas-disease-day/2022

[5] Chagas C. Nova tripanosomiase humana. Estudo sobre a morfologia e o ciclo evolutivo do Schizotrypanum cruzi, n. gen, n. sp. agente etiológico de nova entidade mórbida do homem. Memórias do Instituto Oswaldo Cruz. 1909;**2**(62):159-218

[6] Rassi A Jr, Rassi A, Marin-Neto JA. Chagas disease. Lancet. 2010;**375**(9723): 1388-1402

[7] Darling MI, Donoghue HD. Insights from paleomicrobiology into the indigenous peoples of pre-colonial America - a review. Memórias do Instituto Oswaldo Cruz. 2014;**109**(2):131-139

[8] Teixeira AR, Nitz N, Guimaro MC, Gomes C, Santos-Buch CA. Chagas disease. Postgraduate Medical Journal. 2006;**82**(974):788-798

[9] Ribeiro V, Dias N, Paiva T, Hagstrom-Bex L, Nitz N, Pratesi R, et al. Current trends in the pharmacological management of Chagas disease. International Journal for Parasitology: Drugs and Drug Resistance. 2020;**12**: 7-17

[10] Sales Junior PA, Molina I, Fonseca Murta SM, Sanchez-Montalva A, Salvador F, Correa-Oliveira R, et al. Experimental and clinical treatment of Chagas disease: A review. The American Journal of Tropical Medicine and Hygiene. 2017;**97**(5):1289-1303

[11] De Alba-Alvarado MC, Torres-Gutierrez E, Reynoso-Ducoing OA, Zenteno-Galindo E, Cabrera-Bravo M, Guevara-Gomez Y, et al. Immunopathological mechanisms underlying cardiac damage in Chagas disease. Pathogens. 2023;**12**(2):1-13

[12] Coura JR, Junqueira AC, Fernandes O, Valente SA, Miles MA. Emerging Chagas disease in Amazonian Brazil. Trends in Parasitology. 2002;**18**(4):171-176

[13] Perez-Molina JA, Molina I. Chagas disease. Lancet. 2018;**391**(10115):82-94

[14] Gonzaga BMS, Horita SIM, Beghini DG, Gomes F, Nisimura LM, Dos Santos IB, et al. Effect of benznidazole on cerebral microcirculation during acute Trypanosoma cruzi infection in mice. Scientific Reports. 2022;**12**(1):21048

[15] Bern C, Martin DL, Gilman RH. Acute and congenital Chagas disease. Advances in Parasitology. 2011;**75**:19-47

[16] Jabari S, de Oliveira EC, Brehmer A, da Silveira AB. Chagasic megacolon: Enteric neurons and related structures.

Histochemistry and Cell Biology. 2014;**142**(3):235-244

[17] J B, M BM, Chanda K. An overview on the therapeutics of neglected infectious diseases-Leishmaniasis and Chagas diseases. Frontiers in Chemistry. 2021;**9**:622286

[18] Mansoldo FRP, Carta F, Angeli A, Cardoso VDS, Supuran CT, Vermelho AB. Chagas disease: Perspectives on the past and present and challenges in drug discovery. Molecules. 2020;**25**(22):1-14

[19] Lidani KCF, Andrade FA, Bavia L, Damasceno FS, Beltrame MH, Messias-Reason IJ, et al. Chagas disease: From discovery to a worldwide health problem. Frontiers in Public Health. 2019;**7**:166

[20] Conners EE, Vinetz JM, Weeks JR, Brouwer KC. A global systematic review of Chagas disease prevalence among migrants. Acta tr#opica. 2016;**156**:68-78

[21] Liu Q, Zhou XN. Preventing the transmission of American trypanosomiasis and its spread into non-endemic countries. Infectious Diseases of Poverty. 2015;**4**:60

[22] Villalta F, Rachakonda G. Advances in preclinical approaches to Chagas disease drug discovery. Expert Opinion on Drug Discovery. 2019;**14**(11):1161-1174

[23] Bern C, Messenger LA, Whitman JD, Maguire JH. Chagas disease in the United States: A public health approach. Clinical Microbiology Reviews. 2019;**33**(1):1-42

[24] Suarez C, Nolder D, Garcia-Mingo A, Moore DAJ, Chiodini PL. Diagnosis and clinical Management of Chagas Disease: An increasing challenge in non-endemic areas. Research and Reports in Tropical Medicine. 2022;**13**:25-40

[25] Samuels AM, Clark EH, Galdos-Cardenas G, Wiegand RE, Ferrufino L, Menacho S, et al. Epidemiology of and impact of insecticide spraying on Chagas disease in communities in the Bolivian Chaco. PLoS Neglected Tropical Diseases. 2013;7(8):e2358

[26] Schijman AG, Alonso-Padilla J, Longhi SA, Picado A. Parasitological, serological and molecular diagnosis of acute and chronic Chagas disease: From field to laboratory. Memórias do Instituto Oswaldo Cruz. 2022;**117**: e200444

[27] Irish A, Whitman JD, Clark EH, Marcus R, Bern C. Updated estimates and mapping for prevalence of Chagas disease among adults, United States. Emerging Infectious Diseases. 2022;**28**(7):1313-1320

[28] Mills RM. Chagas disease: Epidemiology and barriers to treatment. The American Journal of Medicine. 2020;**133**(11):1262-1265

[29] Manne-Goehler J, Umeh CA, Montgomery SP, Wirtz VJ. Estimating the burden of Chagas disease in the United States. PLoS Neglected Tropical Diseases. 2016;**10**(11):e0005033

[30] Candia-PumaMA,Machaca-LuqueLY, Roque-Pumahuanca BM, Galdino AS, Giunchetti RC, Coelho EAF, et al. Accuracy of diagnostic tests for the detection of Chagas disease: A systematic review and meta-analysis. Diagnostics (Basel). 2022;**12**(11):1-20

[31] Shikanai Yasuda MA. Emerging and reemerging forms of Trypanosoma cruzi transmission. Memórias do Instituto Oswaldo Cruz. 2022;**117**:e210033

[32] Imai K, Maeda T, Sayama Y, Osa M, Mikita K, Kurane I, et al. Chronic

Chagas disease with advanced cardiac complications in Japan: Case report and literature review. Parasitology International. 2015;**64**(5):240-242

[33] Jackson Y, Pinto A, Pett S. Chagas disease in Australia and New Zealand: Risks and needs for public health interventions. Tropical Medicine & International Health. 2014;**19**(2): 212-218

[34] Basile L, Jansá JM, Carlier Y, Salamanca DD, Angheben A, Bartoloni A, et al. Chagas disease in European countries: The challenge of a surveillance system. Eurosurveillance. 2011;**16**(37):19968

[35] Ayres J, Marcus R, Standley CJ. The importance of screening for Chagas disease against the backdrop of changing epidemiology in the USA. Current Tropical Medicine Reports. 2022;**9**(4):185-193

[36] Alarcón, de Noya B, Díaz-Bello Z, Ruiz-Guevara R, Noya O. Chagas disease expands its epidemiological Frontiers from rural to urban areas. Frontiers in Tropical Diseases. 2022;**3**

[37] Monge-Maillo B, Lopez-Velez R. Challenges in the management of Chagas disease in Latin-American migrants in Europe. Clinical Microbiology and Infection. 2017;**23**(5):290-295

[38] Requena-Mendez A, Moore DA, Subira C, Munoz J. Addressing the neglect: Chagas disease in London, UK. The Lancet Global Health. 2016;**4**(4):e231-e233

[39] Angheben A, Anselmi M, Gobbi F, Marocco S, Monteiro G, Buonfrate D, et al. Chagas disease in Italy: Breaking an epidemiological silence. Eurosurveillance. 2011;**16**(37):19969

[40] Jackson Y, Varcher Herrera M, Gascon J. Economic crisis and increased immigrant mobility: New challenges in managing Chagas disease in Europe. Bulletin of the World Health Organization. 2014;**92**(10):771-772

[41] Vermelho AB, Rodrigues GC, Supuran CT. Why hasn't there been more progress in new Chagas disease drug discovery? Expert Opinion on Drug Discovery. 2020;**15**(2):145-158

[42] Vela A, Coral-Almeida M, Sereno D, Costales JA, Barnabe C, Breniere SF. In vitro susceptibility of Trypanosoma cruzi discrete typing units (DTUs) to benznidazole: A systematic review and meta-analysis. PLoS Neglected Tropical Diseases. 2021;**15**(3):e0009269

[43] Busselman RE, Hamer SA. Chagas disease ecology in the United States: Recent advances in understanding Trypanosoma cruzi transmission among Triatomines, wildlife, and domestic animals and a quantitative synthesis of vector-host interactions. Annual Review of Animal Biosciences. 2022;**10**:325-348

[44] Herwaldt BL. Laboratory-acquired parasitic infections from accidental exposures. Clinical Microbiology Reviews. 2001;**14**(4):659-688 table of contents

[45] Huprikar S, Bosserman E, Patel G, Moore A, Pinney S, Anyanwu A, et al. Donor-derived Trypanosoma cruzi infection in solid organ recipients in the United States, 2001-2011. American Journal of Transplantation. 2013;**13**(9):2418-2425

[46] Luquetti AO, Tavares SB, Siriano Lda R, Oliveira RA, Campos DE, de Morais CA, et al. Congenital transmission of Trypanosoma cruzi in Central Brazil. A study of 1,211 individuals born to infected mothers. Memórias do Instituto Oswaldo Cruz. 2015;**110**(3):369-376

[47] Abras A, Ballart C, Fernandez-Arevalo A, Pinazo MJ, Gascon J, Munoz C, et al. Worldwide control and Management of Chagas Disease in a new era of globalization: A close look at congenital Trypanosoma cruzi infection. Clinical Microbiology Reviews. 2022;**35**(2):e0015221

[48] Antinori S, Galimberti L, Grande R, Ricaboni D, Sala S, Giacomet V, et al. Family cluster of Chagas disease among Bolivian immigrants in Italy: High rate of maternal-fetal transmission. Travel Medicine and Infectious Disease. 2022;**49**:102370

[49] Carlier Y, Torrico F, Sosa-Estani S, Russomando G, Luquetti A, Freilij H, et al. Congenital Chagas disease: Recommendations for diagnosis, treatment and control of newborns, siblings and pregnant women. PLoS Neglected Tropical Diseases. 2011;**5**(10):e1250

[50] Klein MD, Proano A, Noazin S, Sciaudone M, Gilman RH, Bowman NM. Risk factors for vertical transmission of Chagas disease: A systematic review and meta-analysis. International Journal of Infectious Diseases. 2021;**105**:357-373

[51] Paes MC, Saraiva FMS, Nogueira NP, Vieira CSD, Dias FA, Rossini A, et al. Gene expression profiling of Trypanosoma cruzi in the presence of heme points to glycosomal metabolic adaptation of epimastigotes inside the vector. PLoS Neglected Tropical Diseases. 2020;**14**(1):e0007945

[52] Carbajal-de-la-Fuente AL, Sanchez-Casaccia P, Piccinali RV, Provecho Y, Salva L, Meli S, et al. Urban vectors of Chagas disease in the American continent: A systematic review of epidemiological surveys. PLoS Neglected Tropical Diseases. 2022;**16**(12):e0011003

[53] Buhaya MH, Galvan S, Maldonado RA. Incidence of Trypanosoma cruzi infection in triatomines collected at Indio Mountains Research Station. Acta Tropica. 2015;**150**:97-99

[54] Reisenman CE, Lawrence G, Guerenstein PG, Gregory T, Dotson E, Hildebrand JG. Infection of kissing bugs with Trypanosoma cruzi, Tucson, Arizona, USA. Emerging Infectious Diseases. 2010;**16**(3):400-405

[55] Ruijtenberg S, van den Heuvel S. Coordinating cell proliferation and differentiation: Antagonism between cell cycle regulators and cell type-specific gene expression. Cell Cycle. 2016;**15**(2):196-212

[56] Won MM, Kruger T, Engstler M, Burleigh BA. The intracellular amastigote of Trypanosoma cruzi maintains an actively beating flagellum. MBio. 2023;**14**(2):e0355622

[57] Martin-Escolano J, Marin C, Rosales MJ, Tsaousis AD, Medina-Carmona E, Martin-Escolano R. An updated view of the Trypanosoma cruzi life cycle: Intervention points for an effective treatment. ACS Infectious Diseases. 2022;**8**(6):1107-1115

[58] de Souza W. Cell biology of Trypanosoma cruzi. International Review of Cytology. 1984;**86**:197-283

[59] May-Concha IJ, Escalante-Talavera MJ, Dujardin JP, Waleckx E. Does Trypanosoma cruzi (Chagas, 1909) (Kinetoplastida: Trypanosomatidae) modify the antennal phenotype of Triatoma dimidiata (Latreille, 1811) (Hemiptera: Triatominae)? Parasites & Vectors. 2022;**15**(1):466

[60] Coura JR. The discovery of chagas disease (1908-1909): Great successes

and certain misunderstandings and challenges. Revista da Sociedade Brasileira de Medicina Tropical. 2013;**46**(4):389-390

[61] Sanchez-Valdez FJ, Padilla A, Wang W, Orr D, Tarleton RL. Spontaneous dormancy protects Trypanosoma cruzi during extended drug exposure. eLife. 2018;**7**

[62] McGonagle K, Tarver GJ, Cantizani J, Cotillo I, Dodd PG, Ferguson L, et al. Identification and development of a series of disubstituted piperazines for the treatment of Chagas disease. European Journal of Medicinal Chemistry. 2022;**238**:114421

[63] Perez-Molina JA, Crespillo-Andujar C, Bosch-Nicolau P, Molina I. Trypanocidal treatment of Chagas disease. Enfermedades Infecciosas y Microbiologia Clinica (Engl Ed). 2020;**39**:458-470

[64] Boiani M, Piacenza L, Hernandez P, Boiani L, Cerecetto H, Gonzalez M, et al. Mode of action of nifurtimox and N-oxide-containing heterocycles against Trypanosoma cruzi: Is oxidative stress involved? Biochemical Pharmacology. 2010;**79**(12):1736-1745

[65] Hall BS, Bot C, Wilkinson SR. Nifurtimox activation by trypanosomal type I nitroreductases generates cytotoxic nitrile metabolites. The Journal of Biological Chemistry. 2011;**286**(15):13088-13095

[66] Kratz JM, Garcia Bournissen F, Forsyth CJ, Sosa-Estani S. Clinical and pharmacological profile of benznidazole for treatment of Chagas disease. Expert Review of Clinical Pharmacology. 2018;**11**(10):943-957

[67] Patterson S, Wyllie S. Nitro drugs for the treatment of trypanosomatid diseases: Past, present, and future prospects. Trends in Parasitology. 2014;**30**(6):289-298

[68] Mendes F, Perez-Molina JA, Angheben A, Meymandi SK, Sosa-Estani S, Molina I. Critical analysis of Chagas disease treatment in different countries. Memórias do Instituto Oswaldo Cruz. 2022;**117**:e210034

[69] Olivera MJ, Cucunuba ZM, Valencia-Hernandez CA, Herazo R, Agreda-Rudenko D, Florez C, et al. Risk factors for treatment interruption and severe adverse effects to benznidazole in adult patients with Chagas disease. PLoS One. 2017;**12**(9):e0185033

[70] Rassi A Jr, Rassi A, Marcondes de Rezende J. American trypanosomiasis (Chagas disease). Infectious Disease Clinics of North America. 2012;**26**(2):275-291

[71] Hughes D, Andersson DI. Evolutionary trajectories to antibiotic resistance. Annual Review of Microbiology. 2017;**71**:579-596

[72] Araujo SC, de Angelo RM, Barbosa H, Costa-Silva TA, Tempone AG, Lago JHG, et al. Identification of inhibitors as drug candidates against Chagas disease. European Journal of Medicinal Chemistry. 2023;**248**:115074

[73] Abegg CP, Abreu AP, Silva JL, Araujo SM, Gomes ML, Ferreira EC, et al. Polymorphisms of blood forms and in vitro metacyclogenesis of Trypanosoma cruzi I, II, and IV. Experimental Parasitology. 2017;**176**:8-15

[74] Bustamante JM, Craft JM, Crowe BD, Ketchie SA, Tarleton RL. New, combined, and reduced dosing treatment protocols cure Trypanosoma cruzi infection in mice. The Journal of Infectious Diseases. 2014;**209**(1):150-162

[75] Vieira GAL, Silva M, Regasini LO, Cotinguiba F, Laure HJ, Rosa JC, et al. Trypanosoma cruzi: Analysis of two different strains after piplartine treatment. The Brazilian Journal of Infectious Diseases. 2018;**22**(3):208-218

[76] Bahia MT, de Andrade IM, Martins TA, do Nascimento AF, Diniz Lde F, Caldas IS, et al. Fexinidazole: A potential new drug candidate for Chagas disease. PLoS Neglected Tropical Diseases. 2012;**6**(11):e1870

[77] Filardi LS, Brener Z. A rapid method for testing in vivo the susceptibility of different strains of Trypanosoma cruzi to active chemotherapeutic agents. Memórias do Instituto Oswaldo Cruz. 1984;**79**(2):221-225

[78] Reigada C, Saye M, Valera-Vera E, Miranda MR, Pereira CA. Repurposing of terconazole as an anti Trypanosoma cruzi agent. Heliyon. 2019;**5**(6):e01947

[79] Martinez SJ, Romano PS, Engman DM. Precision health for Chagas disease: Integrating parasite and host factors to predict outcome of infection and response to therapy. Frontiers in Cellular and Infection Microbiology. 2020;**10**:210

[80] Dumonteil E, Herrera C, Buekens P. A therapeutic preconceptional vaccine against Chagas disease: A novel indication that could reduce congenital transmission and accelerate vaccine development. PLoS Neglected Tropical Diseases. 2019;**13**(1):e0006985

[81] Michel-Todo L, Reche PA, Bigey P, Pinazo MJ, Gascon J, Alonso-Padilla J. In silico Design of an Epitope-Based Vaccine Ensemble for Chagas disease. Frontiers in Immunology. 2019;**10**:2698

[82] Franco CH, Warhurst DC, Bhattacharyya T, Au HYA, Le H, Giardini MA, et al. Novel structural CYP51 mutation in Trypanosoma cruzi associated with multidrug resistance to CYP51 inhibitors and reduced infectivity. International Journal for Parasitology: Drugs and Drug Resistance. 2020;**13**:107-120

[83] Molina I, Gomez i Prat J, Salvador F, Trevino B, Sulleiro E, Serre N, et al. Randomized trial of posaconazole and benznidazole for chronic Chagas' disease. The New England Journal of Medicine. 2014;**370**(20):1899-1908

[84] Torrico F, Gascon J, Ortiz L, Alonso-Vega C, Pinazo MJ, Schijman A, et al. Treatment of adult chronic indeterminate Chagas disease with benznidazole and three E1224 dosing regimens: A proof-of-concept, randomised, placebo-controlled trial. The Lancet Infectious Diseases. 2018;**18**(4):419-430

[85] Morillo CA, Waskin H, Sosa-Estani S, Del Carmen BM, Cuneo C, Milesi R, et al. Benznidazole and Posaconazole in eliminating parasites in asymptomatic T. Cruzi carriers: The STOP-CHAGAS trial. Journal of the American College of Cardiology. 2017;**69**(8):939-947

[86] Pathak S, Bhardwaj M, Agrawal N, Bhardwaj A. A comprehensive review on potential candidates for the treatment of chagas disease. Chemical Biology & Drug Design. 2023:1-19

[87] de Melo GD, Coatnoan N, Gouault N, Cupif JF, Renault J, Cosson A, et al. Prodrugs as new therapies against Chagas disease: in vivo synergy between Trypanosoma cruzi proline racemase inhibitors and benznidazole. Journal of Global Antimicrobial Resistance. 2022;**28**:84-89

[88] Beltran-Hortelano I, Alcolea V, Font M, Perez-Silanes S. Examination of multiple Trypanosoma cruzi targets

in a new drug discovery approach for Chagas disease. Bioorganic & Medicinal Chemistry. 2022;**58**:116577

[89] Herreros-Cabello A, Callejas-Hernandez F, Girones N, Fresno M. Trypanosoma Cruzi genome: Organization, multi-gene families, transcription, and biological implications. Genes (Basel). 2020;**11**(10):1-26

[90] Quinones W, Acosta H, Goncalves CS, Motta MCM, Gualdron-Lopez M, Michels PAM. Structure, properties, and function of Glycosomes in Trypanosoma cruzi. Frontiers in Cellular and Infection Microbiology. 2020;**10**:25

[91] Callejas-Hernandez F, Herreros-Cabello A, Del Moral-Salmoral J, Fresno M, Girones N. The complete mitochondrial DNA of Trypanosoma cruzi: Maxicircles and Minicircles. Frontiers in Cellular and Infection Microbiology. 2021;**11**:672448

[92] Martinez-Peinado N, Martori C, Cortes-Serra N, Sherman J, Rodriguez A, Gascon J, et al. Anti-Trypanosoma cruzi activity of metabolism modifier compounds. International Journal of Molecular Sciences. 2021;**22**(2):1-16

[93] Shah-Simpson S, Lentini G, Dumoulin PC, Burleigh BA. Modulation of host central carbon metabolism and in situ glucose uptake by intracellular Trypanosoma cruzi amastigotes. PLoS Pathogens. 2017;**13**(11):e1006747

[94] Barison MJ, Rapado LN, Merino EF, Furusho Pral EM, Mantilla BS, Marchese L, et al. Metabolomic profiling reveals a finely tuned, starvation-induced metabolic switch in Trypanosoma cruzi epimastigotes. The Journal of Biological Chemistry. 2017;**292**(21):8964-8977

[95] De-Simone SG, Bourguignon SC, Goncalves PS, Lechuga GC, Provance DW Jr. Metabolic alteration of Trypanosoma cruzi during differentiation of Epimastigote to Trypomastigote forms. Pathogens. 2022;**11**(2):1-10

[96] Saraiva FMS, Cosentino-Gomes D, Inacio JDF, Almeida-Amaral EE, Louzada-Neto O, Rossini A, et al. Hypoxia effects on Trypanosoma cruzi Epimastigotes proliferation, differentiation, and energy metabolism. Pathogens. 2022;**11**(8):1-15

[97] Cannata JJ, Cazzulo JJ. Glycosomal and mitochondrial malate dehydrogenases in epimastigotes of Trypanosoma cruzi. Molecular and Biochemical Parasitology. 1984;**11**: 37-49

[98] Opperdoes FR. Biochemical peculiarities of trypanosomes, African and south American. British Medical Bulletin. 1985;**41**(2):130-136

[99] Coronel C, Rovai LE, Gerez de Burgos NM, Burgos C, Blanco A. Properties of alpha-hydroxyacid dehydrogenase isozymes from Trypanosoma cruzi. Molecular and Biochemical Parasitology. 1981;**4**(1-2):29-38

[100] Montamat EE, Arauzo SS, Blanco A. Subcellular localization of leucine aminotransferase and alpha-hydroxyacid dehydrogenase in Trypanosoma cruzi. Molecular and Biochemical Parasitology. 1987;**22**(2-3):185-193

[101] Chena MA, Elizondo-Jimenez S, Rodriguez-Paez L, Nogueda-Torres B, Baeza-Ramirez I, Wong-Ramirez C. Trypanosoma cruzi: Inhibition of alpha-hydroxyacid dehydrogenase isozyme II by N-allyl and N-propyl oxamates and their effects on intact epimastigotes. Memórias do Instituto Oswaldo Cruz. 2004;**99**(8):831-837

[102] Chena MA, Elizondo S, Rodriguez-Paez L, Nogueda B, Baeza I, Wong C. Trypanocidal activity of N-isopropyl oxamate on cultured epimastigotes and murine trypanosomiasis using different Trypanosoma cruzi strains. Journal of Enzyme Inhibition and Medicinal Chemistry. 2005;**20**(2):189-197

[103] Resendiz-Mora A, Barrera-Aveleida G, Sotelo-Rodriguez A, Galarce-Sosa I, Nevarez-Lechuga I, Santiago-Hernandez JC, et al. Effect of B-NIPOx in experimental Trypanosoma cruzi infection in mice. International Journal of Molecular Sciences. 2022;**24**(1)

[104] Wong-Baeza C, Nogueda-Torres B, Serna M, Meza-Toledo S, Baeza I, Wong C. Trypanocidal effect of the benzyl ester of N-propyl oxamate: A bi-potential prodrug for the treatment of experimental Chagas disease. BMC Pharmacology and Toxicology. 2015;**16**:10

[105] Avila CC, Mule SN, Rosa-Fernandes L, Viner R, Barison MJ, Costa-Martins AG, et al. Proteome-wide analysis of Trypanosoma cruzi exponential and stationary growth phases reveals a subcellular compartment-specific regulation. Genes (Basel). 2018;**9**(8)

[106] Basse F, Sainte-Marie J, Maurin L, Bienvenue A. Effect of benzyl alcohol on phospholipid transverse mobility in human erythrocyte membrane. European Journal of Biochemistry. 1992;**205**(1):155-162

[107] Bringaud F, Riviere L, Coustou V. Energy metabolism of trypanosomatids: Adaptation to available carbon sources. Molecular and Biochemical Parasitology. 2006;**149**(1):1-9

[108] da Silveira AB, Lemos EM, Adad SJ, Correa-Oliveira R, Furness JB, D'Avila RD. Megacolon in Chagas disease: A study of inflammatory cells, enteric nerves, and glial cells. Human Pathology. 2007;**38**(8):1256-1264

[109] de Souza W, de Carvalho TM, Barrias ES. Review on Trypanosoma cruzi: Host cell interaction. International Journal of Cell Biology. 2010;**2010**

[110] Urbina JA. Specific chemotherapy of Chagas disease: Relevance, current limitations and new approaches. Acta Tropica. 2010;**115**(1-2):55-68

Chapter 10

Modern Aspects of Leishmaniasis: Basis of Development New Approaches against Infection

Asli Pinar Zorba Yildiz, Gulnaz Yildirim Koken, Burcak Yavuz, Emrah Sefik Abamor, Ozlem Ayse Tosyali, Serap Yesilkir Baydar, Ikram Ullah, Ahmet Berkay Civan, Melahat Bagirova and Adil M. Allahverdiyev

Abstract

In this review, the basic principles of developing new approaches to leishmaniasis have been stated contrary to the available literature on *Leishmania*. In general, the morphology of parasites, life cycle, clinical forms, correspondence to epidemiology, and distribution according to species in the world were described. It has been expressed in various aspects of the interaction between host and parasite cell receptors. This plays an extremely important role in vaccine and drug development against leishmaniasis. Immunologically, natural immunocytes emphasize the importance of macrophages and dendritic cells in the *Leishmania* parasites' immunopathology. This review will also discourse on the possibilities and necessity for the generation of new treatment technologies for leishmaniasis.

Keywords: Leishmaniasis, vaccine, cytokines, parasite, infection

1. Introduction

Human infection is caused by approximately 21 of 30 species of *Leishmania* parasites that are pathogenic for humans. The species are found in two morphologic forms during their life cycle. In hosts (both human and mammalian), parasites exist within macrophages and monocytes as round to oval non-flagellate morphology. Macrophages can play a crucially important role in *Leishmania* infection for professional phagocytes. The *Leishmania parasites* can be viewed as carefully selecting the optimal phagocyte receptors to promote their survival in the host. Neutrophils are thought to participate in the containment of *Leishmania* parasites within an hour of infection and they are important to be the first cells recruited to the site of infection, and are also dendritic cells (DCs). The main obligation of DCs is the diagnosis and processing of foreign antigens and presentation to T cells. The parasitic surface molecules (LPG, GPI, GP63, *etc.*) give detailed information that plays an important role in infectivity in the pathogenesis of leishmaniasis. The *Leishmania* parasites have a dense covering of glycocalyx, which as a significant role in host-parasite interactions. The glycocalyx is attached to the plasma membrane via GPI (glycophosphoinositol). The GPI anchor molecules (LPG, GP63) have different roles, such as promoting infectivity, helping parasite survival, and important virulence role. The *Leishmania* infection initiation mechanism can be explained by its interaction between the parasite-expressed lipophosphoglycan (LPG) and the host cell-expressed TLR-2. The third complement receptor (CR3), first complement receptor (CR1), mannose receptor (MR), Fc gamma receptors (FcgRs, in particular, FcgRII-B2), and fibronectin receptors (FnRs) have been reported to take place for the facilitator to include *Leishmania* internalization. On the other hand, in this review, we have included the cytokines and signal molecules that play an important role in the immunology of leishmaniasis, and these molecules, especially the interaction between natural and acquired immunity as well.

In the last part, it was stated that the basic principles of vaccine development against leishmaniasis, information about the diagnosis of leishmaniasis and different generations of vaccine types, and the important role of parasite-host interaction in the development of a vaccine. Treatment outcome is a complex phenomenon with the potential of multi-factors such as genetics, immunological response, characteristics, and clinical treatment of the patient. Also, drug quality, duration of therapy, compliance, and parasite characteristics, such as variable intrinsic susceptibility (species) and drug resistance should be considered.

As a result, this literature review titled "Modern Aspects of Leishmaniasis: Basis of Development New Approaches against Infection" provides current information on various aspects of the leishmaniasis problem and suggests new approaches to struggling with the disease.

2. About *Leishmania spp*

Leishmaniasis is a zoonotic disease caused by *Leishmania* protozoa. The genus of *Leishmania* has more than 20 species and they are all obligate intracellular parasites. Leishmaniasis is transmitted to humans by the bites of infected female *phlebotominae* sandflies (genus Lutzomyia) [1], which survive in natural areas such as sylvans, caves, or coves [2, 3]. World Health Organization (WHO) declares leishmaniasis threatens about 350 million adults and children in approximately 90 countries around the world. It is believed that 12 million people are currently infected. Every year about 2 million new cases consist of this illness [3, 4]. Endemic regions for the illness are expressed as the west side of Asia and Africa, India, China, and the Mediterranean region [5].

2.1 Epidemiological and clinical form of old and new world *Leishmania*

Kala-Azar discovered in India by Leishman and Donovan, is endemic in 88 countries. In addition to India, the majority of new cases are seen in Brazil, Somalia, South Sudan, Ethiopia, Kenya, and Sudan, according to the data announced by WHO (2018) [6]. The epidemiological distributions are detailed in **Table 1**.

Leishmaniasis has four main types and each type differs in specific properties [4].

Cutaneous leishmaniasis (CL): Skin ulcers usually form on exposed areas, such as the face, arms, and legs. Healing of the wounds takes a few months but generally leaves scars [4]. The incidence of the cases is seen in Afghanistan, Brazil, Iran, Peru, Saudi Arabia, and Syria with a ratio of 90% [8].

Clinical Forms	Species	Country or Territory
Cutaneous Leishmaniasis	*L. tropica*	Afghanistan, Azerbaijan, Egypt, Ethiopia, Turkey
	L. major	Afghanistan, Azerbaijan, Egypt, Ethiopia India, Iran, Iraq, Kenya, Morocco, Nigeria, Pakistan, Tunisia, and Yemen
	L. infantum	Albania, Bulgaria, China
		Ethiopia, Kenya
	L. aethiopica	Cyprus, Israel
		Belize, Colombia, Mexico
	L. donovani	Argentina, Brazil, Bolivia, Colombia, Mexico, Panama, Paraguay, Peru
	L. mexicana	Argentina, Brazil, Guyana, Peru, and Venezuela
	L. braziliensis	Colombia, Costa Rica, Ecuador, Honduras, Panama
	L. guyanensis	Peru
	L. panamensis	
	L. peruviana	
Mucocutaneous Leishmaniasis	*L. braziliensis*	Argentina, Bolivia, Brazil, Colombia, Mexico, Paraguay, Peru
	L. major	America, Mexico
	L. panamensis	Colombia, Costa Rica, Honduras, Panama
	L. braziliensis guyanensis	Peru
Diffuse cutaneously Leishmaniasis	*L. aethiopica*	Ethiopia, Kenya
	L. Mexicana	America, Costa Rica, Ecuador, Mexico Guatemala
	L. amazonensis	Bolivia, Colombia, Ecuador, Venezuela
Visceral Leishmaniasis	*L. donovani*	Africa, Bangladesh, India, Sudan
	L. infantum	Afghanistan, African Republic, Albania, Brazil, Central Asia, Central Iraq, France, the Mediterranean basin, Tunisia, Turkey
	L. chagasi	New World
Post-kala-azar dermal	*Leishmaniasis L. donovani*	Bangladesh, Ethiopia, India, Nepal, Sudan

Table 1.
Leishmaniasis clinical forms, Leishmania *species and territory [7].*

Diffuse cutaneous leishmaniasis (DCL): The heel expands on the skin. It is a difficult type to treat because of chronic lesions [4].

Mucocutaneous leishmaniasis (MCL): It takes place on mucous membranes of the mouth, nose, and throat damaging or destroying the tissues [4]. The incidence of the cases is seen in Bolivia, Brazil, and Peru with a ratio of 90% [8].

Visceral leishmaniasis (Kala-azar, VL): Interior organs are affected by this type and have no treatment. Symptoms of VL include high said to be high fever, significant loss in weight, increase in sizes of the spleen and liver, and anemia. Sometimes death occurs within 2 years [4]. It is observed in humans but not in other mammals [9]. The incidence of the cases is seen in Bangladesh, Brazil, India, Nepal, and Sudan with a ratio of 90% [8]. Detailed leishmaniasis territory and its' vectors are shown in a table with Clinical Forms (**Table 1**).

2.2 *Leishmania spp.* lifespan

It has two stages: sand fly stage and human stage. At different stages of their life cycle, which includes vertebrates and invertebrates as hosts, parasites exist in several morphologies according to flagellum location and nucleus-kinetoplast location.

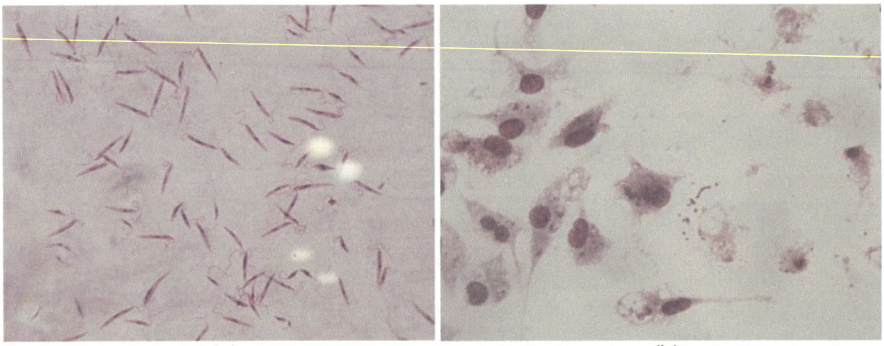

Figure 1.
a. L.infantum *(MONI/EP126) promastigotes (Giemsa staining, x100), b. amastigote form - phagocytosed by macrophage (Giemsa staining, x100) [10].*

Basically, *Leishmania* parasites are divided into two classes: promastigote form and amastigote form.

Promastigote form: Extracellular form of the parasite is called a promastigote. This form of parasite exists in the invertebrate region of the host's (sand fly) body at 270°C. They have a flagellum, and so they are motile. Their cell body length is 15–30 μm with a 5 μm width. The proliferation of the parasites follows longitudinal binary fission (**Figure 1a**).

Amastigote form: The parasite's intracellular form is called an amastigotes. This non-motile form exists in the vertebrate host's body at 37°C. They do not have a flagellum and their cell body length is 3–6 μm with a 1.5–3.0 μm width. The proliferation of the parasites follows longitudinal binary fission (**Figure 1b**) [10].

2.3 Vectors and reservoirs

Human infection is caused by approximately 21 of 30 species of *Leishmania* parasites that are pathogenic for humans [11, 12]. *Leishmania* reservoirs are expanded worldwide [13]. Expansion of the infection is commonly caused by mice, foxes, cats, and especially dogs [14]. Reservoir hosts show changes according to geographical location [15] in American Bradypus, opossums, rodents, and domestic dogs are the main hosts [13], and in India foxes, opossums, black rats, and domestic cats [14], and also humans are known as reservoirs [13]. Several parameters affect reservoir hosts. The factors that affect the system are the ecological properties of the homeland (habitat, geologic structure, and biotope), structure population (age, movement, dispersion, and reproduction), and sociology (feeding and customs) important to understand the behavior and type of the infection.

2.3.1 Interaction with Leishmania *parasites and host cells*

Leishmania specifically selects macrophages of mammalian cells as infected host cells [16, 17]. The transition of the parasite to the extracellular and intracellular environments is affected by different factors such as nutrients, pH, temperature, and availability of oxygen. Nutritional requirements, growth rate and ability to divide, the regulated expression of their surface molecules, and morphology are the factors that

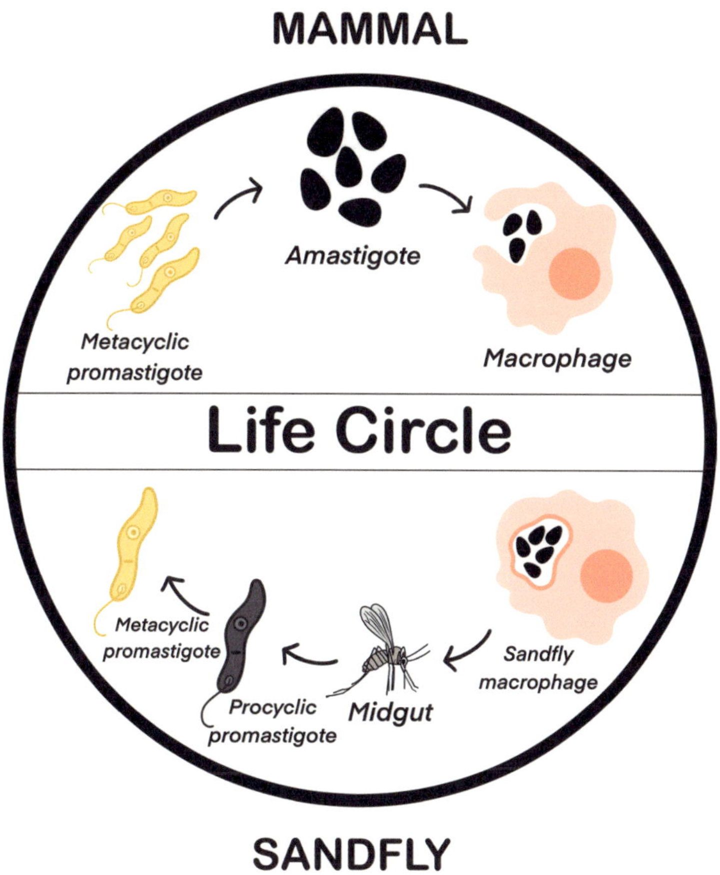

Figure 2.
Life circle of Leishmania *parasites.*

distinguish the developmental forms. The procyclic to metacyclic differentiation of promastigotes (also called metacyclogenesis) and the metacyclic promastigote are the two differentiation events studied with *Leishmania* to amastigote transformation [18] inside the host macrophage (**Figure 2**).

Procyclic phase promastigotes existing in the insect's midgut are not only non-disjunctional but, mammalian-infective, metacyclic phase promastigotes in the thoracic midgut and proboscis of the sandfly as well [19].

The metacyclic promastigotes differentiate into the intracellular flagellate amastigote form by inoculating into a mammalian host through a sandfly bite. This form of the parasite is named the parasitophorous vacuole by residing within a vacuole with lysosomal features [20].

Metacyclic promastigotes become resistant to complement by expressing stage-specific surface molecules. In this respect, it differs from the procyclic forms and is pre-adapted for survival in the mammalian host. Amastigotes are formed in macrophages by multiplying within the parasitophore vacuole. They are also intracellular, immobile forms, having a reduced size and a very reduced flagellum that does not protrude from the flagellum pocket. In addition, amastigotes are acidophiles with an energy metabolism adapted to the low pH of this compartment. They are characterized *in vitro* by low pH, lack of oxygen, and nutritional depletion of tetrahydrobiopterin. The conditions such as low pH, 37°C temperature, and high CO_2 that mimic a phagolysosome-like environment can cause promastigote to amastigote differentiation [18]. Although environmental factors influencing *Leishmania* differentiation are known, little is known about the molecular processes that mediate cellular remodeling. Polycistronic RNAs transcripted *Leishmania* protein codes are not regulated at a transcriptional level, also they identify the stage-specific genes problematic [16]. There are many studies on different *Leishmania* species related to transcoelomic and proteomic approaches for identifying stage-regulated genes and proteins [17]. Some clear-cut stage-specific markers have functions that differ from nutrient acquisition to cellular reshaping and recycling and these markers involve peptidases. Moreover, they have a relationship with the mammalian virulence of *Leishmania* [21–23]. The peptidases are effective in the differentiation of the parasite. Host factors (species, concomitant infections/health, sex, age, behavioral patterns), parasite traits (generation time, dispersion strategies, molecular and biochemical characteristics of its sub-populations), exposure (inoculum size), and local environmental conditions (influenced, e.g., by stress and availability of natural resources) are the main factors that determine the patterns of *Leishmania* infection in any mammalian host species [23].

2.3.2 Receptors

The mechanism of initiation of *Leishmania* infection can be explained by the interaction between the parasite-expressed lipophosphoglycan (LPG) and the host cell-expressed TLR-2 [24, 25]. The third complement receptor (CR3), first complement receptor (CR1), mannose receptor (MR), Fc gamma receptors (FcgRs, in particular, FcgRII-B2), and fibronectin receptors (FnRs) [16] have been reported to be involved in the process. A definitive understanding of the roles of various receptors in parasite survival during natural infection has remained elusive [20]. Previous reports show that TLR-2 may not necessarily be host-protective, as proposed for all TLR anti-pathogen functions [20, 24–26]. However, nine types of TLRs are implicated differentially in infections with different *Leishmania* species [24, 27]. It is indicated that activation of TLRs leads to activation for adaptive immune responses; maturation of antigen-presenting cells and T cell activation can be observed first [24, 28, 29]. A significant role is taken in adaptive immune responses to *Leishmania* infection by CD40 [30, 31].

2.3.3 Host cells

Macrophages can play a crucially important role in *Leishmania* infection as professional phagocytes. The parasites make use of their phagocytic function as a strategy for learning and subsequent replication within the macrophage phagolysosomes as well. Thus, macrophages figure likewise both the host cells for effector cells that kill the parasites and parasite replication. Learning of *Leishmania* by macrophages triggers the production of reactive oxygen species [32] and leads to the generation of nitric oxide (NO) [33] and N-hydroxy-L-arginine (LOHA) [34] as mediators of parasite killing. The macrophage entry mechanism represents, in part, the dynamic nature of the parasite surface. The most abundant surface membrane components are the extracellular promastigote form, which can be found in insects, and the intracellular amastigote form, which is typically found in mammals [6]. Metacyclogenesis, the developmental process leading promastigotes to transform into a virulent form in the sand fly gut, is characterized by further modifications in surface proteins and other glycoconjugates [10, 35]. Different sources of macrophages and different *Leishmania spp*. vary in their surface molecule composition, leading to unique parasite–host receptor interactions for each species-cell pair [2, 7].

Neutrophils are important in that they are the first cells to head to the site of infection with bite of a sand fly. Neutrophil uptake occurs by *Leishmania* parasites 1 hour after infection [36, 37]. Apoptotic neutrophils and neutrophils are more likely to play a role in promoting disease advance, instead of resisting. CR3 (CD18/CD11b) is an integrin expressed on the surface of neutrophils (PMNs) and they play a significant role in the immune defense system. iC3b and pathogen ligands are adhesion factors during phagocyte migration [16].

The main obligation of DCs is the diagnosis and processing of foreign antigens and presentation to T cells [38]. They are considered to be gatekeepers in the defense against invading pathogens. The body has the most efficient antigen-presenting cells (APCs) like skin DCs, Langerhans cells, and dermal DCs [39, 40]. Dermal DCs appear to present antigens directly to T cells during *Leishmania* infection [41]. Afterward, the infection, small numbers of parasites are involved directly by dermal DCs [42], although the majority of the DCs become infected through contact with parasitized neutrophils [43]. After weeks of post-infection, the number of DCs (CD11c (+) cells) in the lesion increases due to their recruitment [44], and those infected DCs can prime native CD4 (þ) and CD8 (þ) T cells [45].

2.3.4 Surface molecules

Among the species of *Leishmania,* the amounts of secreted proteophosphoglycans show differences. This means that different proteophosphoglycans have different functions, but the knowledge about this is still insufficient. In all *Leishmania* species, these GPI-anchored molecules include LPG, glycoinositolphospholipids (GIPLs), glycoproteins 63 (GP63), and the proteophosphoglycan (PPG) [46, 47].

Proteophosphoglycans: The family of these molecules includes several secreted or membrane-anchored proteins lustily modified by phosphoglycan chains [48]. A protein modification like this, called phosphoglycosylation, is common in Protozoa and includes the [6Galβ1,4Manα1PO4]n units, which are combined with serine-containing regions of proteophosphoglycan [47–49].

Lipophosphoglycan: In short, LPG is the main surface glycoconjugate of promastigotes. The most studied glycoconjugate is LPG, which forms a dense glycocalyx covering the entire surface of the parasite and the flagellum with approximately 5×10^6 copies/cell [20]. LPG is predominantly expressed in promastigotes, whereas it is absent in intracellular amastigotes. LPG has been chemically characterized and shown to vary in different species and during promastigote development in the sandfly. This LPG structure consists of four structures: a GPI anchor, a glycan core, a linear phosphoglycan chain (PG), and a terminator oligosaccharide cap (**Figure 3**). The structure and number of phosphoglycan repeat units vary and depend on the stage of differentiation and the species of *Leishmania*. The polymorphisms in its structure are important in allowing *Leishmania* parasites to colonize the host [46].

The GPI anchor includes an alkyl phosphatidylinositol containing either C24 or C26 as the aliphatic chain. The LPG glycan core is a consisting of the structure Gal (α1,6) Gal(α1,3) Galf(β1,3) [Glc(α1)-PO4] Man(α1,3) Man(α1,4)-GlcN(α1). There are 15–40 phosphodisaccharide (Galβ1,4Manα1-PO4) units between a linear PG and the glycan core. Eventually, an oligosaccharide cap structure is in the termination of LPG [46, 50].

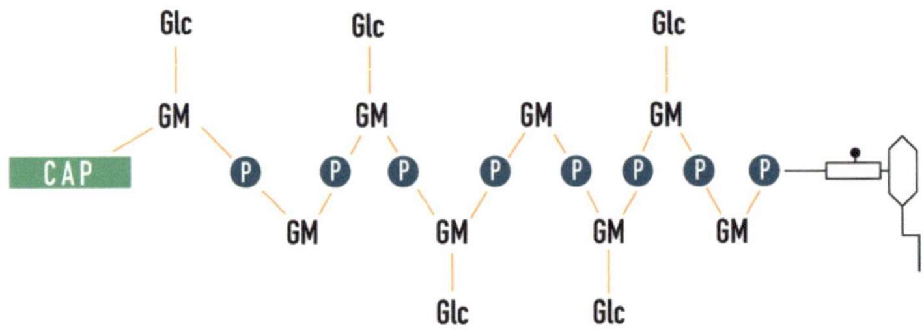

Figure 3.
Structure of LPG.

The molecular functions of LPG are;

1. Inhibiting phagosome-endosome fusion

2. Disruption of macrophage signaling pathways

3. Protection of promastigotes against oxidative burst during phagocytosis

4. Regulation of NO synthesis expression in macrophages

5. Retarding maturation of macrophagic phagolysosomes

6. Prevention of IL12 secretion by macrophages [51, 52].

Glycosylphosphatidylinositols: GPIs are the most abundant molecules, which bind a lot of proteins and carbohydrates settled in the membranes of the *Leishmania* parasites.

Glycoinositolphospholipids: GIPLs, other glycoconjugates are the glycoinositol-phospholipids (GIPLs), which are expressed both in promastigotes and amastigotes (approximately 107 molecules per cell), the replicating form during the infection in the host. GIPLs are also polymorphic like LPG in both glycan and lipid structures, however, a conserved main core are shown in all *Leishmania* species studied to date. It contains the Manα1,4GlcNα1,6 myoinositol1phospholipid structure. In the other trypanosomatids, there is no unsaturated fatty acid component of the lipid moiety [53].

The metalloproteinase GP63 (leishmanolysin): GP63 is the main GPI-anchored zinc-dependent metalloprotease of the cell surface of *Leishmania* parasites and was first discovered in the 1980s. The molecular mass is 58–65 kDa and an average of 5×10^5 GP63 copies are expressed per cell, which makes up about 1% of the total cellular protein [47]. The GP63 has expressed promastigotes however is down-regulated in amastigotes [54]. The GP63 probably plays different roles in both forms of the parasite. The GP63 was found to cleave C3b into iC3b so helping *L. amazonensis* and L. major promastigotes to avoid complement-mediated lysis [55]. Also, the GP63 molecules can bind to macrophages and can easily survive and replicate in them [56, 57]. The role of structural differentiation of GP63 molecules in both amastigotes and promastigotes of *Leishmania* is still unknown [47].

2.4 Cytokines and signaling molecules

A variety of different cytokines are associated with Th1 (gamma interferon [IFN-gamma], interleukin-2 [IL-2]) and Th2 cells (IL-4 and IL-10), and they have important roles in host-parasite infection in leishmaniasis. The cellular immune responses (Th1 type) play a role against the disease [58]. There are four main steps in *Leishmania* infection, as explained below:

In the first step, *Leishmania* promastigotes calmly enter macrophages. The macrophages cannot manage to induce innate immune responses and this result may cause a delayed induction of an adaptive immune response. The delayed adaptive immunity may provide the parasite to replicate inside macrophages. In the second step, the replication of a parasite is prevented by macrophages which finally generate the immune signals. In the third step, amastigote spreads by blasting the macrophages and they infect other macrophages. Amastigotes coat themselves in host IgG and the IgG binds to macrophage FcγR which results in the overproduction of IL-10 cytokine. This cytokine can prevent macrophage responses to IFN γ and also allow the parasites to survive [45].

It is known that the production of IFN-γ induces the macrophages which were infected before. Hence the induced macrophages provide the upregulation of nitric oxide (NO) synthesis. NO has an important role in killing *Leishmania* parasites [59].

The cellular response to leishmaniasis is elicited by the T cell response after infection. First, the amastigotes proliferate and turn into the phagolysosome in the macrophage. Then both the parasites and their antigens can be taken up by antigen-presenting cells (APCs). These APCs transfer them to $CD4^+$ and $CD8^+$ T cells. After that, these cells induce specific T cells for the production of different types of cytokines like TNFα, IL-6, IL-10, IL-12, and IFN-γ. This condition has the ability to activate macrophages to kill amastigotes [60]. Specific $CD8^+$ T cells, which are triggered during infection, have cytolytic antileishmanial activity. Possibly it can do this by inducing the production of IFN-γ and TGF-b. $CD4^+$ T cells are major cytokine-expressing cells that can produce both type 1 and type 2 cytokines [61]. IL-4 was shown to induce Th2 differentiation and lead to IL-4, IL-5, and IL-10 production. IL-10 has a major important role in *Leishmania* disease progression. In contrast, the cytokine IL-12 was shown to be linked to Th1 differentiation, cell proliferation, and secretion of IFN-γ. It supports protective immunity against the disease. A strong and specific cellular immune response against leishmaniasis is interested in long-term protection.

3. Importance of host-parasite interactions in vaccine technology

Type-1, polytypic, and peripheral membrane proteins are important plasma membrane components, reflecting the different microbicidal responses and nutritional environments encountered. Recently, single or multiple surface components missing in *Leishmania* mutants have been developed. Wild-type parasites are more deadly than some mutant parasites. Mutant parasites may have little or no loss of infectivity. Identification of other surface or intracellular components with these mutants would be helpful, as it is necessary for determining virulence in macrophages [62]. Although there are several leishmanial antigens tested for potential vaccine candidates, vaccine candidates whose efficacy and phase studies have been completed are limited [63]. There are some difficulties in the selection of these vaccine candidates. The cellular components of complex organisms, such as protozoa, are highly immunogenic and initiate complex immune processes. Immunogenicity and induction of mixed immune system on the immune system are also quite mixed. Some cellular components may cross-react with the host, causing pathological responses or aggravating infection-related disease. The mouse model of leishmaniasis shows some similarities with human diseases. In addition, there is limited evidence for the protection of vaccine candidates in multiple animal models. Advances in technology in molecular biology and immunological techniques may provide some important insights that answer the challenge. In addition, potential vaccine candidates can be found with the availability of genome sequences with gene encoding [63].

In the last century, vaccination strategies have been developed for those struggling with leishmaniasis [64]. However, no vaccine candidate whose efficacy against leishmaniasis has been completed has been found in phase studies. In general, there are three main categories of vaccines for leishmaniasis;

1. First-generation vaccines

2. Second-generation vaccines

    a. Live attenuated organisms as vaccine candidates

3. Subunit and recombinant vaccine candidates

4. Third-generation vaccines

Fractions of the parasite or whole-killed *Leishmania* with adjuvants or not can generate first-generation vaccines. The vaccines that are committed to treating leishmaniasis symbolize that first-generation vaccines are prepared with killed parasites or parasite fractions. Towards the end of the 1930s, Brazil carried out these vaccines. The big part of these vaccines that become phase III developed against CL [65] and VL [66]. Recombinant proteins, DNA vaccines, and their combinations form the second-generation vaccines against leishmaniasis [67]. Determining the exact ways of the cellular and molecular mechanism of pathogen-host interaction is the most important road to improving an ideal vaccine candidate. Also, researchers consisted of live-attenuated vaccines in search of a safe, stable, and efficient vaccine candidate. For this purpose, the attenuated parasite could be generated based on defined or undefined changing in the parasite. These methods applied to *in vitro* cultures such as gamma irradiation, chemical mutagenesis, and temperature sensitivity were preferred for the formation of attenuated strains [68, 69].

Wolff and colleagues established the concept of DNA vaccination that composes the third-generation vaccines. The colleagues determined that the protein expression was appointed with direct injection of recombinant plasmid DNA into mouse skeletal muscle [70, 71]. According to these findings, DNA vaccines that are produced for preventing infection with *Leishmania* parasites also represent vaccine candidates. In addition to that, these can be used as immunotherapeutic tools. The gene encoding of GP63 was used to produce the first DNA vaccine against *Leishmania* parasites. As a result, it is reported that the mice, immunized with plasmid DNA encoding GP63, developed a strong Th1 response [72].

There have been several studies associated with parasitic antigens and the advantages of vaccine technologies. Vaccination is the most important way to ensure the control of infectious diseases. The achievement of the development of vaccines depends on intellection the biology of between host and parasite interaction. Selection of suitable vaccine candidates, determining the correct adjuvants, and determination of appropriate carriers are also important. Nevertheless, the immunity that is generated from vaccines must be long-standing. Immune regulatory pathways formed after infection and vaccination have been identified but our knowledge is limited to attenuating the advantages of available adjuvants and drugs. Vaccines must be effective against all of the agents that cause certain diseases. The vaccine against leishmaniasis development process is quite slow. However, information related to the construction and testing of new vaccines aimed at preventing and treating *Leishmania* has increased significantly in recent years. The control or treatment of such diseases may be possible with the accumulation of knowledge about the molecular mechanisms of parasite and host immune response. Different points in parasite metabolism are important strategies to prevent and treat the targeted area to increase efficiency and resistance. Immunomodulators are used to mansion and restore homeostasis to contribute to the treatment and may be appropriate to reduce tissue damage [67].

While the developments in exosome technology in recent years have discussed the functionality of cell-free vaccine candidates, the discovery of the exoproteome contents of *Leishmania* parasite reveals the vaccine potential [73].

As a result, even if agents such as pesticides developed against the parasite-vector-reservoir-host relationship produce temporary solutions by breaking the infection chain elements, the ecological cycle will eventually return to the system by gaining resistance. It should not be forgotten that the most important element in the prevention of the disease that will occur with this cycle is vaccination. Both patient survival, public health, psychology, and economic development approaches in health systems are made controllable by preventive medicine and vaccine applications.

4. Medical treatment

Treatment of leishmaniasis is dependent on especially chemical therapies used. Pentavalent antimonial, oral miltefosine, amphotericin B, liposomal amphotericin B, and paromomycin are the most commonly used drugs. There are several problems with these drugs including the cost of drugs, toxicity, length and duration of treatment, route of injection for treatment, and the development of parasite drug resistance [51]. The most used drug was pentavalent antimonial which was the first line of treatment for many years. According to this, increasing the ratio of parasite resistance in endemic regions has limited their usage for treatment [74]. Antileishmanial activity of the pentavalent antimony can be activated by reducing to its trivalent form inside macrophages. Although the mechanism of antimonial effects in the cells is not completely clarified, the inhibition of the glycolytic pathway, fatty acids, and trypanothione reductase is related to antimonial effects [75].

Second-line drugs for the treatment of leishmaniasis are pentamidine, amphotericin B, miltefosine, and paromomycin [76]. Although there is evidence that involves mitochondrial function intervention, the mechanism of pentamidine action is not well known [77]. Inhibition of protein synthesis of the parasite can be provided treatment with paromomycin. This drug is covalently bound to protein, which affects translation and vesicle-mediated trafficking [78]. Another drug for the treatment of leishmaniasis is miltefosine, which affect the cell signal transduction pathway by inhibiting protein kinase B. This pathway has an important role in the biosynthesis of sterols and phospholipids [79]. Ergosterol is a major component of the cellular membrane of *Leishmania*. Amphotericin B binds to ergosterol creating transmembrane channels that release monovalent ions (K^+, Na^+, H^+, and Cl^-) leading to cell death [80]. Various lipid formulations have been introduced leading to rapidly concentrated in organs such as the liver and spleen to reduce the adverse effects of amphotericin B [81, 82].

Several studies have demonstrated that exosomes derived from MSCs have significantly improved the process of healing cutaneous wounds. Exosome formulations were developed to investigate their impact on the healing of cutaneous wounds caused by *Leishmania major* parasite on the skin. The study observed that the exosome formulations had an anti-leishmanial effect when compared to salicylic acid, which is known for its efficacy in wound healing and is commonly used in cosmetic products. Furthermore, *in vitro* wound model experiments showed that exosome formulations had a remarkable ability to inhibit *Leishmania* parasites while promoting wound healing, surpassing the effects of aloe-emodin, which is frequently used in cosmetic applications [83, 84].

5. Diagnostic

VL and KL diagnoses mostly are made with microscopic examinations from Giemsa painted smear preparations prepared from bone marrow and skin lesions. A smear is a simple sample, prepared easily and rapidly that is often the preferred diagnostic method, and finds out *Leishmania* amastigotes directly [85]. The microculture method and NNN medium (Novy-MacNeal-Nicolle) are used for the isolation of parasites [86]. The aspiration or biopsy material with a fine needle is mixed NNN medium for culture and microscopic examination [85]. The microculture method is the other culture method in which the development and identification of parasites are studied within microaerophilic niches developed by Allahverdiyev and his colleagues. These niches can supply optimal conditions for isolation, adaptation, and proliferation. The microculture method, which was compared with the NNN agar method, was found to be more sensitive in a short time [87]. The microculture method makes certain the microaerophilic environment (higher CO_2 concentrations, diminish O_2 concentrations, and pH) is essential for the growth of *Leishmania* parasites. In the following years, this method is used in asymptomatic leishmaniasis, the samples obtained from a blood donor, vaccine development, working mice without sacrificed in the studies, the isolation of stem cells, and the diagnosis of helicobacter [88, 89]. Various using molecular methods such as polymerase chain reaction (PCR), restriction fragment length polymorphism (RFLP), and DNA sequencing are performed for identifying *Leishmania* species in recent years although these methods require special equipment and are needed expertise [90]. It may not available infeasible to determine species easily in some clinical cases with molecular methods [91, 92]. Nowadays it is increased the works targeted different gene regions with DNA sequencing for *Leishmania* species and are also highly sensitive [91]. The other most important method is preferred isoenzyme gel electrophoresis except for PCR, RFLP, and real-time PCR (RT-PCR) used for the identification of *Leishmania* parasites. All these methods have disadvantages based on the number of parasites in the scar or blood samples. Moreover, they require costly technical equipment and specialist [93]. The sensitivity of CL and MCL are 20–30% and 55–70% respectively when using PCR-based methods in biopsy material or lesion aspires [94]. Serological methods are mainly based on a primer, or a secondary monoclonal antibody targeting parasite surface antigens and provide a great advantage for early diagnosis. For the diagnosis of leishmaniasis; serological methods such as enzyme-linked immunoassay (ELISA) test, western blot (WB), rk39 immunochromatographic diagnostic test (ICT), immunofluorescence antibody test (IFAT) are used. The basic principle of these methods is that they should be non-invasive methods based on the detection of antibodies or antigens against the parasite in the patient's serum or urine [95–97]. IFAT, which is a method based on serological and microscopy, provide investigation taken in different concentration serum sample of consisting IgG by staining the detected parasites with fluorescence to determine the presence of parasites. In the study done by Ates et al., the blood bank serum samples were diluted to a 1/128 ratio and measured based on the immunofluorescence effect with the IFAT test for the detection of leishmanial parasites [98]. Affinity reagents, such as antibodies are mainly used as therapeutic, diagnostic, and biological [99] agents for infectious diseases [100]. Polyclonal and monoclonal antibodies are essential tools obtained from hybridomas actually [101].

The hybridomas method is discovered in 1975 by Kohler and Milstein and today, antibody engineering is a rising trend in modern life science technology [99, 100]. The polyclonal and monoclonal antibodies utilization are more proper to diagnose leishmaniasis in terms of specificity. Therefore technology of hybridoma is used typically [90, 100]. The rK39 Kalazar Detect rapid kit is commercially produced by using antibody engineering [98]. However, the kit is specific to the diagnosis of VL, and when compared to VL-KL serum sample, it is not inadequate in the diagnosis of CL. It was reported the sensitivity is less than 20% based on the ELISA method for diagnosis of KL [102]. Diagnostic systems for leishmaniasis based on antibody engineering are very insufficient. In vaccine studies developed against leishmaniasis is especially important the identification components of *Leishmania* parasites. In the production processes of polyclonal and monoclonal antibodies obtained by hybridoma technology, many factors such as the experimental animals used, adjuvant structure, antigen production technique, *etc*. affect the effectiveness of the diagnosis stage. In particular, the combination of antigen and adjuvant that affects the antigen-specific specificity of these antibodies during the immunization phase is very important. At this stage, there are various studies on the development of effective adjuvant systems that are not toxic, do not affect the antigen-specific specificity of hybridomas, do not create an immune response alone, and do not show the risk of cross-reactions [103].

6. Conclusions

For many years, researchers studied and tested potential vaccine candidates with leishmanial antigens. The spread of the disease of *Leishmania* has greatly increased incidence worldwide, therefore, today, we need *Leishmania* vaccines more than yesterday. Additionally, the conditions including lacking sensitive and specific diagnostics techniques, difficulties in obtaining cheap drugs and effective vaccines, emerging drug resistance, and toxicity of chemical drugs conduct us to produce new vaccines to treat leishmaniasis. Furthermore, new drugs, different from those used against human leishmaniasis, are needed. This slow translation of knowledge from the laboratories to the industry is probably the consequence of various factors. However, studies with leishmaniasis have gained in recent years. In particular, the activities of regenerative medicine products such as non-drug-based, cellular, and exosomes, or their synergistic effects with drugs, include new generation designs. In addition, diagnostic studies have gained momentum. The diagnosis of leishmaniasis has been approved by isolating, visualizing, and culturing the parasite from infected tissue, historically [104]. It explains that there is a serious need to develop more expensive, precise, sensitive, rapid, and specific diagnostic tests, especially for the detection of leishmaniasis [105].

Besides these molecular methodology investigations, proteomic studies should go on to find out new diagnostic markers of *Leishmania*. Studies of these markers will also increase our understanding of disease progression on contribute to the search for new drug targets. Every *Leishmania spp*. infection may present different symptoms in the host. The genetic structure of the host also plays an active role in the determination of these symptoms. In this case, it affects the treatment process. The main antimonials, amphotericin B (AmpB), miltefosine, paromomycin, and pentamidine are used in the clinical treatment of VL [106]. High cost, drug resistance, and toxic side effects limit the use of traditional drugs. Therefore, the WHO strongly recommends the investigation and development of novel therapeutic alternatives against leishmaniasis. New synthetic drugs and antileishmanial plant extracts need to be rapidly evaluated both individually or together (combination therapy) in all forms of leishmaniasis by researchers. Recently, researchers, have special attention is given to innovative nanostructures based on unique physicochemical properties. Until today AmBisomes is the only nano-based antileishmanial drug, which has been using in clinically, and recently nano-liposomal AmB gel was approved for the treatment of CL, fungal, and tropical diseases. These nano-based drugs are unquestionably effective but their use remains restricted in some areas due to their high cost [107]. Also, polymeric nanoparticles [108], metallic nanoparticles [109], and plant-based solid lipid nanoparticles [110] used in recent studies have shown promising developments in treatments. Nanocarriers have not only been used for drug delivery but also for vaccine delivery. During the past decades, various types of *Leishmania* antigens (e.g., killed or attenuated whole parasites, synthetic or recombinant peptides, or recombinant live vaccine vectors) have been identified and tested with or without cytokines or other adjuvants for vaccine development to control parasite multiplication and dissemination, both in humans and dogs [111]. However, nowadays, new approaches are being researched for effective and safe vaccines thanks to nanotechnology. The nanocarriers provide to deliver antigens, antigen-adjuvant, or antigen cocktails to APCs that play a profound role in activating the host immune system. These small particles give a useful update on work on future vaccines. Likewise, exosomes produced from various cells among nanocargo carrier candidate structures, which have superior properties in terms of size and structure, can also carry active substances with antileishmanial activity. It has also been observed that combination treatments of cells and chemotherapeutic agents have more successful results in terms of antileishmanial effect compared to stem cell alone or chemical-based treatment options alone [112]. Immunotherapy, which is an emerging trend, has added a different perspective to parasitic diseases such as leishmaniasis as a different and personalized medicine. Especially in the treatment of VL, modulation provided by immunotherapy, and understanding the immunological dimension of the host-parasite relationship, may reduce the parasite burden and prevent drug resistance. Although there are studies showing that immunotherapeutic agents modulate leishmanial activities, the preclinical experiment remained in the size of animal studies [113, 114]. Immunotherapeutic agents, recombinant cytokines, or antibodies developed in this field, which are frequently used and patented, especially in diagnostics, have experienced a serious decline, especially with the Covid-19 pandemic, causing the neglect of two million new cases each year [115].

Science and technology develop day by day but the nature of the world has also changed. The climate change, wars, and immigrants are causing the disease to spread to areas where it has never been identified before. This means that leishmaniasis will not only affect developing countries but also others. Therefore, more improvement is needed in leishmaniasis control. This can be achieved by considering parameters such as correct diagnosis and treatment, good analysis of public health effectiveness, and the natural course of the infection. In the future, researchers also must carefully design appropriate immunization protocols focusing on the parasite genotypes, powerful new adjuvants, development of new antigen-adjuvants in a different way (using advanced bioconjugation chemistries). These considerations can be providing a high level of protection and safety. In addition, designing new target drugs explored with shorter treatment duration, fewer adverse effects, and less risk of drug resistance provides an exciting future direction for rational treatment combinations at low cost.

Acknowledgements

We would like to thank the artist Meryem Demir (sistersprintabless@gmail.com) who contributed to the drawing of **Figures 2** and **3**. These drawings were made in the Procreate program. We know that Mehmet Aydoğdu, who joined us when this study was being written but passed away last year, is watching us from afar. Rest in peace Mehmet.

Conflict of interest

The authors declare no conflict of interest.

Author details

Asli Pinar Zorba Yildiz[1*], Gulnaz Yildirim Koken[2], Burcak Yavuz[3], Emrah Sefik Abamor[4], Ozlem Ayse Tosyali[5], Serap Yesilkir Baydar[6,7], Ikram Ullah[8], Ahmet Berkay Civan[9], Melahat Bagirova[10] and Adil M. Allahverdiyev[10]

1 Vocational of Health School, Department of Medical Services and Techniques, Istinye University, Topkapi Campus, Istanbul, Turkey

2 Sabancı University Nanotechnology Research and Application Center, Istanbul, Turkiye

3 Vocational School of Health Services, Altinbas University, Istanbul, Turkey

4 Department of Bioengineering, Davutpasa Campus Istanbul, Yildiz Technical University, Turkey

5 Faculty of Engineering and Architecture, Biomedical Engineering Department, Beykent University, Ayazaga Campus, Istanbul, Turkey

6 Faculty of Engineering and Architecture, Department of Biomedical Engineering, Istanbul Gelisim University, Istanbul, Turkey

7 Life Sciences and Biomedical Engineering Application and Research Center, Istanbul Gelisim University, Istanbul, Turkey

8 Department of Biotechnology and Genetic Engineering, Hazara University Mansehra, Pakistan

9 Stem Cell, and Tissue Engineering R&D Center, Istinye University, Istanbul, Turkey

10 V. Akhundov National Scientific Research Medical Prophylactic Institute, Baku, Azerbaijan Republic

*Address all correspondence to: aslipinarzorba@gmail.com

References

[1] Roque AL, Jansen AM. Wild and synanthropic reservoirs of Leishmania species in the Americas. International Journal For Parasitology Parasites and Wildlife. 2014;**3**(3):251-262

[2] Handemir E, Öncel T, Kamburgil K. İstanbul sokak söpeklerinde visseral leishmaniasis seroprevalansı. Türkiye Parazitoloji Dergisi. 2004;**28**(3):123-125

[3] World Health Organization. Report of a meeting of the WHO expert committee on the control of Leishmaniases. In: WHO Technical Report Series, 949. Switzerland; 2010

[4] Selvapandiyan A, Duncan R, Mendez J, Kumar R, Salotra P, Cardo LJ, et al. A Leishmania minicircle DNA footprint assay for sensitive detection and rapid speciation of clinical isolates. Transfusion. 2008;**48**(9):1787-1798

[5] Bodur H, Korkmaz M, Akıncı A, Çolpan A, Eren SS, Erbay A. Viseral Layşmanyaz: İki olgu bildirisi. Klinik Dergisi. 2003;**16**(2):95-97

[6] Sasidharan S, Saudagar P. Leishmaniasis: Where are we and where are we heading? Parasitology Research. 2021;**120**(5):1541-1554

[7] Yildiz AP. Leishmania tropica parazitlerinden elde edilen immünojen moleküllere karşı tanıda kullanılmak üzere hibridoma teknolojisine dayalı antikor üretilmesi [thesis]. Istanbul: Yildiz Technical University. 2015

[8] World Health Organization Leishmaniasis 2015 [Internet]. 2015. Available from: http://www.who.int/search/semantic/en/#search=Leishmaniasis&sort=score%20desc&fq=%7B!noshow%3Dtrue%7Dlanguages%3Aen. [Accessed: 2023-02-169]

[9] Madeira MF, Figueiredo FB, Pinto AG, Nascimento LD, Furtado M, Mouta-Confort E, et al. Parasitological diagnosis of canine visceral leishmaniasis: Is intact skin a good target? Research in Veterinary Science. 2009;**87**(2):260-262

[10] Allahverdiyev AM, Cakir KR, Bagirova M, Elcicek S, Baydar SY, Oztel ON, et al. A new approach for the development of a vaccine against visceral leishmaniasis: Lipophosphoglycan and polyacrylic acid conjugates. Asian Pacific Journal of Tropical Medicine. 2017;**10**(9):877-886

[11] Dey A, Singh S. Transfusion transmitted leishmaniasis: A case report and review of the literature. Indian Journal of Medical Microbiology. 2006; **24**(3):165-170

[12] Herwaldt BL. Leishmaniasis. Lancet. 1999;**354**(9185):1191-1199

[13] Scarpini S, Dondi A, Totaro C, Biagi C, MelchiondaF ZD, et al. Visceral Leishmaniasis: Epidemiology, diagnosis, and treatment regimens in different geographical areas with a focus on pediatrics. Microorganisms. 2022; **10**(10):1887

[14] Quinnell RJ, Courtenay O. Transmission, reservoir hosts and control of zoonotic visceral leishmaniasis. Parasitology. 2009; **136**(14):1915-1934

[15] Ashford RW. Leishmaniasis reservoirs and their significance in control. Clinics in Dermatology. 1996; **14**(5):523-532

[16] Ueno N, Wilson ME. Receptor-mediated phagocytosis of Leishmania:

Implications for intracellular survival. Trends in Parasitology. 2012;**28**(8): 335-344

[17] Hsiao CH, Ueno N, Shao JQ, Schroeder KR, Moore KC, Donelson JE, et al. The effects of macrophage source on the mechanism of phagocytosis and intracellular survival of Leishmania. Microbes and Infection. 2011;**13**(12–13): 1033-1044

[18] Dandugudumula R, Fischer-Weinberger R, Zilberstein D. Morphogenesis dynamics in Leishmania differentiation. Pathogens. 2020; **11**(9):952

[19] Bates PA, Rogers ME. New insights into the developmental biology and transmission mechanisms of Leishmania. Current Molecular Medicine. 2004;**4**(6): 601-609

[20] Besteiro S, Williams RA, Coombs GH, Mottram JC. Protein turnover and differentiation in Leishmania. International Journal for Parasitology. 2007;**37**(10):1063-1075

[21] Duque TLP, Andrade-Neto VV, Ennes-Vidal V, Menna-Barreto RFS. Autophagic balance between mammals and protozoa: A molecular, biochemical and morphological review of Apicomplexa and Trypanosomatidae infections. In: Bailly Y, editor. Autophagy - a Double-Edged Sword - Cell Survival or Death? 2nd ed. London: IntechOpen Limited; 2013. pp. 289-319

[22] Mottram JC, Coombs GH, Alexander J. Cysteine peptidases as virulence factors of Leishmania. Current Opinion in Microbiology. 2014;**7**(4): 375-381

[23] Williams RA, Tetley L, Mottram JC, Coombs GH. Cysteine peptidases CPA and CPB are vital for autophagy and differentiation in Leishmania mexicana. Molecular Microbiology. 2006;**61**(3): 655-674

[24] Chandel HS, Pandey SP, Shukla D, Lalsare K, Selvaraj SK, Jha MK, et al. Toll-like receptors and CD40 modulate each other's expression affecting Leishmania major infection. Clinical and Experimental Immunology. 2014;**176**(2):283-290

[25] Srivastava S, Pandey SP, Jha MK, Chandel HS, Saha B. Leishmania expressed lipophosphoglycan interacts with toll-like receptor (TLR)-2 to decrease TLR-9 expression and reduce anti-leishmanial responses. Clinical and Experimental Immunology. 2014;**172**(3): 403-409

[26] Vargas-Inchaustegui DA, Tai W, Xi L, Hogg AE, Corry DB, Soong L. Distinct roles for MyD88 and toll-like receptor 2 during Leishmania braziliensis infection in mice. Infection And Immunity. 2009;**77**(7):2948-2956

[27] Srivastava N, Sudan R, Saha B. CD40-modulated dual-specificity phosphatases MAPK phosphatase (MKP)-1 and MKP-3 reciprocally regulate Leishmania major infection. Journal of Immunology. 2011; **186**(10):5863-5872

[28] Iwasaki A, Medzhitov R. Toll-like receptor control of the adaptive immune responses. Nature Immunology. 2004; **5**(10):987-995

[29] Pasare C, Medzhitov R. Control of B-cell responses by toll-like receptors. Nature. 2005;**438**(7066):364-368

[30] Kamanaka M, Yu P, Yasui T, Yoshida K, Kawabe T, Horii T, et al. Protective role of CD40 in Leishmania major infection at two distinct phases of cell-mediated immunity. Immunity. 1996;**4**(3):275-281

[31] Soong L, Xu JC, Grewal IS, Kima P, Sun J, Longley BJ, et al. Disruption of CD40-CD40 ligand interactions results in enhanced susceptibility to Leishmania amazonensis infection. Immunity. 1996; **4**(3):263-273

[32] Basu MK, Ray M. Macrophage and Leishmania: An unacceptable coexistence. Critical Reviews in Microbiology. 2005;**31**(3):145-154

[33] Liew FY, Millott S, Parkinson C, Palmer RM, Moncada S. Macrophage killing of *Leishmania* parasite *in vivo* is mediated by nitric oxide from L-arginine. Journal of Immunology. 1990; **144**(12):4794-4797

[34] Iniesta V, Gomez-Nieto LC, Corraliza I. The inhibition of arginase by N (omega)-hydroxy-l-arginine controls the growth of Leishmania inside macrophages. The Journal of Experimental Medicine. 2001;**193**(6):777-784

[35] Pace D. Leishmaniasis. The Journal of Infection. 2014;**69**(1):10-18

[36] Belkaid Y, Mendez S, Lira R, Kadambi N, Milon G, Sacks D. A natural model of *Leishmania major* infection reveals a prolonged "silent" phase of parasite amplification in the skin before the onset of lesion formation and immunity. Journal of Immunology. 2001;**165**(2):969-977

[37] Peters NC, Egen JG, Secundino N, Debrabant A, Kimblin N, Kamhawi S, et al. In vivo imaging reveals an essential role for neutrophils in leishmaniasis transmitted by sand flies. Science. 2008;**321**(5891):970-974

[38] Banchereau J, Steinman RM. Dendritic cells and the control of immunity. Nature. 1998;**392**(6673): 245-252

[39] Stebut E. Immunology of cutaneous leishmaniasis: The role of mast cells, phagocytes and dendritic cells for protective immunity. European Journal of Dermatology. 2007;**17**(2):115-122

[40] Stebut E. Cutaneous *Leishmania* infection: Progress in pathogenesis research and experimental therapy. Experimental Dermatology. 2007;**16**(4): 340-346

[41] Ritter U, Mattner J, Rocha JS, Bogdan C, Korner H. The control of *Leishmania* major by TNF *in vivo* is dependent on the parasite strain. Microbes and Infection. 2004;**6**(6): 559-565

[42] Ng LG, Hsu A, Mandell MA, Roediger B, Hoeller C, Mrass P, et al. Migratory dermal dendritic cells act as rapid sensors of protozoan parasites. PLoS Pathogens. 2008;**4**(11): 1000222

[43] Peters NC, Sacks DL. The impact of vector-mediated neutrophil recruitment on cutaneous leishmaniasis. Cellular Microbiology. 2008;**11**(9):1290-1296

[44] von Stebut E, Belkaid Y, Nguyen BV, Cushing M, Sacks DL, Udey MC. *Leishmania* major-infected murine Langerhans cell-like dendritic cells from susceptible mice release IL-12 after infection and vaccinate against experimental cutaneous Leishmaniasis. European Journal of Immunology. 2000; **30**(12):3498-3506

[45] Woelbing F, Kostka SL, Moelle K, Belkaid Y, Sunderkoetter C, Verbeek S, et al. Uptake of *Leishmania major* by dendritic cells is mediated by Fcgamma receptors and facilitates the acquisition of protective immunity. The Journal of Experimental Medicine. 2006;**203**(1): 177-188

[46] de Assis RR, Ibraim IC, Nogueira PM, Soares RP, Turco SJ. Glycoconjugates in New World species of *Leishmania*: Polymorphisms in lipophosphoglycan and glycoinositolphospholipids and interaction with hosts. Biochimica et Biophysica Acta. 2012;**1820**(9): 1354-1365

[47] Novozhilova NM, Bovin NV. Structure, functions, and biosynthesis of glycoconjugates of *Leishmania spp.* cell surface. Biochemistry. Biokhimiia. 2010; **75**(6):686-694

[48] Mule SN, Saad JS, Fernandes LR, Stolf BS, Cortez M, Palmisano G. Protein glycosylation in *Leishmania spp*. Moleculer Omics. 2020;**16**(5):407-424

[49] Kamhawi S. Phlebotomine sand flies and *Leishmania* parasites: Friends or foes? Trends in Parasitology. 2006;**22**(9): 439-445

[50] Bahr V, Stierhof YD, Ilg T, Demar M, Quinten M, Overath P. Expression of lipophosphoglycan, high-molecular-weight phosphoglycan and glycoprotein 63 in promastigotes and amastigotes of *Leishmania mexicana*. Molecular and Biochemical Parasitology. 1993;**58**(1):107-121

[51] Croft SL, Sundar S, Fairlamb AH. Drug resistance in leishmaniasis. Clinical Microbiology Reviews. 2006;**19**(1): 111-126

[52] Yao C, Donelson JE, Wilson ME. The major surface protease (MSP or GP63) of *Leishmania spp.* biosynthesis, regulation of expression, and function. Molecular and Biochemical Parasitology. 2003; **132**(1):1-16

[53] Ralton JE, MJ MC. Delineation of three pathways of glycosylphosphatidylinositol biosynthesis in *Leishmania mexicana.* Precursors from different pathways are assembled on distinct pools of phosphatidylinositol and undergo fatty acid remodeling. The Journal of Biological Chemistry. 1998;**273**(7):4245

[54] Ilg T, Stierhof YD, McConville MJ, Overath P. Purification, partial characterization and immunolocalization of a proteophosphoglycan secreted by *Leishmania mexicana* amastigotes. European Journal of Cell Biology. 1995; **66**(2):205-215

[55] Rogers ME, Ilg T, Nikolaev AV, Ferguson MA, Bates PA. Transmission of cutaneous leishmaniasis by sand flies is enhanced by regurgitation of fPPG. Nature. 2004;**430**(6998):463-467

[56] Ilg T, Stierhof YD, Etges R, Adrian M, Harbecke D, Overath P. Secreted acid phosphatase of *Leishmania mexicana*: A filamentous phosphoglycoprotein polymer. Proceedings of the National Academy of Sciences of the United States of America. 1991;**88**(19):8774-8778

[57] Lovelace JK, Gottlieb M. Comparison of extracellular acid phosphatases from various isolates of *Leishmania*. The American Journal of Tropical Medicine and Hygiene. 1986;**35**(6):1121-1128

[58] Ribeiro-de-Jesus A, Almeida RP, Lessa H, Bacellar O, Carvalho EM. Cytokine profile and pathology in human leishmaniasis. Brazilian Journal of Medical and Biological Research. 1998; **31**(1):143-148

[59] Murray HW, Nathan CF. Macrophage microbicidal mechanisms *in vivo*: Reactive nitrogen versus oxygen intermediates in the killing of intracellular visceral *Leishmania donovani*. The Journal of Experimental Medicine. 1998;**189**(4):741-746

[60] von Stebut E, Udey MC. Requirements for Th1-dependent immunity against infection with *Leishmania major*. Microbes and Infection. 2004;**6**(12):1102-1109

[61] Lagler H, Willheim M, Traunmuller F, Wahl K, Winkler H, Ramharter M, et al. Cellular profile of cytokine production in a patient with visceral leishmaniasis: Gammadelta+ T cells express both type 1 cytokines and interleukin-10. Scandinavian Journal of Immunology. 2003;**57**(3):291-295

[62] Naderer T, Vince JE, McConville M. Surface determinants of *Leishmania* parasites and their role in infectivity in the mammalian host. Current Molecular Medicine. 2004;**4**(6):649-665

[63] Natera S, Machuca C, Padrón-Nieves M, Romero A, Díaz E, Ponte-Sucre A. *Leishmania spp.*: Proficiency of drug-resistant parasites. International Journal of Antimicrobial Agents. 2004;**29**(6):637-642

[64] McAllister MM. Successful vaccines for naturally occurring protozoal diseases of animals should guide human vaccine research. A review of protozoal vaccines and their designs. Parasitology. 2014;**141**(5):624-640

[65] Velez ID, Gilchrist K, Arbelaez MP, Rojas CA, Puerta JA, Antunes CM, et al. Failure of a killed Leishmania amazonensis vaccine against American cutaneous leishmaniasis in Colombia. Transactions of the Royal Society of Tropical Medicine and Hygiene. 2005; **99**(8):593-598

[66] Khalil EA, El Hassan AM, Zijlstra EE, Mukhtar MM, Ghalib HW, Musa B, et al. Autoclaved *Leishmania major* vaccine for prevention of visceral leishmaniasis: A randomized, double-blind, BCG-controlled trial in Sudan. Lancet. 2000; **356**(9241):1565-1569

[67] Khamesipour A, Rafati S, Davoudi N, Maboudi F, Modabber F. Leishmaniasis vaccine candidates for development: A global overview. The Indian Journal of Medical Research. 2006;**123**(3):423-438

[68] Rivier D, Shah R, Bovay P, Mauel J. Vaccine development against cutaneous leishmaniasis. Subcutaneous administration of radio-attenuated parasites protects CBA mice against virulent *Leishmania major* challenge. Parasite Immunology. 1993;**15**(2):75-84

[69] Daneshvar H, Coombs GH, HaganP PRS. *Leishmania mexicana* and *Leishmania major*: Attenuation of wild-type parasites and vaccination with the attenuated lines. The Journal of Infectious Diseases. 2003; **187**(10):1662-1668

[70] Garmory HS, Brown KA, Titball RW. DNA vaccines: Improving expression of antigens. Genet Vaccines Ther. 2003;**1**(1):2

[71] Ivory C, Chadee K. DNA vaccines: Designing strategies against parasitic infections. Genetic Vaccines Therapy. 2004;**2**(1):17

[72] Coler RN, Reed SG. Second-generation vaccines against leishmaniasis. Trends in Parasitology. 2005;**21**(5):244-249

[73] Esteves S, Costa I, Luelmo S, Santarém N, Cordeiro-da-Silva A. *Leishmania* vesicle-depleted exoproteome: What, why, and how? Microorganisms. 2022;**10**(12):2435

[74] Kumar R, Engwerda C. Vaccines to prevent leishmaniasis. Clinical & Translational Immunology. 2014;**3**(3):e13

[75] Zhou Y, Messier N, Ouellette M, Rosen BP, Mukhopadhyay R. *Leishmania*

major LmACR2 is a pentavalent antimony reductase that confers sensitivity to the drug pentosan. The Journal of Biological Chemistry 2004; **279**(36):37445-37451

[76] Golenser J, Domb A. New formulations and derivatives of amphotericin B for treatment of leishmaniasis. Mini-Reviews in Medicinal Chemistry. 2006;**6**(2):153-162

[77] Sun T, Zhang Y. Pentamidine binds to tRNA through non-specific hydrophobic interactions and inhibits aminoacylation and translation. Nucleic Acids Research. 2008;**36**(5):1654-1664

[78] Chawla B, Jhingran A, Panigrahi A, Stuart KD, Madhubala R. Paromomycin affects translation and vesicle-mediated trafficking as revealed by proteomics of paromomycin -susceptible -resistant Leishmania donovani. PLoS One. 2011; **6**(10):e26660

[79] Soto J, Toledo J, Valda L, Balderrama M, Rea I, Parra R, et al. Treatment of Bolivian mucosal leishmaniasis with miltefosine. Clinical Infectious Diseases. 2007;**44**(3):350-356

[80] Baginski M, Czub J. Amphotericin B, and its new derivatives - mode of action. Current Drug Metabolism. 2009;**10**(5): 459-469

[81] Sundar S, Chakravarty J. Leishmaniasis: An update of current pharmacotherapy. Expert Opinion on Pharmacotherapy. 2013;**14**(1):53-63

[82] Sivayogana R, Krishnakumar A, Kumaravel S, Rajagopal R, Ravikanth P. Treatment of Leishmaniasis. In: Calderon LA, editor. Leishmaniasis - General Aspects of a Stigmatized Disease. London: IntechOpen Limited; 2022. pp. 1-11

[83] Koken GY, Abamor ES, Allahverdiyev A, Karaoz E. Combinations of Wharton jelly derived exosomes and salicylic acid: A new hope for eradication of cutaneous leishmaniasis. Fresenius Environmental Bulletin. 2022;**31**: 3241-3256

[84] Koken GY, Abamor ES, Allahverdiyev A, Karaoz E. Wharton jelly derived mesenchymal stem Cell's exosomes demonstrate significant Antileishmanial and wound healing effects in combination with aloe-Emodin: An *in vitro* study. Journal of Pharmaceutical Sciences. 2022;**111**(12): 3232-3242

[85] Uzun S, Gurel MS, Durdu M, Akyol M, Fettahlioglu KB, Aksoy M, et al. Clinical practice guidelines for the diagnosis and treatment of cutaneous leishmaniasis in Turkey. International Journal of Dermatology. 2018;**57**(8): 973-982

[86] Allahverdiyev A, Bagirova M, Uzun S, Alabaz D, Aksaray N, Kocabas E, et al. The value of a new microculture method for diagnosis of visceral leishmaniasis by using bone marrow and peripheral blood. The American Journal of Tropical Medicine and Hygiene. 2005;**73**(2): 276-280

[87] Allahverdiyev A, Uzun S, Bagirova M, Durdu M, Memisoglu HR. A sensitive new microculture method for diagnosis of cutaneous leishmaniasis. The American Journal of Tropical Medicine and Hygiene. 2004;**70**(3): 294-297

[88] Allahverdiyev A, Bagirova M, Elcicek S, Koc RC, Baydar SY, Findikli N, et al. Adipose tissue-derived mesenchymal stem cells as a new host cell in latent leishmaniasis. The

American Journal of Tropical Medicine and Hygiene. 2011;**85**(3):535-539

[89] Allahverdiyev A, Baydar SY, Bagirova M, Findikli N. Microcapillary culture method: A novel tool for *in vitro* expansion of stem cells from scarce sources. Archives of Medical Research. 2012;**43**(6):423-430

[90] Nourizadeh E, Zargar SJ, Alimohammadian MH, Ajdary S, Mahdavi M. Development of monoclonal antibodies against axenic amastigotes of *Leishmania infantum* strain in Iran: Implication for diagnosis of kala-azar. Iranian Journal of Basic Medical Sciences. 2018;**21**(4):388-394

[91] Ozbilgin A, Harman M, Karakus M, Bart A, Toz KO, et al. Leishmaniasis in Turkey: Visceral and cutaneous leishmaniasis caused by *Leishmania donovani* in Turkey. Acta Tropica. 2017; **173**:90-96

[92] Toz SO, Nasereddin A, Ozbel Y, Ertabaklar H, Culha G, Sevil N, et al. Leishmaniasis in Turkey: Molecular characterization of *Leishmania* from human and canine clinical samples. Tropical Medicine & International Health. 2009;**14**(11): 1401-1406

[93] Constantina N, Tsokana LVA, Valiakos G, Spyrou V, Manolakou K, Billinis C. Molecular diagnosis of Leishmaniasis, species identification, and phylogenetic analysis. In: Claborn DM, editor. Leishmaniasis - Trends in Epidemiology, Diagnosis and Treatment. London: IntechOpen Limited; 2014. pp. 161-193

[94] Burza S, Croft SL, Boelaert M. Leishmaniasis. Lancet. 2018;**392**:951-970

[95] Ozensoy S, Ozbel Y, Turgay N, Alkan MZ, Gul K, Gilman-Sachs A, et al. Serodiagnosis and epidemiology of visceral leishmaniasis in Turkey. The American Journal of Tropical Medicine and Hygiene. 1998;**59**(3):363-369

[96] Mohammed EA, Wright EP, Kager PA, Laarman JJ, Pondman KW. ELISA using intact promastigotes for immunodiagnosis of kala-azar. Transactions of the Royal Society of Tropical Medicine and Hygiene. 1985; **79**(3):344-350

[97] Mary C, Lamouroux D, Dunan S, Quilici M. Western blot analysis of antibodies to *Leishmania infantum* antigens: The potential of the 14-kD and 16-kD antigens for diagnosis and epidemiologic purposes. The American Journal of Tropical Medicine and Hygiene. 1992;**47**(6):764-771

[98] Ates SC, Bagirova M, Allahverdiyev A, Baydar SY, Koc RC, Elcicek S, et al. Detection of antileishmanial antibodies in blood sampled from blood bank donors in Istanbul. Future Microbiology. 2012; **7**(6):773-779

[99] Zhang Z, Liu H, Guan Q, Wang L, Yuan H. Advances in the isolation of specific monoclonal rabbit antibodies. Frontiers in Immunology. 2017;**8**:494

[100] Kennedy PJ, Oliveira C, Granja PL, Sarmento B. Monoclonal antibodies: Technologies for early discovery and engineering. Critical Reviews in Biotechnology. 2018;**38**(3):394-408

[101] Buhr DL, Acca FE, Holland EG, Johnson K, Maksymiuk GM, Vaill A, et al. Use of micro-emulsion technology for the directed evolution of antibodies. Methods. 2012;**58**(1):28-33

[102] el Safi SH, Evans DA. A comparison of the direct agglutination test and enzyme-linked immunosorbent assay in

the serodiagnosis of leishmaniasis in the Sudan. Transactions of the Royal Society of Tropical Medicine and Hygiene. 1989; **83**(3):334-337

[103] Yildiz APZ, Koken GY, Abamor ES, Bagırova M, Tosyali OA, Kocagoz T, et al. Polymeric approach to adjuvant system in antibody production against Leishmaniasis based on Hybridoma technology. Iranian Journal of Parasitology. 2022;**17**(4):506-516

[104] Bhattacharyya R, Das K, Sen S, Roy S, Majumder HK. Development of a genus-specific primer set for detection of *Leishmania* parasites by polymerase chain reaction. FEMS Microbiology Letters. 1996;**135**(2–3):195-200

[105] Akhoundi M, Downing T, Votypka J, Kuhls K, Lukes J, Cannet A, et al. *Leishmania* infections: Molecular targets and diagnosis. Molecular Aspects of Medicine. 2017;**57**:1-29

[106] Nagle AS, Khare S, Kumar AB, Supek F, Buchynskyy A, Mathison CJ, et al. Recent developments in drug discovery for leishmaniasis and human African trypanosomiasis. Chemical Reviews. 2014;**114**(22):11305-11347

[107] Gutierrez V, Seabra AB, Reguera RM, Khandare J, Calderon M. New approaches from nanomedicine for treating leishmaniasis. Chemical Society Reviews. 2016;**45**(1):152-168

[108] Karam TK, Ortega S, Ueda Nakamura T, Auzély-Velty R, Nakamura CV. Development of chitosan Nanocapsules containing essential oil of Matricaria Chamomilla L. for the treatment of cutaneous Leishmaniasis. International Journal of Biological Macromolecules. 2020;**162**:199-208

[109] Javed B, Mashwani ZU, Sarwer A, Raja I, Nadhman A. Synergistic response of physicochemical reaction parameters on biogenesis of silver nanoparticles and their action against colon cancer and Leishmanial cells. Artificial Cells, Nanomedicine, and Biotechnology. 2020;**48**:1340-1353

[110] Jesus JA, Sousa IMO, da Silva TNF, Ferreira AF, Laurenti MD, Antonangelo L, et al. Preclinical assessment of Ursolic acid loaded into nanostructured lipid carriers in experimental visceral Leishmaniasis. Pharmaceutics. 2021;**13**:908

[111] Singh B, Sundar S. Leishmaniasis: Vaccine candidates and and perspectives. Vaccine. 2012;**30**(26):3834-3842

[112] Kian M, Mirzavand S, Sharifzadeh S, Kalantari T, Ashrafmansouri M, Nasri F. Efficacy of mesenchymal stem cells therapy in parasitic infections: Are anti-parasitic drugs combined with MSCs more effective? Acta Parasitologica. 2022; **67**(4):1487-1499

[113] Mazire PH, Saha B, Roy A. Immunotherapy for visceral leishmaniasis: A trapeze of balancing counteractive forces. International Immunopharmacology. 2022;**110**:108969

[114] Ikeogu NM, Akaluka GN, Edechi CA, Salako ES, Onyilagha C, Barazandeh AF, et al. Leishmania immunity: Advancing immunotherapy and vaccine development. Microorganisms. 2020;**8**(8):1201

[115] Albuquerque LWN, Ferreira SCA, Dos Santos T, Varjão M, da Silva AE, Duarte AWF, et al. New immunodiagnostic methods for human tegumentary leishmaniasis in the last 10 years: Technological prospecting. Acta tropica. 2023;**242**:106903

Chapter 11

Neglected Bacterial and Parasitic Zoonoses of Tropical Countries

Deepali Kalambhe and Nilam Wavhal

Abstract

Approximately 60% of human infectious diseases are zoonotic. Many of these zoonotic diseases are endemic in developing countries, adversely impacting people's health and livelihood. Most of these endemic zoonoses are neglected because they affect explicitly the socioeconomically poor communities. Due to the endemic status, the diseases are often underreported and remain highly neglected. Despite knowing the fact that neglected zoonotic diseases (NZDs) add to a substantial socioeconomic burden of a country, it is difficult to assess the mortality and morbidity caused by the lack of diagnostic facilities, poor surveillance, inadequate veterinary or medical care, and at times underreported owing to undifferentiated clinical symptoms. However, most of these NZDs are preventable; hence, awareness of their epidemiology, transmission, prevention, and control measures is fundamental. Some of the critically neglected zoonotic diseases, such as anthrax, bovine tuberculosis, brucellosis, leptospirosis, cysticercosis, echinococcosis, toxoplasmosis, and trichinellosis, are discussed in this chapter

Keywords: neglected, anthrax, brucellosis, bovine tuberculosis, leptospirosis, taenia cysticercosis, toxoplasmosis, trichinellosis

1. Introduction

1.1 Synonyms

Charbon, Ragpicker's disease, Splenic fever, Woolsorter's disease.

1.2 Etiology

Anthrax is caused by *Bacillus anthracis*, a rod-shaped, Gram-positive, nonmotile, capsulated, aerobic, or facultatively anaerobic, spore-forming bacterium [1]. The bacterium sporulates after getting exposed to free oxygen. Robert Koch (1876) established Koch's postulates by cultivating a pure culture of *B. anthracis in vitro* and inducing anthrax in animals. Also, the first bacterial vaccine was prepared against anthrax by Louis Pasteur (**Table 1**).

SN	B. anthracis strains	Isolated from and/or used as	Location	Ref.
1	Strain 836	Weapon by USSR	Kirov in 1953	[2]
2	Ames strain	Dead cow	Texas, USA, in 1981	[3]
3	Sterne strain	Avirulent, toxigenic strain for vaccine production	Canada	[4]
4	Vollum	Isolated from cow and used for bioweapon trials in 1942 on Gruinard Island	Oxford, England	[5]

Table 1.
The strains of Bacillus anthracis with different evolutionary histories or origins.

1.3 Epidemiology

B. anthracis has a wide geographical distribution. It caused the death of 30,000–60,000 animals in 1923 in South Africa due to this disease [6]. While in North America, Western Europe, and Australia, anthrax is reported sporadically. Anthrax is absent in northern and central Europe; however, enzootic occurrence has been documented in Greece, Spain, Southern Italy, Turkey, and Albania, whereas it is endemic in Asia, including eastern India, South Korea, the Philippines, Mongolia, and the mountainous region of western China [1, 7]. The outbreaks in African countries occur every summer with increased years of heavy rainfall [1, 7]. Anthrax spores are the potential bioterrorism agent which resulted in five deaths and the suffering of 30,000 people in the USA in 2001 [1].

1.4 Host range and reservoir

Soil, fodder, bone meal, infected excreta, blood, and infected discharges are the potential reservoirs of anthrax bacilli. The bacilli spread through contaminated streams, insects, and feces of infected birds, feral cats, dogs, and other carnivores [7]. Compared to sheep and goats, cattle are more frequently infected as they ingest higher doses of bacilli from contaminated soil as cattle graze by pulling pasture out of the ground with roots. In contrast, sheep and goats browse plants and shrubs off the ground level [8]. Anthrax occurs less frequently in horses, pigs, and dogs, whereas cats are relatively resistant. Anthrax is mainly transmitted to herbivores by ingesting contaminated fodder or improperly processed feed and inhaling spores. Carnivores and omnivores can become infected through ingestion of infected carcasses or contaminated meat, as well as direct contact with body secretions or contaminated fomites. Direct animal-to-animal transmission is rare, and there is no evidence of transmission through milk. Direct exposure to anthrax spores is necessary for the disease to occur, which can happen through contact with infected animals during agricultural or animal husbandry operations, handling of animal carcasses, or inhalation of spores in dust clouds created from handling animal products like hides, skins, bone, blood meal, and meat meal.

1.5 Pathogenesis

B. anthracis possesses two important virulence factors, the capsule and the toxin complex, encoded by plasmids pXO2 and PXO1. The capsule helps the bacterium evade the host immune system and establish itself in host tissues, while the toxin complex comprises three lethal proteins to the host. Anthrax outbreaks have been associated with significant climate changes, such as heavy rain after a prolonged drought or warm weather [7, 9]. Sporulation of *B. anthracis* occurs rapidly when the environmental temperature is over 53°F (12°C) [10]. Anthrax spores have a high surface hydrophobicity, leading to their clumpy, concentrated nature in standing water and concentration on soil surfaces after the water evaporates. These relationships between anthrax and climate may help predict anthrax years [7, 9].

1.6 Disease

1.6.1 Disease in animals

Infected animals exhibit congestion, hemorrhages, high fever, dyspnea, edema, depression, anorexia, convulsions, staggering gait, diarrhea/dysentery, abortion, blood-stained milk, and absence of rigor mortis. In herbivores, the disease is primarily hyperacute and fatal, with sudden death occurring within 10–24 h due to septicemia and toxemia. The gastrointestinal form is the most common. Cutaneous anthrax can occur in animals through the bite of mechanical vectors or wound contamination, but death usually occurs before eschars/carbuncles develop. The disease can be fatal in carnivores, or the animal can recover. Intestinal form is occasional, and death is due to airway occlusion. Carbuncular lesions may develop on the tongue or oropharynx.

1.6.2 Disease in man

Human anthrax has a variable incubation period (usually 2–5 days) which is potentially fatal.

- *Cutaneous form (malignant pustule/eschar):* The spores enter through cuts or abrasions in the skin and form a papule which becomes necrotic and later ruptures to painless black eschar or carbuncle (that resolves within 2–6 weeks) surrounded by an edematous zone. The secondary bacterial infection leads to pus formation. In septicemic cases, symptoms include fever (40°C), chills, headache, nausea, anorexia, dyspnea, cyanosis, and collapse preceding death.

- *Pulmonary form (Woolsorter's disease):* The spores enter through inhalation while handling raw wool, hides, bones, blood meal, and meat meal. Symptoms include fever, dyspnea, pneumonia, emphysema, and cardiac failure. The septicemic complication is highly fatal.

- *Intestinal form:* Characteristic eschar or malignant carbuncle occurs on the oropharynx, stomach, duodenum, and upper ileum. The spores enter by ingesting infected meat, milk, or other foodstuffs. The symptoms include nausea, vomiting, anorexia, fever, abdominal pain, watery to bloody diarrhea, and tenderness in the right upper and lower quadrants.

1.7 Diagnosis

In the case of an animal suspected of dying of anthrax, the carcass should not be opened to prevent contamination of the surrounding area with spores. If the carcass has been mistakenly opened, the dark unclotted blood and massive hemorrhagic spleen will be visible. A quick and reliable diagnosis can be made by staining blood smears from ear clippings (in all animals, including wild animals), laryngeal edema (in dogs and pigs), or mesenteric lymph nodes (in sheep, goats, cattle, and horses) with polychrome methylene blue; the bacterial capsule appears reddish-purple on microscopic examination, while the bacilli take up a deep blue color. The pathogen can be isolated from clinical material on blood agar to study the characteristic morphology of bacilli and the "medusa head" appearance of colonies. Laboratory animals, such as guinea pigs (subcutaneous (s/c)) and mice (intraperitoneal (i/p)), can be inoculated with clinical material (0.5 ml) to confirm Koch's postulates and the pathogenicity of the bacilli (death of the animal by pathogenic bacilli occurs within 30–40 h of inoculation). Ascoli's precipitation test uses anthrax hyperimmune serum against attenuated anthrax spores to detect residual anthrax antigens in tissues/hides. Polymerase chain reaction (PCR) can detect even a single cell of *B. anthracis* and differentiate it from other closely related species.

1.8 Treatment

Penicillin (V or G) is the drug of choice for 5–7 days by oral, intramuscular (i/m), or intravenous (i/v) route. Streptomycin may also act synergistically with penicillin. Other drugs used are tetracycline, gentamicin, erythromycin, and chloramphenicol.

1.9 Prevention and control

It is crucial to interrupt the infection cycle by stopping the source of infection. Contaminated feed and the source of infection should be promptly disposed of. The introduction of new animals to the affected farms should be prevented. If insects (flies) are believed to be spreading the disease, measures should be taken to control their population [11]. In cases where there is a delay in the disposal of the anthrax carcass and infected materials, applying 5% formaldehyde and covering the area with double-thickness plastics are recommended. The formalin-treated carcass can be left in place for a few days before disposal, as it will maintain an anaerobic environment inside. Special attention is required to disinfect areas or items contaminated with anthrax, such as floors, rooms, fertilizers, meat, hides, and wool. Regular disinfectants or heat (60°C for a few minutes) can eliminate the vegetative form of bacteria shortly after the animal has died. Strong disinfectants like Peracetic acid (3% solution), 5% Lysol, formalin, or sodium hydroxide (5 to 10%) are helpful. Dirty shoes can be disinfected with ethylene oxide, while hides and wool can be sterilized by gamma irradiation. Contaminated clothes should be treated with 10% formaldehyde. If human skin is contaminated, the affected area must be disinfected [7]. The live attenuated *B. anthracis* strain Sterne 34F2 vaccine is the most effective vaccine against anthrax in animals. Vaccination should be done 2–4 weeks before a potential anthrax outbreak, followed by a second dose 2–4 weeks after the first dose. Suppose anthrax cases are detected in a specific area for the first time. In that case, animals that have come into contact with the infected ones should be treated with hyperimmune serum or vaccinated. Typically, after the vaccination of cows, the milk should not be consumed for 72 h, and the animals are not slaughtered for 45 days. Human anthrax cases should be promptly treated, and the disease should be notified to local health authorities.

2. Brucellosis

2.1 Synonyms

(*In man:* Undulant fever, Malta fever; *In animals*: Contagious abortion, Infectious abortion, Epizootic abortion; *In cattle:* Bang's disease; and *In male sheep*: Ram epididymitis).

2.2 Etiology

Brucella genus belongs to the α-2-Proteobacteriacae family, which is responsible for causing Brucellosis in both animal and human species. These Gram-negative, intracellular nonsporulating coccobacilli are aerobes, but some species require 5–10% carbon dioxide (CO2) for survival. Out of the recognized *Brucella* species, seven are terrestrial (*Brucella abortus, Brucella melitensis, B. suis, Brucella ovis, B. canis, Brucella neotomae, and Brucella microti*) [12, 13], while two are marine (*Brucella ceti and Brucella pinnipedialis*) [14, 15]. In addition, three new species (*Brucella inopinata, B. papionis, and B. vulpis*) have been isolated from human breast implants, baboons, and red foxes, respectively, and a new lineage of *Brucella* (BO2 strain) has been identified [16]. Besides, 36 atypical *Brucella* species have been isolated from frogs [17, 18].

2.3 Host range and epidemiology

Brucella organisms can be found in cattle, buffaloes, sheep, and goats. Cattle and buffalo are the primary hosts for *B. abortus*, but under certain conditions, *Brucella* species can cross the species barrier and infect new susceptible hosts [19]. This interhost transmission seriously threatens public health, particularly with the highly virulent and zoonotic *B. melitensis and B. suis strains. B. ovis* can infect sheep, but the infection does not typically last long in ewes and gets eliminated before the next lambing [20]. Swine brucellosis is primarily a problem in domesticated pigs, caused by *Brucella suis*, and can lead to chronic reproductive issues in both sexes.

2.4 Transmission

- *In animals:* Bovines catch an infection while grazing on contaminated pastures or barns. Infection can also transmit via contact with infected animals, ingesting contaminated feed, fodder, and water, or through uterine secretions and aborted materials. Using infected milking cups, feeding pooled colostrum to newborn calves, and artificial insemination can also contribute to the spread of the disease. Bringing infected animals into a healthy herd can also introduce the risk of infection. In sheep and goats, brucellosis is highly contagious due to close contact in dense flocks, mingling at animal fairs, overcrowding in winter, and exposure to different flocks from different owners. *B. suis* can survive for long periods in hog lots and furrowing pens, increasing the risk of transmission. In India, the spread of the disease has been attributed to a lack of vaccination for female calves, a ban on cow slaughter, and a lack of awareness about protective measures.

- *Humans:* Humans are at risk of contracting brucellosis, typically through handling infected animal tissues and body fluids, consuming raw milk and milk products, or inhaling contaminated aerosols.

2.5 Pathogenicity

The ability of *Brucella* species to cause disease is determined by its capacity to adhere to, invade, and replicate within host cells. *Brucella* bacterium can prevent phagosome-lysosome fusion and spread to other host cells. It causes chronic infections by prolonged survival and replication in phagocytic macrophages or acute reproductive tract pathology and abortion by extensive replication in nonphagocytic epithelial cells, such as placental trophoblasts, in natural animal hosts. In humans, *Brucella* colonizes different organs, with a preference for the lymphoreticular system. The disease is more apparent in adults and pregnant animals than young animals of either sex because a concentration of sex hormones and erythritol sugar increases with age and sexual maturity, which are required for the growth and multiplication of the *Brucella* pathogen.

2.6 Disease

2.6.1 Disease in animals

Bovine brucellosis is a longlasting infection with *B. abortus* causing abortion, infertility, repeat breeding, retention of placenta, stillbirth, epididymitis, and orchitis. Asymptomatic bovines play a significant role in maintaining a hidden infection within a herd. Asymptomatic females become carriers after the first abortion and transmit the infection to other healthy animals. Among small ruminants, goats are more susceptible than sheep, as they can excrete the organism for a more extended period. Lactating ewes are also more susceptible to infection than sheep raised for meat [21]. In female sheep and goats, brucellosis causes abortion during the last trimester of pregnancy, weak offspring, and retention of fetal membranes. In males, acute orchitis, epididymitis, and infertility can occur. Carrier males can spread the infection through semen, as the bacteria can be present in their testicles, epididymis, and secondary sex organs. Arthritis has been reported in both sexes, but it is not shared. Males are less susceptible to infection than females due to the lower concentration of erythritol sugar in their bodies [22]. Infected boars carry bacteria in semen, becoming a transmission source [23].

2.6.2 Brucellosis in humans

The most common symptoms are undulant fever, joint pain, and night sweats. Other symptoms may include spondyloarthropathy, epididymal-orchitis, infertility, spondylitis, acute polyarthritis, upper and low back pain, and fatigue. In rare cases, *Brucella* infection may lead to abortion in pregnant women. Children with brucellosis may experience joint pain, low backache, fatigue, and night sweats. Neurobrucellosis is a severe disease that affects the nervous system, can occur untreated, and may even cause transient ischemic attacks [24].

2.7 Diagnosis

Animals are typically screened for brucellosis using the Rose Bengal Plate Test (RBPT) and the serum tube agglutination test (STAT). A positive test in small ruminants is considered when agglutination occurs at a titer of 1:20 (40 international units (IU)) or higher. According to the Centers for Disease Control and Prevention

(CDC), a titer of 1:80 or greater is clinically significant in humans. However, a 4-fold or greater increase in titer between acute and convalescent phase sera is required to diagnose acute infection. The complement fixation test (CFT) is a recommended test for brucellosis control and surveillance programs and for international trade [25]. Enzyme-linked immunosorbent assay (ELISA) is a sensitive and rapid method for diagnosing brucellosis, with the added advantage of diagnosing the disease in both endemic and low-incidence areas. The Milk Ring Test (MRT) is a rapid agglutination test that detects immunoglobulins such as immunoglobulin M (IgM) and immunoglobulin A (IgA) attached to fat globules in whole milk or cream. It is the method of choice in dairy herds for inexpensive screening of individual or pooled milk samples in conjunction with other tests. The 2-mercaptoethanol serum tube agglutination test (2ME-STAT) and Coombs test are other critical diagnostic tests for detecting immunoglobulin G (IgG) antibodies in chronic brucellosis cases. Molecular techniques such as polymerase chain reaction (PCR) are promising methods for rapid and accurate diagnosis of brucellosis.

2.8 Treatment

Animals infected with brucellosis cannot be effectively treated, and treatment is not recommended. For humans, the recommended treatment is a combination of rifampicin and doxycycline, taken once daily for 6 weeks.

2.9 Prevention and control

The test and slaughter of positive animals successfully eradicate brucellosis in many developed countries. However, it is not a feasible option in developing countries like India due to the economic loss it would cause to farmers and due to the cultural and religious significance of cattle. In place of this, vaccination, test, and quarantine policies, improved housing practices, proper disposal of infected materials, thorough disinfection of contaminated animal premises, and mandatory calf hood vaccination are recommended. The World Organization for Animal Health (OIE) has recommended the *Brucella* S19 and RB51 vaccines for the prevention of bovine brucellosis, with the RB51 vaccine having been successfully used in the United States since 1996. Positive bulls should be culled and segregated. It is essential to avoid consuming undercooked and unpasteurized milk and milk products, and people who handle animal tissues should use protective gear such as rubber gloves, goggles, gowns, or aprons.

3. Bovine tuberculosis

3.1 Synonyms

Great white plague, Pearl disease, Scrofula, Tuberculous, caseous pneumonia.

3.2 Etiology and pathogenicity

Mycobacterium bovis is part of the *Mycobacterium tuberculosis* complex (MBTC), which also includes other species such as Mtb, *M. caprae, M. microti, M. africanum, M. canettii, Mycobacterium pinnipedii, M. bovis, Mycobacterium leprae*, and *M. mungi*. Mycobacteria are aerobic, nonmotile, noncapsulated, nonspore-forming, and have straight or slightly curved rods. The survival of tubercle bacilli in the environment differs greatly depending on temperature, sunlight, and relative humidity, ranging from a few days to 2 years. *M. bovis* can be inactivated by heat, direct sunlight, and dry conditions. They can be killed at a temperature of 65°C or higher for at least 30 min and by ultraviolet (UV) light. However, *M. bovis* (*M. bovis*) is resistant to prolonged freezing and can persist in slurry and soil for at least 6 months at ordinary temperatures [26]. *Mycobacterium* are known to be resistant due to their high lipid content to several chemicals and disinfectants. While quaternary ammonium compounds, hexachlorophene, and chlorhexidine can have a bacteriostatic effect on it, formaldehyde vapor, chlorine compounds, 70% ethanol, hydrogen peroxide, alkaline glutaraldehyde, and 5% phenol are effective in killing the bacteria. *M. bovis* are highly pathogenic mycobacteria that cause TB in humans and animals. *M. bovis* is the leading cause of TB in cattle [27].

3.3 Epidemiology

Developed countries have controlled the spread of the disease in cattle by implementing test-and-slaughter control programs. In contrast, bovine tuberculosis (bTB) continues to be widespread in developing countries such as India, where humans and cattle live close to each other, and unpasteurized milk consumption is typical. *Mycobacterium orygis* (*M. orygis*) is a new subspecies of the *M. tuberculosis* complex (MTBC) that causes tuberculosis in animals and humans and has been reported in several countries, including India, Pakistan, Bangladesh, and Nepal [28–31]. In 2016, 147,000 new cases of zoonotic TB and 12,500 deaths were reported globally [32].

3.4 Host range and reservoir

M. bovis and *M. tuberculosis* belong to the *M. tuberculosis* complex (MTBC). *M. bovis* causes bovine tuberculosis (bTB) in animals, while *M. tuberculosis* causes tuberculosis (TB) in humans [33]. Cattle are the primary carriers of *M. Bovis*. Besides cattle, goats, pigs, buffalo, dogs, primates, badgers, deer, possums, and bison can also serve as reservoirs of *M. bovis.*

3.5 Transmission

Ingestion of raw milk is the primary transmission route of *M. bovis* from cattle to humans. Individuals working in close contact with livestock are at risk of transmitting infection between cattle and humans and vice versa. Inhalation of cough droplets from infected cattle causes a typical pulmonary TB [34–37].

3.6 Disease

3.6.1 Disease in cattle

The superficial lymph nodes are usually swollen in infected animals. The affected udder progressively becomes more rigid and swollen. The milk of infected animals is thin and watery with yellow flakes. Chronically infected animals become emaciated, with a dry and rough coat, sunken and dull eyes, diarrhea, unpredictable appetite, and fluctuating body temperature. In some cases, the animal may snore due to the involvement of the retropharyngeal lymph node. In cases of cutaneous TB, there may be lumpy swelling, sometimes with cording, on the lower part of the front legs and rarely on the hind legs.

3.6.2 Disease in man

Clinical tuberculosis occurs in three stages in humans.

- *Primary tuberculosis:* Lung infection leads to the formation of tubercles with center-containing bacteria. When the center of the tubercle breaks, it turns into a necrotic, cheese-like substance called a caseous lesion, but eventually, it may heal and harden by forming calcium deposits.

- *Secondary tuberculosis:* Inactive bacteria in the primary infection become active again, producing chronic tuberculosis. The bacteria move to the upper respiratory tract and bronchial tubes, causing severe coughing, fever, weight loss, anorexia, fatigue, chest pain, and greenish or bloody sputum production.

- *Extrapulmonary tuberculosis*: In secondary tuberculosis, the bacteria spread quickly to other body parts such as the lymph nodes, kidneys, long bones, genital tract, brain, and meninges. Renal tuberculosis can lead to tissue death and scarring in the kidneys, pelvis, ureters, and bladder. Genital tuberculosis impacts reproductive functions in males and females. Tuberculosis in bones and joints, especially the vertebral column, can result in loss of sensation and paralysis. Tuberculous meningitis can cause mental deterioration, permanent mental retardation, blindness, and deafness. *M. bovis* can cause a condition called scrofula in children. It occurs when the infection spreads to the cervical and, less commonly, axillary lymph nodes, primarily through ingestion of contaminated food.

3.7 Diagnosis

Isolation and identification of the pathogen remain the only confirmatory test, but the growth of *M. bovis* may take 6–8 weeks. In animals, the histological examination of the tubercle from suspected animals or carcasses enables rapid diagnosis of acid-fast bacilli. Delayed-type hypersensitivity (DTH) assays, such as Single intradermal tuberculin, Stormont, and Short thermal tests, are helpful. Inoculation of suspected milk samples into the thighs of guinea pigs produces typical lesions in the liver, spleen, and lymph nodes. Multiplex PCR and gamma-interferon (IFN-γ) assays are more sensitive than skin tests but are costly. A combination of intradermal skin test (ST) and ELISA has enhanced sensitivity compared to individual tests. In humans, chest X-rays, roentgenographs, and the Mantoux test have diagnostic importance.

3.8 Treatment

In men, tuberculosis (TB) is a treatable disease that is usually controlled with a 6-month duration of antibiotics, like rifampicin and isoniazid. However, drug-resistant TB requires longer and more complex treatment. Compared to the traditional 6 months, treatment options have been shortened to only 1 or 3 months.

3.9 Prevention and control

- *In animals:* The test-and-slaughter policy is the most effective method to eradicate bTB, but it is only feasible in developed countries. Due to public and religious issues, a test-and-slaughter policy may not be possible in India. Good surveillance and reporting systems are essential for screening and controlling bovine TB in animal populations. The sanitary inspection of carcasses at abattoirs can reduce transmission at the animal-human interface. Animal sheds should be spacious and ventilated to avoid transmission of infection between animals. Establish reference laboratories to confirm diagnosis and research on the potential role of other domestic and wild animals as disease reservoirs and vaccination.

- *In man:* Condemnation of milk from infected herds, regular health checks for occupational groups at risk, such as butchers and farmers regarding *M. bovis*, promotion of milk pasteurization, health education, effective implementation of BCG vaccination, and preventive chemotherapy.

4. Leptospirosis

4.1 Synonyms

Cane cutter's disease, Harvest fever, Infectious jaundice, Mud fever, Rice field worker's disease, Seven-day fever, Swamp fever, Swine herd's disease, Weil's disease

4.2 Etiology

Leptospirosis is caused by *Leptospira interrogans* (*L. interrogans*) complex, which has over 20 serogroups and more than 200 serovars. Previously, all saprophytic species of *Leptospira* were classified under *Leptospira biflexa*, while *L. interrogans* were referred to as all pathogenic species [38, 39]. *Leptospirae* are small, highly motile, thin, flexible, and filamentous, made up of delicate spirals with hook-shaped ends. *Leptospirae* cannot survive in dry environments, heat, acids, and primary disinfectants but can sustain alkali pH up to 7.8. This bacterium can only be visualized with silver impregnation staining, immune peroxidase staining, or immunofluorescence under a dark field microscope (**Table 2**).

4.3 Epidemiology

Leptospirosis has high incidence rates in Southeast Asia, Oceania, the Indian subcontinent, the Caribbean, and Latin America [41]. The occurrence of the disease is significantly affected by changes in climate, flooding, inadequate sanitation, and the presence of reservoir hosts such as rats. The annual incidence in these regions can range from 10 to 100 cases per 100,000, which increases during outbreaks and in high-risk populations [42]. In recent years, there have been changes in the epidemiology of leptospirosis, with sporadic outbreaks occurring in nonendemic regions such as Canada, continental USA, and Europe, often associated with water-sport activities in natural settings contaminated with pathogenic leptospires [41, 43–45] or changing climatic patterns [41], in recreational settings such as adventure races [45], endurance events [46], and water-sporting events. Leptospirosis is considered a waterborne

Serovar	Maintenance host	Incidental host
L. bratislava	Pig	Horse, Dog
Leptospira canicola	Dog	Pig, Cattle
L. grippotyphosa	Rodent	Cattle, Pig, Horse, Dog
L. hardjo	Cattle	Human
L. interohemorrhagie	Brown cat	Domestic animals and human
L. pomona	Pig, Cattle	Sheep, Horse, Dogs

Table 2.
Maintenance and incidental hosts for important serovars of Leptospira interrogans [40].

disease in the Asia-Pacific region, and the outbreaks in Indonesia (2003), India (2005), Sri Lanka (2008), and the Philippines (2009) have been linked to major urban flooding [42, 47]. Lack of proper sanitation and climatic conditions contribute significantly to human leptospirosis. The disease is also prevalent in rural areas, where agricultural activities such as farming and animal husbandry are potential risk factors.

4.4 Transmission

Leptospirosis is primarily transmitted through contact with the urine of infected animals or through contact with skin abrasions. Moist and damp areas, such as riverbanks or muddy livestock-rearing areas, are most likely to carry the bacteria. It is speculated that leptospirosis is transmitted through the semen of infected animals. Humans are accidental hosts, typically becoming infected through direct or indirect contact with infected animals, tissues, body fluids, or urine of acutely infected or asymptomatic carrier animals. Animal carriers and environmental sources play an essential role in the transmission of leptospirae.

4.5 Host range and reservoirs

Leptospirosis primarily infects animals, but humans are "dead-end" hosts. The disease has been reported in domestic animals (cattle, buffalo, sheep, goats, pigs, and horses), wild animals (elephants, deer, and monkeys), and rodents (rats, mice, bats, rabbits, hares, and squirrels). Carnivores (dogs, cats, jackals, foxes, mongooses, skunks, civets, and raccoons) and porcupines, insectivores, and frogs may also carry leptospirae. Birds, including domestic poultry, are resistant to the disease; wading birds can act as passive carriers of the infection. Infected rodents and mammals are the primary natural reservoirs of the disease, with the pathogen surviving and being shed in urine, particularly in herbivores. The pathogen can survive for weeks in soil and water frequently contaminated by urine from carriers, particularly in alkaline pH conditions. Fish, reptiles, and birds have also been identified as potential disease carriers.

4.6 Disease

4.6.1 Disease in animals

The symptoms and severity of the disease can vary depending on the animal species.

- *Cattle:* In the acute form of the disease, cattle may show a sudden onset of fever, anorexia, jaundice, anemia, hemoglobinuria, depression, and abortion during the third trimester of pregnancy. In the subacute form, "milk drop syndrome" is expected due to mastitis resulting in reduced milk yield, thick flaking, and yellow-to-blood coloration of milk. Chronic cases may result in abortions, stillbirths, weak calves, and retained placenta cases.

- *Swine:* Leptospirosis in swine is usually mild or inapparent, with only one or a few affected pigs showing acute signs of anorexia, fever, and diarrhea. Chronic cases may result in late pregnancy abortion or weak piglets that usually fail to survive and recover but become renal shedders for at least 6 months.

- *Dogs:* Leptospirosis can cause elevated body temperature, depression, deep sunken eyes, anorexia, muscle tenderness, vomiting, intussusception, foul breath, ulcerated gums, and extensive jaundice that may lead to death. The acute form of the disease, known as "Stuttgart disease," is characterized by vomiting, rapid dehydration, collapse, necrosis, and sloughing of the buccal mucosa and tongue, the occasional passage of blood-stained feces, and high mortality.

- *Horses:* Leptospirosis in horses is rare and usually mild, but it can cause pyrexia, icterus, periodic ophthalmia, and abortion.

- *Sheep:* The common signs include abortion, fever, agalactia, dyspnea, jaundice, hematuria, and sudden death.

- *Goats:* Mostly asymptomatic but shed leptospires in the urine for short periods or may develop jaundice, hemoglobinuria, and abortions.

4.6.2 Disease in man

The disease is manifested in two phases after an incubation period of 7: 12 days

- *Early or Leptospiaremic phase:* The disease is manifested as a flu-like illness characterized by abrupt onset of high fever, chills, headache, muscle pain, vomiting, and eye redness. Most individuals recover fully from the mild form, even without medication. Untreated infection may progress to the second stage.

- *Second or Immune phase/Weil's syndrome:* Untreated disease worsens to kidney and liver failure. Jaundice results from liver failure. Anemia occurs due to widespread hemorrhages, which can lead to coma and death, particularly in older patients or with more virulent strains of the disease. Conjunctival suffusion, "red eye," is a constant and unique symptom. In rare cases, severe forms of the disease may present as atypical pneumonia, aseptic meningitis, or myocarditis. The mortality rate of severe forms ranges from 5 to 10%, which is significant.

4.7 Diagnosis

A tentative diagnosis of the disease can be made based on the clinical symptoms that suggest possible infection, especially in individuals from high-risk groups and endemic areas. However, a confirmatory diagnosis is necessary and can be made as follows

4.7.1 Direct examination of samples

Microscopic techniques, such as dark field microscopy (400x) and silver staining, can visualize leptospires in impression smears or tissue sections.

4.7.2 Isolation of leptospires

Conventional methods for detecting leptospires in clinical or pathological materials, especially blood, include culture, animal inoculation, and culture following animal inoculation.

i. **Culture:** The isolation rate of leptospires from clinical specimens such as blood, urine, cerebrospinal fluid (CSF), kidney, liver, and brain from aborted fetuses, uterine swabs from abortion cases, and semen is shallow. Media for culturing leptospires are media containing serum (Korthof's medium, Stuart's medium, and Fletcher's semisolid medium), media containing bovine albumin fraction V and Tween 80 (EMJH (Ellinghausen-McCullough-Johnson-Harris) medium, protein-free medium, Ellis medium), and chemically defined media (Burgess medium and T80 medium).

ii. **Animal inoculation:** It is carried out to increase the concentration of *Leptospira* cells. In gerbils, a 10^6 leptospire inoculum usually induces a fatal reaction in 3–5 days. Inoculation of a hamster (3 weeks old) with 0.5^{-1} ml of a sample through the intraperitoneal route induces jaundice, resulting in a fatal infection. Leptospires can be recovered from guinea pigs (1 week old) that died after 21 days of inoculation with 0.5^{-1} ml of the infected material through the intraperitoneal route.

4.7.3 Common serological diagnostic tests

i. **Microscopic agglutination test (MAT):** MAT is the World Health Organization (WHO) standard reference test for the fast, specific, and routine diagnosis of leptospirosis. It employs mixing equal volumes of a series of serum dilutions and either live or formalized *Leptospira* culture. A titer of 1:100 or more indicates present or past infection, and the titer may be higher in vaccinates.

ii. **Macroscopic agglutination test:** This test is similar to the MAT, but the agglutination reaction is visible to the naked eye. It is less sensitive than the MAT and is not recommended for routine diagnosis.

iii. **Enzyme-linked immunosorbent assay (ELISA):** This test is highly sensitive and specific and can detect IgG and IgM antibodies separately.

iv. **The indirect hemagglutination (IHA) test:** This test involves sensitizing sheep or human red blood cells with *Leptospira* antigens, which agglutinate antibodies in the test serum. A positive result is indicated by an agglutination reaction equivalent to 2+ or more.

v. **Complement fixation test (CFT):** This test involves inactivating the serum and titrating the complement in the presence of antigen to be used in the test.

A positive result is indicated by reduced complement activity due to antibodies in the serum.

vi. **The sensitized erythrocyte lysis (SEL) test**: This test involves mixing twofold dilutions of test serum with sensitized sheep erythrocytes and complement and observing for hemolysis in the presence of complement.

vii. Other tests that may be used include the growth inhibition test (GIT), immunoperoxidase test, chemiluminescent test, and DNA hybridization with biotin-labeled leptospiral DNA.

4.7.4 Diagnostic tests for rapid or early detection

Several other sensitive and specific tests are available for detecting leptospires. However, they are not routinely used as they are more complex or expensive than conventional methods and may require specialized equipment or expertise. These include the Immunofluorescence test, Polymerase chain reaction (PCR), Microcapsule agglutination test (MCAT), Radioimmunoassay (RIA), Passive hemagglutination (PHA) test, and Rapid microscopic agglutination test (RMAT).

4.8 Treatment

Antibiotic treatment should be initiated as soon as possible once symptoms appear. Ampicillin, doxycycline, erythromycin, penicillin, tetracycline, and streptomycin can treat leptospirosis. Treatment and vaccination of beef herds are recommended to prevent abortion. While in dairy cattle, only infected animals should be treated to prevent the spread of infection.

4.9 Prevention and control

The risk of leptospirosis can be reduced by avoiding water contaminated with animal urine or contact with infected animals, proper draining and cleaning of yards, pens, sheds, and kennels with cresol or sodium hypochlorite (1:4000), avoidance of stagnation of water, urine, and feces, and burial or burning of infected carcasses, aborted fetuses, placentas, and bedding. Occupational workers should wear protective clothing or footwear. Any skin cuts should be covered with waterproof dressing while swimming in freshwater. Preventing rodents from invading residential areas and water sources reduces the risk of infection. Vaccination against the bacteria can protect pet dogs and the household from leptospirosis, while human immunization provides a certain degree of protection. Available vaccines for domestic animals can decrease the severity of the disease, although they cannot provide complete protection as the immunity is serovar-specific. Pigs are typically vaccinated every 6 months, while annual vaccination is usually sufficient for dogs, cattle, and sheep. Proper quarantining and testing new animals before introducing them to a herd or flock would help remove carrier animals. Educating the general public, especially high-risk groups, about leptospirosis and avoiding recreational activities in contaminated water are necessary for disease prevention.

5. Hydatidosis

5.1 Etiology

The adult tapeworms (cestode) of *Echinococcus granulosus* and *Echinococcus multilocularis* occur in the small intestine of canids (definitive host). Larval stages of *E. granulosus* (hydatid) and *E. multilocularis* (metacestode) occur in tissues of the liver, lung, and other organs of other mammals (intermediate host), including humans. Infection with the larval stages of *E. granulosus* in, the intermediate host, causes "cystic echinococcosis" or "hydatidosis," which causes significant economic losses and public health issues. In contrast, infection with metacestode causes severe disease, referred to as "alveolar echinococcosis."

A hydatid cyst is a big sac filled with liquid and lined by germinal epithelium, which produces small scolices that are either separate or clumped together in brood capsules. Anything inside the cyst other than the liquid, such as the scolices and brood capsules, is sometimes called "Hydatid Sand." If the cyst wall breaks open from the outside, hydatid sand can also form inside the cyst [48]. The fluid inside a hydatid cyst is typically pale yellow and contains 17–200 mg of protein per 100 ml. The hydatid cyst has an outer connective tissue covering beneath the germinal epithelium. Both large and daughter cysts contain germinal layers from which scolices develop. Each protoscolex can grow into one adult tapeworm in the final host.

5.2 Life cycle

An adult tapeworm of *E. granulosus* passes eggs in the feces of the definitive host (Canids). Eggs hatch in the small intestine of an intermediate host when ingested through contaminated feed and water. Hatched eggs release six-hooked oncospheres that penetrate the intestinal wall and migrate through the circulatory system into various organs, especially the liver, and lungs, where they develop into a thick-walled hydatid cyst from the oncospheres. When a definitive host ingests organs infested with cysts, the protoscolices evaginate from the cyst and attach to intestinal mucosa to develop into the adult stages in 32 to 80 days, and this slow-growing hydatid cyst usually takes 6–12 months to become an infective mature stage which has two layers: inner germinal epithelium and an outer membrane. Brood capsules detach from the germinal epithelium and exist freely in the hydatid fluid. Daughter cysts are formed inside or outside the mother cyst [48]. The multilocular, unilocular, and sterile cysts are frequently noted in sheep, horses, and cattle. As a thin-walled cyst embedded in the organ grows, it leads to a local reaction, whereas a thick fibrous capsule is formed around the cyst in horses. Humans act as dead-end hosts because dogs do not have access to eat hydatid cysts containing flesh.

5.3 Epidemiology

Hydatidosis is a zoonotic infection that occurs worldwide. It is most commonly found in Mediterranean countries, Southern South America, the Middle East, Iceland, New Zealand, Australia, and Southern Africa. In endemic areas, the incidence of cystic echinococcosis (CE) varies from 1 to 220 cases per 100,000 people, whereas the incidence of alveolar echinococcosis (AE) ranges from 0.03 to 1.2 cases per 100,000 people [49]. In India, the prevalence of *E. granulosus* infection in the stray dog population varies from 4.35% in Karnataka [50], 33.3% in Andhra Pradesh [51], and 5.22–6.57% prevalence in Maharashtra [52].

5.4 Pathogenicity of human hydatidosis

Echinococcus granulosus causes cystic echinococcosis (CE) while *Echinococcus multilocularis* (rare, most virulent) produces alveolar echinococcosis [49]. In 63% of echinococcosis cases, cysts have been reported in the liver and 25% in the lungs [49]. The symptoms of cystic echinococcosis in the liver include obstructive jaundice, abdominal pain, rupture of cyst into the abdominal or peritoneal cavity, urticaria, and/or severe anaphylactic reaction due to the pressure effect of the cyst in the liver and due to the presence of cysts in the lungs causes chronic cough, dyspnea, pleuritic chest pain, and hemoptysis. Anaphylaxis due to the rupture of the cyst may lead to death; however, if the person survives, the released daughter cysts may again grow in other parts of the body [48]. The cerebral involvement is signified by headache, dizziness, and diminished consciousness [49].

Intermediate hosts usually show no visible symptoms. Most often, cysts are discovered only at slaughter. Definitive hosts (canids) are also asymptomatic, even in the presence of thousands of adult tapeworms [48].

5.5 Diagnosis

Diagnosis is based on the detection of adult worm segments (three segments, namely tiny rostellum, six-hooked scolices, and the kidney-shaped ovary) and eggs (an oval shape with a thick shell and radial striation (embryophore)) in the feces [53]. Necropsy can reveal tapeworms attached to the small intestine as slender papillae. Intestinal scrapping, sedimentation, and counting techniques at necropsy also detect intestinal *E. multilocularis* in definitive hosts [54]. Hydatids are rarely suspected in intermediate hosts, and diagnosis is usually postmortem. Imaging tests such as ultrasound, computed tomography (CT) scan, magnetic resonance imaging (MRI), and serological assays such as complement fixation and immunoelectrophoresis are more commonly used in man. The Casoni test is a hypersensitivity reaction that occurs within 15 min after inoculating fluid of hydatid cyst in the suspected individual [53]. Recent diagnostic trends include peroxidase micro-ELISA and Ab-ELISA, which are used for bovine fertile hydatid cysts [53].

5.6 Treatment

There is no specific treatment for hydatid cysts in domestic animals [55]. Praziquantel is a highly effective drug for treating *Echinococcus* tapeworms in dogs and cats [48]. Surgical removal is the best treatment for hydatid cysts in humans, but the disease can reoccur even after surgery. Anthelmintics like praziquantel, albendazole, and mebendazole effectively treat hydatid cysts in humans [54].

5.7 Prevention and control

Dog deworming, thorough meat inspection, and public awareness are crucial to break the transmission cycle between the definitive and intermediate hosts. Prevent access of dogs to abattoirs. In some countries, purgative anthelmintiics, like arecoline hydrochloride, are used to expel the entire tapeworm from infected dogs [48]. It is crucial to adopt good personal hygiene practices before and after handling food and dog to prevent the transmission of eggs to humans.

6. Taeniasis

6.1 Etiology

Taeniasis/cysticercosis is a neglected tropical disease highly endemic in many sub-Saharan African, Southeast Asia, and Latin American countries. The socioeconomic impact of cysticercosis is immense as it affects the health and livelihood of farming communities by reducing the market value of pigs (and cattle) and rendering pork/beef unsafe for human consumption. Taeniasis is an intestinal infection caused by pork tapeworm (*Taenia solium*), beef tapeworm (*Taenia saginata*), and Asian tapeworm (*Taenia asiatica*).

6.2 Life cycle

Humans are the only definitive host for *Taenia* tapeworms, whereas cattle serve as an intermediate host for *T. saginata*, and pigs are the intermediate host for *Theridion solium* and *Torenia asiatica* species. *Taenia* eggs are released in human feces and survive for days to months in the environment. Intermediate hosts catch infection when grazing on pastures/soil contaminated with eggs or gravid proglottids. The animal's intestinal eggs hatch to produce oncospheres that invade the intestinal wall and reach the striated muscles via blood circulation. The larval form (cysticerci) of *Taenia* tapeworm encysts in muscles where it remains alive for several years. Infection in humans occurs after consuming raw or undercooked meat infected with tapeworm larvae. The larvae develop into adult tapeworms in the human intestine, attaching themselves to their scolex and residing for years. The mature tapeworms release segments called gravid proglottids, which detach from the worm and are excreted in the feces.

6.3 Epidemiology

The infections in men are subjective to poor personal hygiene, sanitary conditions, food habits, and cooking pattern. These infections are common in regions where people are habituated to eating insufficiently cooked or smoked meat (pork/beef). Eating contaminated raw leafy green vegetables with human excreta containing eggs of *T. solium* can also cause infection in vegetarians.

6.4 Disease

6.4.1 Disease in man

It is manifested mainly in three forms namely Taeniasis, Cysticercosis, and Neurocysticercosis.

a. *Taeniasis:* It is an infestation with adult tapeworms. Most people with tapeworm infections have no symptoms or mild symptoms. Patients with *T. saginata* taeniasis often experience more symptoms than those with *T. solium or T. asiatica* infections because the *T. saginata* tapeworm is larger (up to 10 m) than the other two tapeworms (usually 3 m). Symptoms include abdominal pain, loss of appetite, weight loss, nausea, diarrhea, or constipation.

b. *Cysticercosis:* It is an infestation with larvae/cysticerci. *T. saginata* does not cause cysticercosis in humans. It is not clear if *T. asiatica* causes cysticercosis in humans or not. However, infection with *T. solium* cysticerci can result in human cysticercosis, which causes variable clinical symptoms, including visible or palpable nodules beneath the skin.

c. *Neurocysticercosis:* It is caused when the larvae of *T. solium* encyst in the central nervous system (CNS), including the brain. It causes chronic headaches, blindness, and epileptic seizures, and sometimes it can be fatal.

6.4.2 Disease in animals

Signs and symptoms of cysticercosis in pigs (porcine cysticercosis): Typically, there are no symptoms in pigs. At examination, the heavily infected pigs can show cysts on their tongue.

6.5 Diagnosis

Diagnosis in man is based on demonstrating proglottids and eggs in the feces. Neurocysticercosis can be confirmed through a CT scan, magnetic resonance imaging (MRI), and immunological tests (ELISA and RIA), while ophthalmoscopic examination helps to know about ocular cysticercosis.

6.6 Treatment

Oral administration of antthelmintics like praziquantel and niclosamide is effective against taeniasis in adults and children. Surgical removal of cysts is advisable in cases with intraventricular cysts causing obstruction, hydrocephalus, and ocular cysticercosis.

6.7 Prevention and control

- (i) Seeking medical help to treat tapeworm infestation in people. (ii) Prohibiting open defecation and promoting using toilets/latrines to avoid environmental contamination and infection of pigs and other people. (iii) Adopting good farming practices and preventing pigs from scavenging in contaminated areas. (iv) Vaccinating pigs/cattle and treating them simultaneously with appropriate antiparasitic drugs. (v) Inspecting meat to detect an infestation of parasitic cysts and discarding infected meat. (vi) Avoiding consumption of raw or undercooked pork. Always cook meat to at least 145–160° F (63–71°C) at its thickest part. (vii) Thorough cleaning of vegetables under running water and proper cooking. (viii) Promoting good hygiene practices such as washing hands with soap and water after using the toilets. (ix) Educating the people about the disease.

7. Toxoplasmosis

7.1 Etiology

Toxoplasmosis is caused by a hemoprotozoan parasite called *Toxoplasma gondii*.

7.2 Life cycle

Toxoplasma gondii has a complex life cycle; it reproduces asexually and sexually [56]. Cats and other felids are the only definitive hosts, while other mammals, including man and birds, are intermediate hosts. The sexual cycle of the parasite takes place in the intestinal epithelium of the definitive host, while the asexual cycle occurs in both the definitive and intermediate hosts [57].

7.2.1 Enteroepithelial cycle

Cats acquire the infection by consuming tissue cysts in chronically infected intermediate hosts or ingesting oocysts in food or water. After ingestion of tissue cysts, the cyst wall is digested by gastric juices resulting in the release of bradyzoites. Bradyzoites invade the intestinal epithelium to convert it into an actively multiplying tachyzoite stage. Some tachyzoites undergo five different developmental stages inside the epithelium to reproduce asexually by endodyogeny. Two daughter cells are created, which undergo schizogony to differentiate into micro- and macrogametocytes within two days of infection. The gametes fuse to form a zygote, which subsequently secretes a cyst wall to develop into oocysts. Oocysts rupture the intestinal epithelial cells and are excreted in feces. Oocysts undergo sporulation outside the host's body to become infective for other hosts. Cats with toxoplasmosis typically show no signs of the disease. The shortest prepatent period (PP), i.e., the time from infection until the shedding of oocysts, is 3 to 10 days after ingestion of tissue cysts. In contrast, it is 13 days or more after consuming tachyzoites and 18 days or more after oocyst ingestion [57]. Almost all cats shed oocysts after tissue cysts' ingestion, whereas less than 30–50% of cats shed oocysts after ingesting tachyzoites or oocysts [58].

7.2.2 Extraintestinal cycle

When the intermediate host ingests oocysts, sporozoites are released into the gut lumen and pass through the gut epithelium to enter cells in the lamina propria. If the intermediate host ingests tissue cysts, the released bradyzoites behave like sporozoites. Both sporozoites and bradyzoites transform into tachyzoites that enter a host cell, dividing rapidly until the cell bursts. Tachyzoites continue to invade adjacent cells or travel elsewhere in the body through the bloodstream. As the host's immunity develops, the replication of tachyzoites decreases, resulting in the conversion of tachyzoites into a slowly dividing bradyzoite (tissue cysts) which do not typically produce a host reaction. The parasite's life cycle is completed when felidae ingests the flesh of an intermediate host containing tissue cysts.

7.3 Epidemiology

The prevalence of *T. gondii* varies in different geographical areas and among different ethnic groups, with warm and humid climates being more conducive to its spread [59, 60]. *T. gondii* infections are widespread and estimated to affect up to one-third of the world's human population [59]. The disease has been documented in numerous countries globally [60, 61]. The prevalence of latent toxoplasmosis in pregnant women globally is 33.8%, with the highest prevalence in South America and the lowest in the Western Pacific region [62]. Developed countries such as France have seen a decrease in *Toxoplasma* infection rates due to changes in food habits and hygiene measures [63, 64]. Toxoplasmosis causes reproductive disorders in various hosts, resulting in economic losses to the sheep industry worldwide [58, 61]. Goats are highly susceptible to clinical toxoplasmosis, while pigs are unaffected.

7.4 Transmission

High temperature and humidity favor the survival of *T. gondii* oocysts in the environment. Rodents are considered reservoir hosts, significantly transmitting the disease to domestic animals and humans. Cats are a crucial part of the transmission cycle of *T. gondii*, as they are the only species capable of shedding oocysts in their feces. The congenital transmission from an infected mother to her child has been reported in humans during pregnancy. Human infection can also result from ingesting food or water contaminated with oocysts [65] and consuming raw or undercooked meat containing tissue cysts. Infection can also be transmitted by transfusion of blood or tissues from infected animals harboring tachyzoites or bradyzoites.

7.5 Disease

7.5.1 Disease in man

- *Congenital toxoplasmosis*: If the mother has a primary infection or is a carrier of a chronic infection, the cysts can infect the fetus during late pregnancy. The mother may not experience symptoms. Severe cases can result in abortion, while surviving fetuses may exhibit symptoms such as fever, enlarged spleen and liver, and developmental delays. Delayed manifestations of toxoplasmosis in children include cataracts, eye inflammation, anemia, and mental retardation.

- *Acquired toxoplasmosis:* In 25% of cases, the disease produces no noticeable symptoms. However, the disease can be severe in people with weakened immune systems. Symptoms may range from fever and body pain to life-threatening encephalitis. Common manifestations of the disease include fever, swollen lymph nodes, high levels of lymphocytes in the blood, unexplained eye lesions, pregnancy complications, heart inflammation, and brain inflammation.

7.5.2 Toxoplasmosis in animals

Toxoplasma gondii can infect cattle, sheep, goats, pigs, dogs, and horses. Symptoms may include respiratory, enteric, and nervous system issues and fevers. Abortion and congenital transmission only occur in sheep.

7.6 Diagnosis in man and animals

Isolation of parasite is carried out by inoculating laboratory mice with fetal brain and placental cotyledons. Several serological tests are available for the detection of *T. gondii* antibodies, including the Feldman dye test, indirect hemagglutination test, complement fixation test, modified agglutination test, latex agglutination test, direct agglutination test, indirect fluorescent antibody test, and enzyme-linked immunosorbent assay.

7.7 Treatment

There is no effective treatment or prophylaxis for farm animals. However, sulfonamides, pyrimethamine, and clindamycin can be therapeutic in dogs and cats.

7.8 Prevention and control

Proper biosecurity measures should be implemented at farms. Aborted materials and contaminated water should be discarded immediately to avoid consumption by domestic or feral cats. Pet cats should be kept indoors to prevent them from hunting infected rodents. Avoid feeding raw/undercooked meat to cats. Vaccination of cats should be done. An infection can be prevented in sheep by vaccinating with the live-attenuated tachyzoite S48 strain vaccine, licensed for sheep in New Zealand, the UK, Ireland, and France. Infection in humans can be prevented by adequate cooking and thorough meat freezing. Pregnant women should avoid direct and indirect contact with cats. Education for health professionals and people, in general, is also necessary.

8. Trichinellosis

8.1 Etiology

Trichinellosis or trichinosis is caused by a roundworm (nematode) called "*Trichinella*." There are nine species and 12 genotypes of *Trichinella*. *T. spiralis* is the most common species causing human disease. However, other species, such *as T. pseudospiralis, T. nativa, T. murelli, T. nelsoni, T. britovi, Trisinuata papuae, and T. zimbabwensis*, are also implicated in human infection.

8.2 Epidemiology and transmission

Human trichinellosis is mainly linked to the consumption of infected pork, often reported in Central and South America, Asia, and Europe [66]. Domestic pork and related products are the critical sources of *Trichinella* infection in humans, primarily obtained from pigs raised under free-ranging practices [67]. Raw horse and dog meat consumption in countries like France and China has led to *Trichinella* outbreaks [68, 69]. Hunters risk infection when consuming raw meat from game animals [70]. Illegal importation of uncontrolled meat from endemic to non-endemic countries resulted in outbreaks in Denmark, Germany, Italy, Spain, and the United Kingdom [71–73]. In countries such as Israel, Lebanon, and Syria, where pork consumption is forbidden by the Judaic and Muslim religions, outbreaks of trichinellosis have only been observed in specific populations who consumed pork from wild boars [74, 75].

8.3 Life cycle

Adult worms and larvae develop within a single vertebrate host, which can serve as both a definitive and an intermediate host. In order to complete its life cycle,

Trichinella requires a second host. In the domestic life cycle of the parasite, pigs and rodents are frequently involved. In sylvatic cycles, wild animals, such as bears, moose, and wild boars, are the primary reservoirs. In the initial stage of trichinellosis, *Trichinella* larvae are present in the muscle of hosts. When a new host ingests infected muscle tissue, larvae are released during digestion, enter the small intestine, and move to the jejunum and ileum to mature into adult roundworms. A single adult female worm produces around 1500 newborn larvae. The larvae leave the intestine and enter the blood circulation to reach muscle tissues, where they mature and become coiled within the muscle fibers. In some cases, larvae are encapsulated due to the host's cellular response and form a host–parasite complex called the nurse cell. The larvae can survive within the nurse cell for months or years, receiving nutrients and oxygen from an increased vascular supply. Eventually, the encapsulated cyst becomes calcified, leading to the death of the larva. It takes 17 to 21 days from exposure to the appearance and encystment of larvae in muscles. Infected animals are partially immune to subsequent infections due to intense and persistent immunity.

8.4 Disease

Disease symptoms depend on the infecting dose, the individual's susceptibility, and the species of *Trichinella* involved. The disease's initial phase is known as the "enteral phase," which appears as early as 1 week after ingesting the infective dose. It is characterized by abdominal discomfort and diarrhea lasting a few days. The parenteral phase of the disease may occur within 1 to 2 weeks following infection, or it may be delayed for several weeks as more significant numbers of worms migrate and accumulate in the musculature. Symptoms of the parenteral phase include periorbital edema, myalgia, headache, fever, macro-papular rash, and conjunctival and subungual hemorrhages. Complications of trichinellosis may lead to myocarditis and encephalitis due to migration of larvae to the heart musculature or the central nervous system.

8.5 Diagnosis

The compression method is the oldest and the most common direct detection method for *Trichinella larvae* in meat samples. A minimum of 1 gram of tissue must be examined to achieve a theoretical sensitivity of 1 larva per gram, which is considered the threshold for infection to pose a public health risk. The magnetic stirrer method is the "gold standard" for detecting *Trichinella larvae* in pooled samples [76]. ELISA can test animals for anti-*Trichinella* antibodies in their serum or meat juice (10^8) due to its high sensitivity for detecting as little as one larva per 100 grams of muscle tissue [77]. The most commonly infected animal muscle tissues are the diaphragm crus, tongue, and masseter muscle [76].

8.6 Treatment

The recommended dosage for albendazole is 400 mg twice daily for 8 to 14 days or mebendazole (200 to 400 mg) thrice a day for 3 days, followed by 400 to 500 mg three times a day for 10 days. Both treatments are suitable for adults and children but are not advocated for pregnant women or children under the age of 2 years [78]. In pregnant women and children, a single dose of pyrantel (10 to 20 mg/kg body weight) for 2 to 3 days is effective against worms in the gut but does not affect newborns and muscle larvae [79]. Prednisone (30 to 60 mg/day) for 10 to 15 days is a standard chemotherapy choice for severe symptoms.

8.7 Prevention and control

Trichinellosis is a 100% foodborne parasitic disease that can be prevented by thoroughly cooking meat to an internal temperature of 71°C (160°F) or higher. Freezing meat at −15°C (5°F) for at least 3 weeks can also kill *Trichinella* larvae. Additionally, avoiding consuming raw or undercooked wild game meat, especially pork, can reduce the risk of infection. In some countries, mandatory inspection and testing of pork products have controlled the incidences of trichinellosis.

9. Conclusion

Neglected zoonotic diseases mainly affect existing populations of low socioeconomic status residing in urban slums and villages and those engaged in poor animal husbandry practices. According to disability-adjusted life years (DALYs) tracked by WHO, OIE, 6 out of 20 infectious zoonotic diseases are neglected. NTDs globally affect more than 1.4 billion people, mainly poor and marginalized populations in low-resource settings. Understanding NTDs is essential to reduce human health risks by controlling animal infections. The primary concern with NTDs is the critical gap between public health needs and veterinary responsibilities, the paucity of research grants for NTDs, the negligence of policymakers, limited diagnostic capacity, and the need for coordinated control and prevention programs.

Conflict of interest

The authors declare no conflict of interest.

Author details

Deepali Kalambhe* and Nilam Wavhal
Centre for One Health, Guru Angad Dev Veterinary and Animal Sciences University, Ludhiana, Punjab, India

*Address all correspondence to: drdeepalikalambhe@gmail.com

References

[1] Fasanella A, Garofolo G, Galante D, Quaranta V, Palazzo L, Lista F, et al. Severe anthrax outbreaks in Italy in 2004: Considerations on factors involved in the spread of infection. The New Microbiologica. 2010;**33**(1):83-86

[2] Wikipedia. *Bacillus anthracis*. [Accessed: February 15, 2021]

[3] Demicheli V, Rivetti D, Deeks JJ, Jefferson T, Pratt M. The effectiveness and safety of vaccines against human anthrax: A systematic review. Vaccine. 1998;**16**(9-10):880-884

[4] Cummings RT, Salowe SP, Cunningham BR, Wiltsie J, Park YW, Sonatore LM, et al. A peptide-based fluorescence resonance energy transfer assay for *Bacillus anthracis* lethal factor protease. Proceedings of the National Academy of Sciences of the United States of America. 2002;**99**(10):6603-6606

[5] Wikipedia. Vollum strain. 2021. [Accessed: February 8, 2021]

[6] Wilson JM, Brediger W, Albright TP, Smith-Gagen J. Reanalysis of the anthrax epidemic in Rhodesia, 1978-1984. PeerJ. 2016;**4**:e2686

[7] Constable P, Hinchcliff KW, Done S, Gruenberg W. Veterinary Medicine. A textbook of the diseases of cattle, horses, sheep, pigs and goats. 11th ed. Amsterdam: Elsevier; 2016

[8] Hornitzky M, Muller J. Anthrax. Canberra, Australia: Australian Government Department of Agriculture, Water, and the Environment; 2010. pp. 1-15

[9] Goossens PL. Animal models of human anthrax: The Quest for the Holy Grail. Molecular Aspects of Medicine. 2009;**30**(6):467-480

[10] Hugh-Jones M, Blackburn J. The ecology of *Bacillus anthracis*. Molecular Aspects of Medicine. 2009;**30**(6):356-367

[11] WHO. Anthrax in Humans and Animals. Geneva, Switzerland: WHO Press; 2008. pp. 1-198

[12] Moriyon OB. International committee on systemic prokaryotes. Subcommittee on the taxonomy of Brucella. In: Int J Syst Evol Microbiol. Minutes of the meeting September 17, 2003. Vol. 56. Pamplona, Spain; 2006. pp. 1173-1175

[13] Scholz HC, Hubalek Z, Nesvadbova J, Tomaso H, Vergnaud G, Le Flèche P, et al. Isolation of Brucella microti from soil. Emerging Infectious Diseases. 2008;**14**(8):1316-1317

[14] Cloeckaert A, Verger JM, Grayon M, Paquet JY, Garin-Bastuji B, Foster G, et al. Classification of Bruella spp. isolated from marine mammals by DNA polymorphism at the omp2locus. Microbes and Infection. 2001;**3**(9):729-738

[15] Foster G, Osterman BS, Godfroid J, Jacques I, Cloeckaert A. Brucellacetisp. nov. International Journal of System Evolution and Microbiology. 2007;**57**(11):2688-2693

[16] Scholz HC, Nockler K, Gollner C, Bahn P, Vergnaud G, Tomaso H, et al. Brucella inopinata species, isolated from breast implant infection. International Journal of Systematic and Evolutionary Microbiology. 2010;**60**:801-808

[17] Al Dahouk S, Köhler S, Occhialini A, Jiménez de Bagüés MP,

Hammerl JA, Eisenberg T, et al. Brucella spp. of amphibians comprise genomically diverse motile strains competent for replication in macrophages and survival in mammalian hosts. Scientific Reports. 2017;**7**:44420

[18] Scholz HC, Revilla-Fernández S, Al Dahouk SA, Hammerl JA, Zygmunt MS, Cloeckaert A, et al. *Brucella vulpis* sp. nov., isolated from mandibular lymph nodes of red foxes (*Vulpes vulpes*). International Journal of Systematic and Evolutionary Microbiology. 2016;**66**(5):2090-2098

[19] Maansi, Upadhyay AK. Epidemiological status of brucellosis in animals and human of Uttar Pradesh and Uttarakhand. International Journal of Basic and Applied Agricultural Research. 2015;**13**(1):92-94

[20] PAHO/WHO. Zoonotic and Communicable Diseases Common to Man, Animals, and Wildlife. Scientific Technical Publication No. 580. Washington, DC: An American health regional office of the WHO; 2001. pp. 44-67

[21] Corbel MJ, Brinley Morgan WJ. In: Krieg NR, Holt TG, editors. Bergey's Manual of Systematic Bacteriology. Vol. Vol. 1. Baltimore and London: Williams & Wilkins; 1984. Genus Brucella Meyer and Shaw 1920,173. pp. 377-88

[22] Hirsh D, Zee Y. Veterinary Microbiology. 2nd ed. Oxford: Wiley; 1999

[23] Godfroid J, Käsbohrer A. Brucellosis in the European Union and Norway at the turn of the twenty-first century. Veterinary Microbiology. 2002;**90**(1-4):135-145

[24] Bingöl A, Togay-Işikay C. Neurobrucellosis as an exceptional cause of transient ischemic attacks. European Journal of Neurology. 2006;**13**(5):544-548

[25] Manual OIE. Chapter 2.1.4. Brucellosis (Brucellaabortus, *B. melitensis* and *B. suis*) (infection with *B. abortus*, *B. melitensis* and *B. suis*). In: OIE Manual of Diagnostic Tests and Vaccines for Terrestrial Animals. Paris; 2016. pp. 1-44

[26] McCallan L, McNair J, Skuce R, Branch B. A Review of the Potential Role of Cattle Slurry in the Spread of Bovine Tuberculosis. Belfast, UK: Agri-food and Biosciences Institute; 2014

[27] Mukundan H, Chambers M, Waters R, Larsen MH, editors. Immunopathogenesis of Mycobacterium bovis infection of cattle. In: Tuberculosis, Leprosy and Mycobacterial Diseases of Man and Animals: The Many Hosts of Mycobacteria; Oxfordshire, UK: CABI; 2015. p. 136

[28] Dawson KL, Bell A, Kawakami RP, Coley K, Yates G, Collins DM. Transmission of Mycobacteriumorygis (M. tuberculosis complex species) from a tuberculosis patient to a dairy cow in New Zealand. Journal of Clinical Microbiology. 2012;**50**(9):3136-3138

[29] Marcos LA, Spitzer ED, Mahapatra R, Ma Y, Halse TA, Shea J, et al. Mycobacteriumorygis lymphadenitis in New York, USA. Emerging Infectious Diseases. 2017;**23**(10):1749-1751

[30] Rahim Z, Thapa J, Fukushima Y, van der Zanden AGM, Gordon SV, Suzuki Y, et al. Tuberculosis caused by Mycobacteriumorygis in dairy cattle and captured monkeys in Bangladesh: A new scenario of tuberculosis in South Asia. Transbound Emerging Diseases. 2017;**64**(6):1965-1969

[31] Van Ingen J, Rahim Z, Mulder A, Boeree MJ, Simeone R, Brosch R, et al.

Characterization of Mycobacteriumorygis as M. tuberculosis complex subspecies. Emerging Infectious Diseases. 2012;**18**(4):653-655

[32] WHO. FAO and the union. Zoonotic tuberculosis. 2017

[33] Charles OT, James HS, Michael JG. Book. Mycobacterium bovis Infection in Animals and Humans. 2nd ed. Hoboken, NJ, USA: Blackwell Publishing; 2006

[34] Bhembe NL, Jaja IF, Nwodo UU, Okoh AI, Green E. Prevalence of tuberculous lymphadenitis in slaughtered cattle in Eastern Cape, South Africa. International Journal of Infected Diseases. 2017;**61**:27-37

[35] Hlokwe TM, Said H, Gcebe N. Mycobacterium tuberculosis infection in cattle from the eastern Cape Province of South Africa. BMC Veterinary Research. 2017;**13**(1):299

[36] Krishnaswami KV, Mani KR. Mycobacterium tuberculosis human is causing zoonotic tuberculosis among cattle. Indian Journal of Public Health. 1983;**27**(2):60-63

[37] Thoen CO, Karlson AG, Himes EM. Mycobacterial infections in animals. Reviews of Infectious Diseases. 1981;**3**(5):960-972

[38] Kmety E, Dikken H. Classification of the Species Leptospirainterrogans and History of Its Serovars. Gronigen, The Netherlands: University Press; 1993

[39] Plank R, Dean D. Overview of the epidemiology, microbiology, and pathogenesis of Leptospira spp. in humans. Microbes and Infection. 2000;**2**(10):1265-1276

[40] Ahmed N, Devi SM, Valverde M, Vijayachari P, Machangu RS, Ellis WA, et al. Multilocus sequence typing method for identification and genotypic classification of pathogenic Leptospira species. Annals of Clinical Microbiology and Antimicrobes. 2006;**5**:28

[41] Pappas G, Papadimitriou P, Siozopoulou V, Christou L, Akritidis N. Theglobalizationofleptospirosis:Worldwide incidence trends. International Journal of Infectious Diseases. 2008;**12**(4):351-357

[42] Victoriano A, Smythe L, Gloriani-Barzaga N, et al. Leptospirosis in the Asia Pacific region. BMC Infectious Diseases. 2009;**9**:147

[43] Ciceroni L, Stepan E, Pinto A, Pizzocaro P, Dettori G, Franzin L, et al. Epidemiological trend of human leptospirosis in Italy between 1994 and 1996. European Journal of Epidemiology. 2000;**16**(1):79-86

[44] Morgan J, Bornstein SL, Karpati AM, Bruce M, Bolin CA, Austin CC, et al. Outbreak of leptospirosis among triathlon participants and community residents in Springfield, Illinois, 1998. Clinical Infectious Diseases. 2002;**34**(12):1593-1599

[45] Stern EJ, Galloway R, Shadomy SV, Wannemuehler K, Atrubin D, Blackmore C, et al. Outbreak of leptospirosis among adventure race participants in Florida, 2005. Clinical Infectious Diseases. 2010;**50**(6):843-849

[46] Teichmann D, Göbels K, Simon J, Grobusch MP, Suttorp N. A severe case of leptospirosis acquired during an iron man contest. European Journal of Clinical and Microbiological Infectious Diseases. 2001;**20**(2):137-138

[47] McCurry J. Philippines struggles to recover from typhoons. Lancet. 2009;**374**(9700):1489

[48] Urqhart GM, Avmour J, Duncan JL, Dunn AM, Jennings FW. Veterinary

Parasitology. 2nd ed. Hoboken, NY: Blackwell Publishing; 1995. pp. 122-129

[49] Atasaliki TM, Altuntas N, Sulu E, Senol T, Kir A. Review of cases with cystic hydatid lung disease in a tertiary referral hospital located in an endemic region: a 10 years' experience. Respiration. 2000;**67**(5):539-542

[50] Prathiush PR, D'Souza PE, Gowda AKJ. Diagnosis of E. granulosus infection in dogs by a coproantigen sandwich ELISA. Veterinary. 2008;**78**:297-305

[51] ReddyCRRM, MorasiahIL, ParthaviG, SomasundaraRao M. Epidemiology of hydatid disease in Kurnool. The Indian Journal of Medical Research. 1958;**56**:1205-1220

[52] Ingole RS, Khakse HD, Jadhao MG, Ingole SR. Prevalence of Echinococcus infection in dogs in Akola district of Maharashtra (India) by Copro- PCR. Veterinary Parasitology Regional Studies in Reports. 2018;**13**:60-63

[53] Mandal SC. Veterinary Parasitology at a Glance. 1st ed. Lucknow, India: International Book Distributing Company; 2006

[54] Taylor MA, Coop R, Wall RL. Veterinary Parasitology. 3rd ed. Oxford: Blackwell Publishing; 2007

[55] Drug Administration and Control authority of Ethiopia (DACA). Standard Treatment Guidelines for Veterinary Practice. 1st ed. Addis Ababa, Ethiopia: Champer Printing House; 2006. pp. 43-44

[56] Jokelainen P. Wild and Domestic Animals as Hosts of *T. gondii* in Finland. Finland: Faculty of Veterinary Medicine, University of Helsinki; 2013. pp. 15-28

[57] Dubey JP. The history of *Toxoplasma gondii*-the first 100 years. The Journal of Eukaryotic Microbiology. 2008;**55**(6):467-475

[58] Dubey JP. Toxoplasmosis in pigs-the last 20 years. Veterinary Parasitology. 2009;**164**(2-4):89-103

[59] Tenter AM, Heckeroth AR, Weiss LM. Toxoplasma gondii: From animal to humans. International Journal for Parasitology. 2000;**30**(12-13):1217-1258

[60] Pal AB, Gari G, Tuli G. Toxoplasmosis in animals and humans – Its diagnosis, epidemiology and control. International Journal of Livestock Research. 2014;**4**(2):22-25

[61] Buxton D, Maley SW, Wright SE, Rodger S, Bartley P, Innes EA. Toxoplasma gondii and ovine toxoplasmosis: New aspects of an old story. Veterinary Parasitology. 2007;**149**(1-2):25-28

[62] Rostami A, Riahi SM, Gamble HR, Fakhri Y, NourollahpourShiadeh M, Danesh M, et al. Global prevalence of latent toxoplasmosis in pregnant women: A systematic review and metaanalysis. Clinical Microbiology Infections. 2020;**20**:S1198

[63] Nogareda F, Le Strat Y, Villena I, De Valk H, Goulet V. Incidence and prevalence of *Toxoplasma gondii* infection in women in France, 1980-2020: Model-based estimation. Epidemiology and Infection. 2014;**142**(8):1661-1670

[64] Picone O, Fuchs F, Benoist G, Binquet C, Kieffer F, Wallon M, et al. Toxoplasmosis screening during pregnancy in France: Opinion of an expert panel for the CNGOF. Journal of Gynecology Obstetrics Human Reproductive. 2020;**16**:101814

[65] Dubey JP. Advances in the life cycle of *Toxoplasma gondii*. International Journal for Parasitology. 1998a;**28**(7):1019-1024

[66] Pozio E. World distribution of Trichinella spp. infections in animals and humans. Veterinary Parasitology. 2007;**149**(1-2):3-21

[67] International Commission on Trichinellosis. Trichinella and Trichinellosis. Available from: http://www.trichinellosis.org [Accessed: May 9, 2023]

[68] Boireau P, Vallée I, Roman T, Perret C, Mingyuan L, Gamble HR, et al. Trichinella in horses: A low frequency infection with high human risk. Veterinary Parasitology. 2000;**93**(3-4):309-320

[69] Liu M, Boireau P. Trichinellosis in China: Epidemiology and control. Trends in Parasitology. 2002;**18**(12):553-556

[70] Møller LN, Petersen E, Kapel CM, Melbye M, Koch A. Outbreak of trichinellosis associated with consumption of game meat in West Greenland. Veterinary Parasitology. 2005;**132**:131-136

[71] Gallardo MT, Mateos L, Artieda J, Wesslen L, Ruiz C, García MA, et al. Outbreak of trichinellosis in Spain and Sweden due to consumption of wild boar meat contaminated with Trichinella britovi. Euro Surveillance. 2007;**12**(3):E070315.1

[72] Nöckler K, Wichmann-Schauer H, Hiller P, Müller A, Bogner K-H. Trichinellosis outbreak in Bavaria caused by cured sausage from Romania. Euro Surveillance. 2007;**12**:EO70823.2

[73] Stensvold CR, Nielsen HV, Molbak K. A case of trichinellosis in Denmark, imported from Poland. Euro Surveillance. 2007;**12**:E070809.3

[74] Hefer E, Rishpon S, Volovik I. Trichinosis outbreak among Thai immigrant workers in the Hadera sub-district. Harefuah. 2004;**143**(9):656-660

[75] Marva E, Markovics A, Gdalevich M, Asor N, Sadik C, Leventhal A. Trichinellosis outbreak. Emerging Infectious Diseases. 2005;**11**:1979-1981

[76] Gamble HR, Bessonov AS, Cuperlovic K, Gajadhar AA, Van Knapen F, Noeckler K, et al. International Commission on trichinellosis: Recommendations on methods for the control of Trichinella in domestic and wild animals intended for human consumption. Veterinary Parasitology. 2000;**93**(3-4):393-408

[77] Office International des Épizooties. chapter 2.2.9. Trichinellosis. In: Manual of Standards for Diagnostic Tests and Vaccines. 5th ed. Paris, France: Office International des Épizooties; 2004

[78] Horton J. The use of antiprotozoan and anthelmintic drugs during pregnancy and contraindications. Journal of Infectology. 1993;**26**(1):104-105

[79] Dupouy-Camet J, Bruschi F. Management and diagnosis of human trichinellosis. In: Dupouy-Camet J, Murrell KD, editors. FAO/WHO/OIE Guidelines for the Surveillance, Management, Prevention and Control of Trichinellosis. Paris: World Organisation for Animal Health Press; 2007. pp. 37-68

Section 4

Viral Zoonoses

Chapter 12

Emerging and Neglected Viral Zoonoses in Europe

Tatjana Vilibić-Čavlek, Vladimir Savić, Snježana Židovec-Lepej, Maja Bogdanić, Vladimir Stevanović and Ljubo Barbić

Abstract

Zoonotic diseases are an important public health problem worldwide. Two large groups of zoonotic viruses include arboviruses and rodent-borne viruses. Avian influenza, SARS-CoV-2, hepatitis E, and recently re-emerged monkeypox are also medically important viral zoonoses. Tick-borne encephalitis is the most important tick-borne disease in Europe with a growing incidence. West Nile infections are continuously reported as small or large outbreaks. Although the number of Usutu virus infections showed an increasing trend, this arbovirus is still neglected as well as Toscana, Tahyna, and Bhanja viruses. The number of Crimean-Congo hemorrhagic fever cases is increasing in the recent years. Hantaviruses are the most important rodent-borne viruses. Orthohantavirus Puumala is responsible for more than 90% of hemorrhagic fever with renal syndrome cases in Europe; however, Dobrava orthohantavirus is also recorded. Lymphocytic choriomeningitis is a neglected viral zoonosis with unknown prevalence. Avian influenza outbreaks in poultry are on the rise over the past two decades, with a consequent increase in human infections. The SARS-CoV-2 pandemic has highlighted the importance of coronaviruses in human diseases. Hepatitis E virus is an emerging virus with zoonotic genotype 3 the most frequently detected in Europe. The epidemiology of monkeypox has changed with considerable human-to-human transmission, predominantly among men who have sex with men.

Keywords: viral zoonoses, Europe, arboviruses, rodent-borne viruses, influenza, SARS-CoV-2, hepatitis E, monkeypox

1. Introduction

Zoonoses represent an important public health problem worldwide. It is estimated that 60% of known infectious diseases and up to 75% of newly emerging diseases are zoonotic in origin [1]. Some zoonotic diseases are still neglected, mainly due to a lack of commercially available diagnostic tests. The most important emerging and neglected viral zoonoses in Europe are presented in **Table 1**.

Tick-borne encephalitis virus (TBEV) is one of the most important human tick-borne viral zoonoses in Europe and Asia. From 2012 to 2020, a significant increase

Virus(es)	Reservoir(s)	Main vector	Main clinical symptoms in humans
Arboviruses			
TBEV	Rodents	*Ixodes* spp.	Febrile headache, Meningitis, encephalitis
WNV	Birds	*Culex* spp.	WNV fever, meningitis, encephalitis, myelitis
USUV	Birds	*Culex* spp.	USUV fever, meningitis, encephalitis
TOSV	Unknown	*Phlebotomus* spp.	Flu-like disease, meningitis
TAHV		*Aedes vexans*	Flu-like disease, meningitis
BHAV	Hares, hedgehogs	*Haemaphysalis* spp.	Flu-like disease, meningitis
CCHFV	Rodents, livestock	*Hyalomma* spp.	Hemorrhagic fever
Rodent-borne viruses			
Hantaviruses	Rodents		HFRS, HPS
LCMV	*Mus musculus, Mus domesticus*		Flu-like disease, meningitis
Respiratory viruses			
AIV	Birds		Conjunctivitis, flu
SARS-CoV-2	Bats, humans		Flu-like disease, pneumonia
Other zoonotic viruses			
HEV	Pigs, wild boar		Hepatitis
MPXV	Rodents		Fever, rash, lymphadenopathy

TBEV = tick-borne encephalitis virus; WNV=West Nile virus; USUV=Usutu virus; TOSV = Toscana virus; TAHV = Tahyna virus; BHAV=Bhanja virus; CCHFV=Crimean-Congo hemorrhagic fever virus; LCMV = lymphocytic choriomeningitis virus; AIV = avian influenza virus; HEV = hepatitis E virus; MPXV = monkeypox virus; HFRS = hemorrhagic fever with renal syndrome; HPS = hantavirus pulmonary syndrome.

Table 1.
Emerging and neglected viral zoonoses in Europe.

in TBEV cases was recorded in the European Union/European Economic Area (EU/EEA) countries with 19 countries reporting 29.974 cases of TBE. The Czech Republic, Germany, and Lithuania reported 52.9% of all cases. TBE cases showed a seasonal distribution with the majority detected from April to November. In many countries, a bimodal distribution was observed with the first peak occurring in early July, and a second, usually smaller peak, at the end of September. Cases were predominantly males (59.5%) [2].

West Nile virus (WNV) is the most widely distributed mosquito-borne viral zoonosis in southern, eastern, and western Europe. Since 2012, WNV cases were continuously reported in small or large outbreaks. The largest outbreak so far was recorded in 2018, when the number of WNV cases exceeded the total number of infections reported between 2010 and 2017 [3]. Since 2008, the WNV lineage 2 has spread over central Europe and the eastern Mediterranean region and has become endemic causing significant outbreaks in humans and animals. WNV lineage 1 re-emerged in Italy in 2021 with a trend of rapid expansion. Comparative analysis of WNV lineage 1 and 2 suggested that WNV-1-infected patients might have an increased risk to develop severe neuroinvasive disease [4].

Although the number of human Usutu virus (USUV) infections is growing, this virus is still neglected in many European countries. To date, over 100 cases of acute human USUV infections have been described in Europe, including 30 patients with neuroinvasive disease. Most human clinical cases were reported in Italy because of active USUV circulation in this country [5]; however, cases of neuroinvasive disease were also reported in Croatia (2013, 2018) [6, 7], France (2016) [8], Hungary (2018) [9], and Austria (2019) [10].

Although Toscana virus (TOSV) is a frequent cause of aseptic meningitis in southwestern Europe, TOSV infection is not a notifiable disease in the EU/EEA. So far, more than 800 autochthonous and imported human cases were reported in residents of Mediterranean countries and in tourists and travelers returning from endemic areas [11]. In some European countries such as France and Italy, TOSV is among the three most common causes of meningitis in the summer months [12].

There are very limited data on the distribution and prevalence of Tahyna orthobunyavirus (TAHV) in the human population as well as the information on the public health significance of its natural foci in Europe. The TAHV disease is neglected and underreported [13]. Similarly, data on the human Bhanja bandavirus (BHAV) infections are very scarce.

Crimean-Congo hemorrhagic fever virus (CCHFV) is an emerging tick-borne arbovirus that causes severe disease with high fatality rates. In the EU/EEA and its neighboring countries, sporadic cases, as well as outbreaks of CCHF were reported in Albania, Bulgaria, Georgia, Greece, Kosovo, Russia, Spain, Ukraine, and Turkey. The number of cases is increasing in the recent years [14].

Puumala (PUUV) and Dobrava (DOBV) are the most frequent orthohantaviruses that cause hemorrhagic fever with renal syndrome (HFRS) in Europe. In the period 2016–2020, the overall HFRS notification rate varied between 0.4 and 1.0 cases/10.000 population, with no obvious long-term trend. Most cases were infected by PUUV (98.3%), and people aged 25 years and older accounted for 92% of cases [15]. Tula orthohantavirus has recently been molecularly confirmed as a human pathogen, resulting in a very mild form of HFRS [16].

Lymphocytic choriomeningitis virus (LCMV) is a neglected rodent-borne virus with very few reports of human infections. The disease has been underreported due to the restricted availability of serological testing, which makes it challenging to estimate the incidence. However, seroprevalence data suggest that the virus is present in Europe with seroprevalence rates of up to 15% in the general population [17]. However, in some highly endemic countries, seropositivity was high (37.5% in Slovakia and 36% in Croatian Vir Island) [18].

Avian influenza virus (AIV) is mainly an occupational (re-)emerging infection in humans in Europe. AIV of subtype H7N7 was detected in 86 humans who handled affected poultry and in three of their family members in the Netherlands in 2003 [19]. Although numerous human H5N1 infections occurred mainly in Asia and Africa, few human cases of H5N1 infection were recently reported in a poultry keeper and poultry workers in the United Kingdom [20].

Severe acute respiratory syndrome coronavirus 2 (SARS-CoV-2) is a novel coronavirus that caused over 6.9 million deaths worldwide by May 2023. The epidemiological situation of coronavirus disease (COVID-19) is continually evolving [21, 22].

Hepatitis E virus (HEV) infection is a global health problem, yet a clinically underdiagnosed cause of acute and chronic hepatitis. The zoonotic HEV3 genotype is the most common cause of infections in Europe [23]. In the past decade, a 10-fold increase in reported cases was observed in EU/EEA countries. Males above 50 years of age represent the majority of acute HEV cases [24].

Monkeypox virus (MPXV) represents a new global health emergency. Although the majority of cases of monkeypox were previously only identified in Africa, the current outbreak is being reported in many regions, including Europe. The first non-endemic outbreak of human monkeypox occurred in the United States (USA) in 2003 with 47 documented cases, but no community transmission, that was traced to imported infected West African rodents. Thereafter, sporadic cases of travel-associated MPXV infections were reported in Israel, the United Kingdom (UK), and the USA with limited secondary spread [25, 26]. In 2022, many countries in previously non-endemic regions reported multiple cases of monkeypox associated with considerable human-to-human transmission, starting with a cluster of cases in the UK in May 2022 [27]. Men who have sex with men (MSM) and bisexual men were predominantly affected in the 2022 outbreak [28].

2. Emerging and neglected arboviruses

Arboviruses are a diverse group of more than 500 viruses transmitted by arthropods (ticks, mosquitoes, sandflies). In nature, arboviruses are maintained in a cycle involving vertebrate hosts and hematophagous arthropods. Humans represent incidental or dead-end hosts for the majority of arboviral infections (**Figure 1**). However, human-to-human transmission through contact with infectious blood or body fluids is documented for CCHFV (**Figure 2**).

2.1 Tick-borne encephalitis virus

TBEV is a tick-borne flavivirus of the family *Flaviviridae*, genus *Flavivirus*, tick-borne encephalitis serocomplex. There are three main subtypes of TBEV: European, Far-East, and Siberian, which are distributed in a wide area from Europe to Japan. Two novel subtypes, the Baikalian subtype (Irkutsk region, Buryat

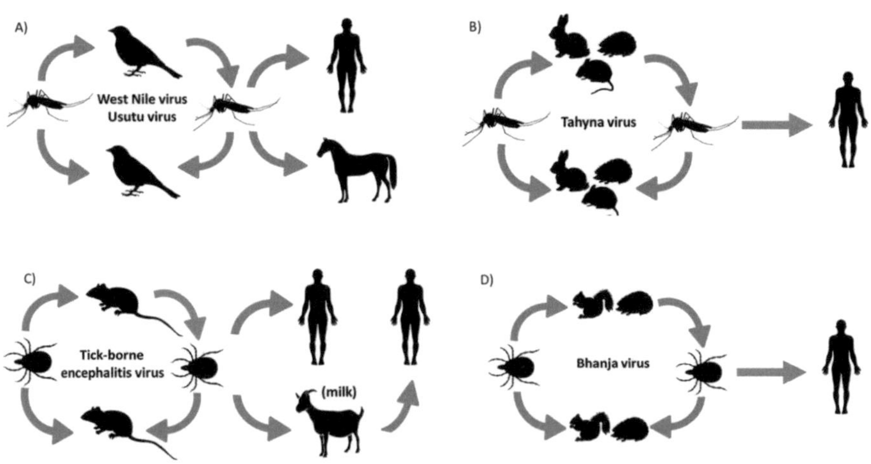

Figure 1.
Transmission cycle of mosquito-borne (A) and tick-borne arboviruses (B-D).

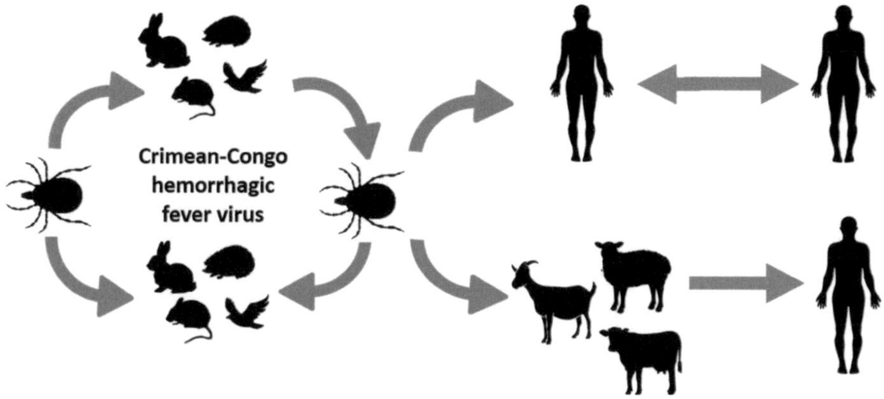

Figure 2.
Transmission cycle of Crimean-Congo hemorrhagic fever virus.

Republic, and Trans-Baikal Territory of Eastern Siberia) and the Himalayan subtype (Qinghai-Tibet Plateau, China), were discovered recently [29–31]. The virus is maintained in nature in a cycle involving ticks of the *Ixodes* spp. and small mammals such as rodents (genera *Apodemus* and *Myodes*). The larvae and nymphs mainly feed on small- and medium-sized mammals, and adults on large animals such as ungulates. Ticks could also be TBEV reservoirs since the virus can be transmitted transovarially and transstadially [32]. The most common mode of transmission to humans is by the bite of an infected tick; however, approximately 1% of infections are caused by food-borne transmission (mainly consumption of unpasteurized goat milk) [33]. Seroprevalence studies from endemic regions indicate that a significant proportion of TBEV infections (70–98%) remain asymptomatic. In general, children typically have a milder form of the disease than adults [29]. The European TBE is usually a biphasic disease. The first phase corresponds to viremia and manifests as fever, fatigue, malaise, headache, muscle, and joint pain. After an improvement of a few days, the second phase occurs characterized by central nervous system (CNS) involvement. The most common presentation of neuroinvasive disease in children is meningitis. In adults, meningitis, meningoencephalitis, and meningoencephalomyelitis occur in 50%, 40%, and 5–10% of patients, respectively [34]. The Siberian TBE also results in a generally mild disease associated with a non-paralytic form of encephalitis. The Far-East subtype of TBEV causes the most severe monophasic form of TBE. The case-fatality rate for the European subtype of TBEV is 0.5–2%, compared to 20% for the Far-East subtype [29]. Analysis of local and systemic cytokine responses in TBE patients revealed a complex network of early innate immune response cytokines, Th1, Th2, Th9, Th22, Th17, and anti-inflammatory cytokines characterized by significantly increased cerebrospinal fluid (CSF) concentrations of IL-6 and IFN-γ [35]. Since the virus has already been cleared from the blood and is very exceptionally present in the CSF at the time of neurological symptoms, isolation of TBEV from blood and detection of viral RNA by reverse transcriptase polymerase chain reaction (RT-PCR) in blood or CSF have a limited diagnostic value [36]. Diagnosis is usually confirmed by the detection of specific IgM and IgG antibodies in the serum and CSF. Determination of IgG avidity may be helpful in cases with atypical serological responses [37]. Vaccination is the most effective method of TBE prevention in endemic areas.

2.2 West Nile virus

WNV is a mosquito-borne flavivirus of the family *Flaviviridae*, genus *Flavivirus*, Japanese encephalitis serocomplex. There are several genetic lineages of which lineages 1 and 2 are the most important [38]. WNV is transmitted in an enzootic cycle between birds and mosquitoes, mainly *Culex* spp. Most human infections occur after the bite of infected mosquitoes. Interhuman transmission may occur through blood transfusion and organ transplantation from an infected and viremic donor [39]. In addition, rare cases of transplacental transmission and transmission through breastfeeding were also described [40]. The majority of human WNV infections are asymptomatic. About 20% of patients present with a non-specific febrile disease (WNV fever) and < 1%, and mainly elderly and immunocompromised patients develop WNV neuroinvasive disease (meningitis, encephalitis, myelitis). Rare clinical presentations of WNV infection include retinitis [41], cerebellitis [42], cauda equina arachnoiditis [43], and opsoclonus-myoclonus syndrome [44]. WNV meningitis manifests as fever, headache, and nuchal rigidity and is clinically indistinguishable from viral meningitis caused by other etiologies. WNV encephalitis is characterized by altered mental status, seizures, focal neurologic deficits, or movement disorders. WNV myelitis is clinically identical to myelitis caused by poliovirus (acute flaccid paralysis) and can progress to respiratory paralysis needing mechanical ventilation. The mortality in neuroinvasive disease is 10% [45]. Cytokine immune responses to WNV in neuroinvasive disease are characterized by increased concentrations of innate and early acute phase responses (IL-6) and Th1 type immune responses (IFN-γ) cytokines in the CSF with Th2, Th17, and pro-inflammatory cytokines in the periphery [46]. Due to short-term and low-level viremia, diagnosis of WNV is usually confirmed by serology. Since IgM antibodies may persist in some patients even years after primary infections, IgG determination could differentiate current from previous infections in these cases. Due to possible cross-reactivity with other flaviviruses, the virus neutralization test (VNT) is still a "gold standard" confirmatory test for the diagnosis of WNV [47]. Prevention of WNV includes preventing mosquito bites using insect repellents, wearing long-sleeved shirts and pants, treating clothing and gear, and controlling mosquitoes indoors and outdoors. Vaccine against WNV is available only for horses [48].

2.3 Usutu virus

USUV is a mosquito-borne flavivirus of the family *Flaviviridae*, genus *Flavivirus*, Japanese encephalitis serocomplex. Birds are the natural reservoirs of USUV, while ornithophilic mosquitoes of the *Culex* spp. are the main vectors. Some bird species such as sparrows (*Passer domesticus*), gray owls (*Strix nebulosi*), and blackbirds (*Turdus merula)* are particularly vulnerable to USUV infection and have a high mortality rate [49]. The virus is transmitted to humans by the bite of infected female mosquitoes. There are eight genetic lineages, five European (Europe 1–5) and three African (Africa 1–3) [50]. The zoonotic potential of USUV has confirmed in a growing number of human cases. Like WNV, the majority of human infections are asymptomatic or present as a non-specific febrile disease (USUV fever). Immunocompromised and elderly patients may develop USUV neuroinvasive disease (meningitis, encephalitis) [51]. USUV Europe 2 lineage is the most prevalent genetic lineage detected in humans [52]. The serological diagnosis of USUV is challenging due to cross-reactivity with other flaviviruses, in particular between USUV and WNV highlighting the need for VNT. Using an RT-PCR, viral RNA can be detected in blood and CSF; however, the sensitivity is low [53]. Since there is no vaccine available, preventing mosquito bites is the best way for USUV prevention.

2.4 Toscana virus

TOSV is a sandfly-borne phlebovirus of the family *Phenuiviridae*, genus *Phlebovirus*. So far, there is no evidence of a vertebrate species acting as a reservoir in the TOSV natural cycle. The virus is transmitted to humans through the bite of an infected female sandfly of the genus *Phlebotomus* (*P. perniciosus* and *P. perfiliewi*) [54]. To date, three genetic lineages A, B, and C of TOSV have been identified. Lineage A included strains initially discovered in Italy, whereas lineage B consisted of strains isolated first in Portugal and in Spain [55]. TOSV lineage C strains were reported in Croatia and Greece [56, 57]. TOSV infections have been recorded in residents of or travelers to Mediterranean countries. Furthermore, human seroprevalence studies conducted in Italy, Turkey, and Greece indicated continuing TOSV circulation. In northern Africa, the TOSV-neutralizing antibody seroprevalence rates are much higher (22–33%) than that observed in southwestern Europe (up to 10% in highly endemic areas) [54]. The majority of TOSV infection are asymptomatic or presented as mild febrile disease, which causes the number of cases to be underestimated and underreported. However, some patients develop neuroinvasive disease, mainly meningitis but in rare cases, fatal encephalitis has been reported [58]. Literature data on immune responses during TOSV infection are limited with one study reporting increased concentrations of IL-6, IFN-γ, and IL-10 in the CSF compared with serum in a limited case series [59]. Indirect immunofluorescence (IFA) and enzyme-immunoassay (EIA) are commonly used serological tests for the diagnosis of TOSV. Cross-reactions can occur between viruses antigenically close to TOSV such as Naples phlebovirus. VNT is recommended for confirmation because it is the most specific serological assay. Although the virus can be isolated in the acute phase from blood or CSF, TOSV RNA detection using real-time RT-PCR is the test of reference for direct diagnostic purposes [11].

2.5 Tahyna orthobunyavirus

TAHV is a mosquito-borne bunyavirus of the family *Peribunyaviridae*, genus *Orthobunyavirus*, California encephalitis serogroup. The vertebrate hosts for TAHV are hares, rabbits, hedgehogs, and rodents, while culicine mosquitoes, *Aedes vexans*, are the main vectors [60]. The disease caused by TAHV ("Valtice fever") was described in the 1960s after the virus was isolated from humans with acute flu-like illness in the Czech Republic [61]. Natural foci of TAHV occur in flooded lowland habitats, sometimes including suburban areas [62]. TAHV infections were reported in continental Europe, Asia, and Africa; however, the incidence of the disease is underestimated and underreported. The majority of TAHV infections are asymptomatic. Human disease caused by TAHV usually presents as a flu-like illness occurring in late summer and early autumn, mainly in children. Despite its association with neurovirulence (meningitis), TAHV infection remains a neglected disease, with rare reports of human clinical infections in the recent decades [61, 63]. However, up to 60–80% of seroprevalence rates have been documented in humans from endemic countries such as the Czech Republic [64]. Diagnosis is confirmed by the detection of TAHV RNA or specific antibodies.

2.6 Bhanja bandavirus

BHAV is a tick-borne bunyavirus of the family *Phenuiviridae*, genus *Bandavirus*. The vertebrate hosts for BHAV are sheep, goats, cattle, African hedgehogs (*Atelerix albiventris),* and African ground squirrels (*Xerus erythropus*), while metastriate ixodid ticks of the *Haemaphysalis* spp. are the main vectors. Human infections occur after a bite of an infected tick. Although BHAV is widely distributed in sub-Saharan Africa, central Europe, the Mediterranean basin, countries of the Middle East, and India, the virus is still neglected with only a few human clinical cases reported [65]. Laboratory BHAV infections were characterized by a low-grade fever, headache, muscle and joint pain, and photophobia that lasted 48 hours [66, 67]. Neuroinvasive infections presented with meningoencephalitis and pareses were also recorded [68]. Diagnosis of BHAV can be confirmed by the detection of viral RNA and/or specific antibodies [69].

2.7 Crimean-Congo hemorrhagic fever virus

CCHFV is a tick-borne bunyavirus of the family *Nairoviridae*, genus *Orthonairovirus*. Phylogenetic analysis of the S-segment CCHFV genome suggests seven major clades: clade I (Africa 2), clade II (Africa 1), clade III (Europe 2), clade IV (Africa 3), clade V (Europe 1), clade VI (Asia 1), and clade VII (Asia 2) [70]. The endemicity of CCHFV is closely associated with the geographical distribution of the reservoirs and vectors, ixodid ticks of the *Hyalomma* spp. Among ticks, the virus is transmitted transstadially and transovarially. CCHFV is transmitted to humans by bites of infected ticks or by direct contact with blood or tissues of viremic patients or viremic livestock [14]. The disease is endemic in all of Africa, the Middle East, Asia, and South-Eastern Europe. Abattoir workers, butchers, and farmers represent high-risk professions for CCHFV [70]. Seroprevalence studies indicate that the majority of CCHF infections (>80%) are asymptomatic or mild. The disease is usually milder in children. Hemorrhagic manifestations are present in severe cases, ranging from petechiae, epistaxis, and ecchymoses around the venipuncture sites to severe hemorrhages from different organs. The mortality rate may reach 40% [14]. In the acute phase of the disease, virus isolation (BSL-4), detection of viral RNA using RT-PCR, and antigen detection confirm the diagnosis of CCHF. IgM and IgG antibodies are detectable after the fifth day of the disease using EIA or IFA [71]. An inactivated vaccine propagated in the mouse brain is used in Bulgaria [72].

3. Emerging and neglected rodent-borne viruses

Orthohantaviruses and arenaviruses are important rodent-borne zoonotic viruses. Small rodents such as voles, rats, and mice are the natural reservoir. The chronically infected rodents shed the virus in urine, droppings, and saliva. Humans are mainly infected by inhalation of contaminated aerosols. Andes virus is the only rodent virus known to spread between humans (**Figure 3**) [73].

3.1 Orthohantaviruses

Orthohantaviruses are rodent-borne viruses of the family *Hantaviridae*, genus *Orthohantavirus*. Old World orthohantaviruses Hantaan (HTNV), DOBV, and Seoul (SEOV) cause HFRS in Europe and Asia, while New World orthohantaviruses cause

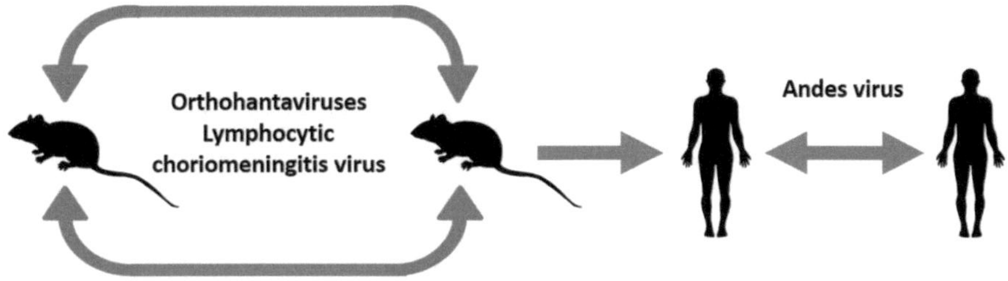

Figure 3.
Transmission cycle of rodent-borne viruses.

hantavirus pulmonary syndrome (HPS) in the Americas. Nephropathia epidemica (NE) is a mild form of HFRS, caused by PUUV in Europe [74]. HTNV was known to be hosted by striped field mice (*Apodemus agrarius*), PUUV by bank voles (*Clethrionomys glareolus*), DOBV by yellow neck mice (*Apodemus flavicollis*), and SEOV by rats (*Rattus rattus*, *Rattus norvegicus)* [75]. SEOV is the only hantavirus with a global distribution, but also the most underestimated and often missed pathogenic orthohantavirus [16]. Infected rodents excrete the virus in urine, feces, and saliva, and humans are mostly infected by inhaling the aerosolized contaminated rodent excreta [15]. In addition, studies suggest that human-to-human transmission of the Andes virus may be possible [76]. In Europe, human outbreaks are associated with the occurrence of mast years, i.e., years with abundant oak and beech seed resulting in an abundance of rodents [15]. Human hantavirus infections usually occur in rural areas such as forests, fields, and farms, but transmission occurs in urban areas as well. The main clinical symptoms of HFRS include acute kidney failure, acute shock and vascular leakage. The mortality in NE is less than 0.5% compared to 15% in HFRS caused by HTNV/DOBV and 40% in HPS [77]. The diagnosis of hantavirus infections in endemic areas is often based on clinical symptoms and the presence of specific IgM and IgG antibodies [78].

3.2 Lymphocytic choriomeningitis virus

LCMV is a zoonotic rodent-borne virus of the family *Arenaviridae*, genus *Mammarenavirus*. The common house mouse (*Mus musculus*, *Mus domesticus*) is the natural rodent host and reservoir for the LCMV. Humans become infected through mucosal exposure to aerosols contaminated with rodent excreta, direct contact with rodents, or rodent bites. Pregnant women infected with LCMV during pregnancy may transmit the virus transplacentally to the fetus [17]. LCMV probably circulates globally due to the cosmopolitan distribution of its reservoirs. However, the true prevalence of LCMV infections is unknown, as many of them are mild or asymptomatic. Phylogenetic analyses of LCMV showed this virus to be highly diverse. Four main lineages were identified with most of the strains clustered within lineage 1 [79]. In immunocompetent individuals, acquired LCMV infection may be asymptomatic in one-third of cases or present as a self-limited febrile illness. However, the disease can progress into meningitis or meningoencephalitis, with an overall mortality of less than 1% [80]. However, in organ transplant recipients, the infection can result in multisystem organ failure resembling the Lassa hemorrhagic fever with a very high fatality rate [81]. LCMV is also an important fetal teratogen. Hydrocephalus, periventricular calcifications, and chorioretinitis are the main characteristics of congenital infection. About 35% of congenitally infected children die, and 70% of them had long-term neurologic sequelae [82]. An RT-PCR has been developed for the detection of LCMV RNA in blood and CSF [83]. EIA and IFA can detect LCMV IgM and IgG antibodies; however, these tests are limited to several laboratories. The diagnosis is more complicated in congenitally infected children since the majority do not harbor the virus at the time of birth. Serology is most commonly used for the diagnosis of congenital LCMV infection; however, transplacentally transferred maternal IgG antibodies frequently complicate the diagnosis [17].

4. Emerging and neglected respiratory viruses

An increasing number of avian influenza outbreaks in domestic poultry during the past two decades caused particularly by the H5N1 subtype, and consequently led to at least 874 confirmed human cases and 458 deaths caused by this subtype in 23 countries across Asia, Africa, Europe, and Americas [84]. Several zoonotic coronaviruses have emerged in the past two decades. The SARS-CoV occurred in November 2002 in China and spread to over 30 countries by July 2003, resulting in more than 8.098 confirmed cases, including 774 deaths. Middle East respiratory syndrome coronavirus (MERS-CoV) emerged in 2012 in Saudi Arabia. In total, 27 countries have reported MERS-CoV cases since 2012, leading to more than 2.580 cases and 858 deaths. SARS-CoV-2 is the third coronavirus with a pandemic potential that emerged in late 2019 in China [85].

4.1 Avian influenza virus

AIVs, belonging to the type A influenza virus, contain a segmented RNA genome. They can be divided into subgroups according to differences in their surface glycoproteins. So far, 16 HA subtypes (H1-H16) and nine NA subtypes (N1-N9) are known and each AIV has one HA and one NA subtype that can occur in any of the 144 possible combinations (from H1N1 to H16N9). All HA and all NA subtypes can be found in wild aquatic birds, which are considered influenza A natural hosts in which AIVs generally do not cause disease [86]. On the other hand, very few HA and NA subtypes are established in other birds and mammals, including humans, causing disease in these hosts [87] such as seasonal influenza in humans contemporarily caused by H1N1 and H3N2 subtypes. Human infections with AIVs occur most often after unprotected contact with infected birds or surfaces contaminated with AIVs. People involved in culling AIV-infected poultry flocks are at particular risk of the infection [88]. Live bird markets in countries with enzootic avian influenza are also places where human infections commonly occur [89]. Although AIVs can be present in poultry commodities from infected birds, consumption of contaminated food has not been substantiated to cause human infections [90]. Symptoms largely vary from asymptomatic, mild upper respiratory symptoms, and conjunctivitis in the vast majority of reported infections with subtypes other than H5 or H7 [91] up to flu-like-illness with severe symptoms, including inflammation of the lower respiratory tract, respiratory distress, and multiple organ dysfunctions in case of infections with H5N1 and H7N9 subtypes [92, 93]. The fatality rates caused by these two subtypes are 53 and 39%, respectively. Diagnosis using real-time RT-PCR primarily targeting the M1 matrix gene is adopted in most laboratories followed by subsequent subtyping using subtype-specific PCR primers and probes. Serological tests have several limitations and should not be considered for initial detection [94]. There are no approved vaccines for preventing avian influenza in humans although candidate vaccine AIVs have been developed for pandemic preparedness purposes.

4.2 SARS-CoV-2

SARS-CoV-2 is a rapidly evolving RNA virus of the family *Coronaviridae*, genus *Betacoronavirus*. The ECDC differentiates variants of concern (VOC), variants of interest (VOI), or variants under monitoring [21]. Until late 2021, before the emergence of Omicron, VOC such as Alpha and Delta were mainly associated with increased transmissibility and modest degrees of immune escape. However, current evidence suggests that immune escape properties were the main driver for the displacement of Delta by Omicron [95]. The genome sequencing showed 96% concordance between human SARS-CoV-2 strains and SARS-CoV-like strains isolated from bats indicating that SARS-CoV-2 originates from bats. Similar coronaviruses were found in Malayan pangolins (*Manis javanica*) suggesting their possible role as intermediate hosts. Further studies confirmed that different animal species are susceptible to SARS-CoV-2 such as farmed minks, zoo animals, and companion animals [96, 97]. Human-to-human SARS-CoV-2 transmission occurs primarily through respiratory droplets and aerosols produced during coughing or sneezing. Patients aged ≥50 years are at a higher risk of severe COVID-19 [85]. The proportion of individuals with asymptomatic infection is unclear. Patients with mild illness may have a fever, cough, sore throat, headache, muscle pain, and loss of taste and smell. More severe cases present with pneumonia that can progress to acute respiratory distress syndrome. The case fatality rates are less than 2% [98]. RT-PCR is considered the gold standard for detecting COVID-19 infection. Serological tests enhance the capacity to diagnose SARS-CoV-2 and have broad clinical applications, including analyzing the immune response and identifying asymptomatic cases [99].

5. Other zoonotic viruses

5.1 Hepatitis E virus

HEV is a zoonotic virus of the family *Hepeviridae*, genus *Orthohepevirus*. Among the eight HEV genotypes in the *Orthohepevirus* A species identified so far, HEV1, HEV2, HEV3, and HEV4 are the most common genotypes causing human infections. HEV1 and HEV2 are prevalent in developing countries and can cause large-scale outbreaks originating from contaminated water. In contrast, HEV3 and HEV4 are zoonotic, and transmission to humans occurs mainly through contaminated raw or undercooked meat from infected animals (pigs, wild boars). HEV3 and HEV4 are distributed mostly in the developed countries [100]. Clinical manifestations of HEV infections include acute hepatitis, acute-on-chronic liver disease, chronic hepatitis, cirrhosis, and liver failure. Although the majority of HEV infections are acute and self-limiting, chronic HEV infections may occur in immunocompromised patients such as solid-organ transplant recipients [101]. In addition, HEV can cause severe hepatitis in pregnant women, especially in the third trimester, with a fatality rate of up to 20% [102]. HEV RNA and anti-HEV IgM antibodies can be detected in serum at the time of diagnosis, followed by anti-HEV IgG antibodies [100]. HEV vaccine has been developed and is licensed in China, but is not yet available elsewhere [103].

5.2 Monkeypox virus

MPXV is a zoonotic poxvirus of the family *Poxviridae*, genus *Orthopoxvirus*. Based on geography, disease severity, and sequence homology, MPXV strains were grouped into two genetic clades, the Central African/Congo Basin (CB) and West African (WA) clades. Some reports suggested that WA clade is associated with a milder disease [104]. The natural reservoirs of MPXV are small rodents. Transmission to humans occurs in direct contact with infected animals, through animal bites and scratches, as well as the handling and eating of infected animal meat. Human-to-human transmission may occur in prolonged direct contact with lesions and bodily fluids of patients, or indirect contact with objects such as bedding and clothing [105]. The clinical features of monkeypox include prodromal symptoms (fever, headache, malaise, chills, myalgia) lymphadenopathy, and a pleomorphic, often umbilicated skin rash [26]. However, in the most recent outbreak, several atypical presentations were observed. In MSM patients, genital lesions were present that subsequently spread to other parts of the body. Generally, monkeypox is a self-limited illness with a resolution over 2–4 weeks [106]. Detection of viral DNA in skin lesions using a PCR is a preferred test for diagnosis of MPXV. Oropharyngeal, anal, or rectal swabs are also suitable for testing in the absence of cutaneous lesions. Serology is not useful as it does not distinguish between different orthopoxviruses [105]. Since most cases of monkeypox are self-limiting, no specific antiviral therapy is indicated [107]. The vaccine protects against monkeypox and other orthopoxviruses, including smallpox and vaccinia [105].

6. Conclusions

Arthropod-borne and rodent-borne viral zoonoses are widely distributed in European countries and represent an important public health threat. While some (re-)emerging arboviruses such as TBEV and WNV are monitored continuously, USUV, TOSV, TAHV, and BHAV are still neglected and underreported. Orthohantaviruses are a significant cause of HFRS in Europe, while the incidence of LCMV is unknown. HEV is also a well-recognized emerging zoonotic virus in many European countries. Along with the above-mentioned zoonoses, the recent MPXV outbreak in non-endemic regions highlights the need for the “One Health approach” to prevent future zoonotic diseases.

Acknowledgements

This manuscript is supported by the project of the Croatian Science Foundation, IP-2016-06-7456: Prevalence and molecular epidemiology of emerging and re-emerging neuroinvasive arboviral infections in Croatia; CRONEUROARBO.

Author details

Tatjana Vilibić-Čavlek[1,2*], Vladimir Savić[3], Snježana Židovec-Lepej[4], Maja Bogdanić[1], Vladimir Stevanović[5] and Ljubo Barbić[5]

1 Croatian Institute of Public Health, Zagreb, Croatia

2 School of Medicine University of Zagreb, Zagreb, Croatia

3 Croatian Veterinary Institute, Zagreb, Croatia

4 University Hospital for Infectious Diseases "Dr Fran Mihaljević", Zagreb, Croatia

5 Faculty of Veterinary Medicine, University of Zagreb, Croatia

*Address all correspondence to: tatjana.vilibic-cavlek@hzjz.hr

References

[1] World Health Organization. Zoonotic Disease: Emerging Public Health Threats in the Region. Geneva, Switzerland: WHO; 2023. Available from: https://www.emro.who.int/fr/about-who/rc61/zoonotic-diseases.html

[2] Van Heuverswyn J, Hallmaier-Wacker LK, Beauté J, Gomes Dias J, Haussig JM, Busch K, et al. Spatiotemporal spread of tick-borne encephalitis in the EU/EEA, 2012 to 2020. Euro Surveillance. 2023;**28**:2200543. DOI: 10.2807/1560-7917.ES.2023.28.11.2200543

[3] Bakonyi T, Haussig JM. West Nile virus keeps on moving up in Europe. Euro Surveillance. 2020;**25**:2001938. DOI: 10.2807/1560-7917.ES.2020.25.46.2001938

[4] Barzon L, Pacenti M, Montarsi F, Fornasiero D, Gobbo F, Quaranta E, et al. Rapid spread of a new West Nile virus lineage 1 associated with increased risk of neuroinvasive disease during a large outbreak in northern Italy, 2022: One health analysis. Journal of Travel Medicine. 2022:taac125. DOI: 10.1093/jtm/taac125

[5] Pacenti M, Sinigaglia A, Martello T, De Rui ME, Franchin E, Pagni S, et al. Clinical and virological findings in patients with Usutu virus infection, Northern Italy, 2018. Euro Surveillance. 2019;**24**:1900180. DOI: 10.2807/1560-7917.ES.2019.24.47.1900180

[6] Santini M, Vilibic-Cavlek T, Barsic B, Barbic L, Savic V, Stevanovic V, et al. First cases of human Usutu virus neuroinvasive infection in Croatia, August-September 2013: Clinical and laboratory features. Journal of Neurovirology. 2015;**21**:92-97. DOI: 10.1007/s13365-014-0300-4

[7] Vilibic-Cavlek T, Savic V, Sabadi D, Peric L, Barbic L, Klobucar A, et al. Prevalence and molecular epidemiology of West Nile and Usutu virus infections in Croatia in the 'One health' context, 2018. Transboundary and Emerging Diseases. 2019;**66**:1946-1957. DOI: 10.1111/tbed.13225

[8] Simonin Y, Sillam O, Carles MJ, Gutierrez S, Gil P, Constant O, et al. Human Usutu virus infection with atypical neurologic presentation, Montpellier, France, 2016. Emerging Infectious Diseases. 2018;**24**:875-878. DOI: 10.3201/eid2405.171122

[9] Nagy A, Mezei E, Nagy O, Bakonyi T, Csonka N, Kaposi M, et al. Extraordinary increase in West Nile virus cases and first confirmed human Usutu virus infection in Hungary, 2018. Euro Surveillance. 2019;**24**:1900038. DOI: 10.2807/1560-7917.ES.2019.24.28.1900038

[10] Graninger M, Hubmer S, Riederer F, Kettner S, Hauk M, Auf T, et al. The first case of Usutu virus neuroinvasive disease in Austria, 2021. Open Forum Infectious Diseases. 2022;**9**:ofac255. DOI: 10.1093/ofid/ofac255

[11] Ayhan N, Charrel RN. An update on Toscana virus distribution, genetics, medical and diagnostic aspects. Clinical Microbiology and Infection. 2020;**26**:1017-1023. DOI: 10.1016/j.cmi.2019.12.015

[12] European Centre for Disease Prevention and Control. Toscana Virus Infection. Stockholm, Sweden: European Centre for Disease Prevention and Control; 2023. Available from:

https://www.ecdc.europa.eu/en/toscana-virus-infection

[13] Vilibic-Cavlek T, Barbic L, Mrzljak A, Brnic D, Klobucar A, Ilic M, et al. Emerging and neglected viruses of zoonotic importance in Croatia. Pathogens. 2021;**10**(1):73. DOI: 10.3390/pathogens10010073

[14] European Centre for Disease Prevention and Control. Factsheet about Crimean-Congo Haemorrhagic Fever. Stockholm, Sweden: European Centre for Disease Prevention and Control; 2023. Available from: https://www.ecdc.europa.eu/en/crimean-congo-haemorrhagic-fever/facts/factsheet

[15] European Centre for Disease Prevention and Control. Hantavirus Infection. Annual Epidemiological Report for 2020. Stockholm, Sweden: European Centre for Disease Prevention and Control; 2020. Available from: https://www.ecdc.europa.eu/sites/default/files/documents/Hantavirus-AER-2020.pdf

[16] Clement J, Ahlm C, Avšič-Županc T, Botten J, Chandran K, Jonsson CB, et al. Meeting report: Eleventh international conference on hantaviruses. Antiviral Research. 2020;**176**:104733. DOI: 10.1016/j.antiviral.2020.104733

[17] Vilibic-Cavlek T, Savic V, Ferenc T, Mrzljak A, Barbic L, Bogdanic M, et al. Lymphocytic choriomeningitis - emerging trends of a neglected virus: A narrative review. Tropical Medicine and Infectious Disease. 2021;**6**:88. DOI: 10.3390/tropicalmed6020088

[18] Dobec M, Dzelalija B, Punda-Polic V, Zoric I. High prevalence of antibodies to lymphocytic choriomeningitis virus in a murine typhus endemic region in Croatia. Journal of Medical Virology. 2006;**78**:1643-1647. DOI: 10.1002/jmv.20749

[19] Fouchier RA, Schneeberger PM, Rozendaal FW, Broekman JM, Kemink SA, Munster V, et al. Avian influenza a virus (H7N7) associated with human conjunctivitis and a fatal case of acute respiratory distress syndrome. PNAS. 2004;**101**:1356-1361

[20] Oliver I, Roberts J, Brown CS, Byrne AM, Mellon D, Hansen R, et al. A case of avian influenza a(H5N1) in England, January 2022. Euro Surveillance. 2022;**27**:2200061. DOI: 10.2807/1560-7917.ES.2022.27.5.2200061

[21] World Health Organization. Coronavirus (COVID-19) Dashboard. Geneva, Switzerland: WHO; 2023. Available from: https://covid19.who.int/

[22] ECDC. COVID-19 situation updates. Stockholm, Sweden: ECDC; 2023. Available from: https://www.ecdc.europa.eu/en/covid-19/situation-updates

[23] Willauer AN, Sherman KE. Hepatitis E virus: Has anything changed? Current Opinion in Gastroenterology. 2023;**39**:169-174. DOI: 10.1097/MOG.0000000000000918

[24] European Centre for Disease Prevention and Control. Facts about Hepatitis E. Stockholm, Sweden: European Centre for Disease Prevention and Control; 2023. Available from: https://www.ecdc.europa.eu/en/hepatitis-e/facts

[25] Reed KD, Melski JW, Graham MB, Regnery RL, Sotir MJ, Wegner MV, et al. The detection of monkeypox in humans in the Western hemisphere. The New England Journal of Medicine. 2004;**350**:342-350. DOI: 10.1056/NEJMoa032299

[26] Rajsri KS, Rao M. A review of Monkeypox: The new global health emergency. Venereology. 2022;**1**:199-211. DOI: 10.3390/venereology1020014

[27] Center for Disease Control and Prevention. 2022 Monkeypox Outbreak Global Map. Poxvirus. Atlanta, Georgia: Center for Disease Control and Prevention; 2023. Available from: https://www.cdc.gov/poxvirus/monkeypox/response/2022/world-map.html

[28] Hatami H, Jamshidi P, Arbabi M, Safavi-Naini SAA, Farokh P, Izadi-Jorshari G, et al. Demographic, epidemiologic, and clinical characteristics of human monkeypox disease pre- and Post-2022 outbreaks: A systematic review and meta-analysis. Biomedicine. 2023;**11**:957. DOI: 10.3390/biomedicines11030957

[29] Ruzek D, Avšič Županc T, Borde J, Chrdle A, Eyer L, Karganova G, et al. Tick-borne encephalitis in Europe and Russia: Review of pathogenesis, clinical features, therapy, and vaccines. Antiviral Research. 2019;**164**:23-51. DOI: 10.1016/j.antiviral.2019.01.014

[30] Sukhorukov GA, Paramonov AI, Lisak OV, Kozlova IV, Bazykin GA, Neverov AD, et al. The Baikal subtype of tick-borne encephalitis virus is evident of recombination between Siberian and far-eastern subtypes. PLoS Neglected Tropical Diseases. 2023;**17**:e0011141. DOI: 10.1371/journal.pntd.0011141

[31] Dai X, Shang G, Lu S, Yang J, Xu J. A new subtype of eastern tick-borne encephalitis virus discovered in Qinghai-Tibet plateau, China. Emerging Microbes & Infections. 2018;7:74. DOI: 10.1038/s41426-018-0081-6

[32] Bournez L, Umhang G, Moinet M, Richomme C, Demerson JM, Caillot C, et al. Tick-borne encephalitis virus: Seasonal and annual variation of epidemiological parameters related to nymph-to-larva transmission and exposure of small mammals. Pathogens. 2020;**9**:518. DOI: 10.3390/pathogens9070518

[33] Buczek AM, Buczek W, Buczek A, Wysokińska-Miszczuk J. Food-borne transmission of tick-borne encephalitis virus-spread, consequences, and prophylaxis. International Journal of Environmental Research and Public Health. 2022;**19**:1812. DOI: 10.3390/ijerph19031812

[34] Bogovič P, Lotrič-Furlan S, Avšič-Županc T, Korva M, Kastrin A, Lusa L, et al. Comparison of clinical, laboratory and immune characteristics of the monophasic and biphasic course of tick-borne encephalitis. Microorganisms. 2021;**9**:796. DOI: 10.3390/microorganisms9040796

[35] Zidovec-Lepej S, Vilibic-Cavlek T, Ilic M, Gorenec L, Grgic I, Bogdanic M, et al. Quantification of antiviral cytokines in serum, cerebrospinal fluid and urine of patients with tick-borne encephalitis in Croatia. Vaccine. 2022;**10**:1825. DOI: 10.3390/vaccines10111825

[36] Bogovic P, Strle F. Tick-borne encephalitis: A review of epidemiology, clinical characteristics, and management. World Journal of Clinical Cases. 2015;**3**:430-441. DOI: 10.12998/wjcc.v3.i5.430

[37] Vilibic-Cavlek T, Barbic L, Stevanovic V, Petrovic G, Mlinaric-Galinovic G. IgG avidity: An important serologic marker for the diagnosis of tick-borne encephalitis virus infection. Polish Journal of Microbiology. 2016;**65**:119-121. DOI: 10.5604/17331331.1197285

[38] Rizzoli A, Jimenez-Clavero MA, Barzon L, Cordioli P, Figuerola J, Koraka P, et al. The challenge of West Nile virus in Europe: Knowledge gaps and research priorities. Euro Surveillance. 2015;**20**:21135. DOI: 10.2807/1560-7917.es2015.20.20.21135

[39] Mrzljak A, Dinjar-Kujundzic P, Santini M, Barbic L, Kosuta I, Savic V, et al. West Nile virus: An emerging threat in transplant population. Vector Borne and Zoonotic Diseases. 2020;**20**:613-618. DOI: 10.1089/VBZ.2019.2608

[40] Hinckley AF, O'Leary DR, Hayes EB. Transmission of West Nile virus through human breast milk seems to be rare. Pediatrics. 2007;**119**:e666-e671. DOI: 10.1542/peds.2006-2107

[41] Konjevoda S, Dzelalija B, Canovic S, Pastar Z, Savic V, Tabain I, et al. West Nile virus retinitis in a patient with neuroinvasive disease. Revista da Sociedade Brasileira de Medicina Tropical. 2019;**52**:e20190065. DOI: 10.1590/0037-8682-0065-2019

[42] Natarajan N, Varman M. West Nile virus cerebellitis in a healthy 10-year-old child. The Pediatric Infectious Disease Journal. 2007;**26**:767. DOI: 10.1097/INF.0b013e3180cc2c3f

[43] Santini M, Zupetic I, Viskovic K, Krznaric J, Kutlesa M, Krajinovic V, et al. Cauda equina arachnoiditis - a rare manifestation of West Nile virus neuroinvasive disease: A case report. World Journal of Clinical Cases. 2020;**8**:3797-3803. DOI: 10.12998/wjcc.v8.i17.3797

[44] Papageorgiou E, Xanthou F, Dardiotis E, Tsironi EE. Dancing eyes syndrome from West Nile virus encephalitis. Postgraduate Medical Journal. 2020;**96**:442. DOI: 10.1136/postgradmedj-2020-137827

[45] Centers for Disease Control and Prevention. West Nile virus. Atlanta, Georgia: Centers for Disease Control and Prevention; 2023. Available from: https://www.cdc.gov/westnile/index.html

[46] Zidovec-Lepej S, Vilibic-Cavlek T, Barbic L, Ilic M, Savic V, Tabain I, et al. Antiviral cytokine response in neuroinvasive and non-neuroinvasive West Nile virus infection. Viruses. 2021;**13**:342. DOI: 10.3390/v13020342

[47] Vilibic-Cavlek T, Kristofic B, Savic V, Kolaric B, Barbic L, Tabain I, et al. Diagnostic significance of immunoglobulin G avidity in symptomatic and asymptomatic West Nile virus infection. Revista da Sociedade Brasileira de Medicina Tropical. 2018;**51**:591-595. DOI: 10.1590/0037-8682-0482-2017

[48] Ng T, Hathaway D, Jennings N, Champ D, Chiang YW, Chu HJ. Equine vaccine for West Nile virus. Developmental Biology (Basel). 2003;**114**:221-227

[49] Cadar D, Simonin Y. Human Usutu virus infections in Europe: A new risk on horizon? Viruses. 2022;**15**:77. DOI: 10.3390/v15010077

[50] Cadar D, Lühken R, van der Jeugd H, Garigliany M, Ziegler U, Keller M, et al. Widespread activity of multiple lineages of Usutu virus, Western Europe, 2016. Euro Surveillance. 2017;**22**:30452. DOI: 10.2807/1560-7917.ES.2017.22.4.30452

[51] Grottola A, Marcacci M, Tagliazucchi S, Gennari W, Di Gennaro A, Orsini M, et al. Usutu virus infections in humans: A retrospective analysis in the municipality of Modena, Italy. Clinical Microbiology and Infection. 2017;**23**:33-37. DOI: 10.1016/j.cmi.2016.09.019

[52] Vilibic-Cavlek T, Petrovic T, Savic V, Lj B, Tabain I, Stevanovic V, et al. Epidemiology of Usutu virus: The European scenario. Pathogens. 2020;**9**:E699

[53] Nikolay B, Weidmann M, Dupressoir A, Faye O, Boye CS, Diallo M, et al. Development of a Usutu virus specific real-time reverse transcription PCR assay based on sequenced strains from Africa and Europe. Journal of Virological Methods. 2014;**197**:51-54. DOI: 10.1016/j.jviromet.2013.08.039

[54] Ayhan N, Prudhomme J, Laroche L, Bañuls AL, Charrel RN. Broader geographical distribution of Toscana virus in the Mediterranean region suggests the existence of larger varieties of sand fly vectors. Microorganisms. 2020;**8**:114. DOI: 10.3390/microorganisms8010114

[55] Baggieri M, Marchi A, Bucci P, Nicoletti L, Magurano F. Genetic variability of the S segment of Toscana virus. Virus Research. 2015;**200**:35-44. DOI: 10.1016/j.virusres.2015.01.013

[56] Ayhan N, Alten B, Ivovic V, Martinkovic F, Kasap OE, Ozbel Y, et al. Cocirculation of two lineages of Toscana virus in Croatia. Frontiers in Public Health. 2017;**5**:336. DOI: 10.3389/fpubh.2017.00336

[57] Papa A, Paraforou T, Papakonstantinou I, Pagdatoglou K, Kontana A, Koukoubani T. Severe encephalitis caused by Toscana virus, Greece. Emerging Infectious Diseases. 2014;**20**:1417-1419. DOI: 10.3201/eid2008.140248

[58] Bartels S, de Boni L, Kretzschmar HA, Heckmann JG. Lethal encephalitis caused by the Toscana virus in an elderly patient. Journal of Neurology. 2012;**259**:175-177. DOI: 10.1007/s00415-011-6121-y

[59] Vilibic-Cavlek T, Zidovec-Lepej S, Ledina D, Knezevic S, Savic V, Tabain I, et al. Clinical, virological, and immunological findings in patients with Toscana neuroinvasive disease in Croatia: Report of three cases. Tropical Medicine and Infectious Disease. 2020;**5**:144. DOI: 10.3390/tropicalmed5030144

[60] Camp JV, Kniha E, Obwaller AG, Walochnik J, Nowotny N. The transmission ecology of Tahyna orthobunyavirus in Austria as revealed by longitudinal mosquito sampling and blood meal analysis in floodplain habitats. Parasites & Vectors. 2021;**14**:561. DOI: 10.1186/s13071-021-05061-1

[61] Mravcová K, Camp JV, Hubálek Z, Šikutová S, Vaux AGC, Medlock JM, et al. Ťahyňa virus-a widespread, but neglected mosquito-borne virus in Europe. Zoonoses and Public Health. 2023;**70**(5):371-382. DOI: 10.1111/zph.13042

[62] Hubálek Z. Mosquito-borne viruses in Europe. Parasitology Research. 2008;**103**(Suppl. S1):S29-S43. DOI: 10.1007/s00436-008-1064-7

[63] Vilibic-Cavlek T, Stevanovic V, Savic V, Markelic D, Sabadi D, Bogdanic M, et al. Detection of Tahyna Orthobunyavirus-neutralizing antibodies in patients with neuroinvasive disease in Croatia. Microorganisms. 2022;**10**:1443. DOI: 10.3390/microorganisms10071443

[64] Hubálek Z. History of arbovirus research in the Czech Republic. Viruses. 2021;**13**:2334. DOI: 10.3390/v13112334

[65] Hubálek Z. Biogeography of tick-borne Bhanja virus (bunyaviridae) in

Europe. Interdisciplinary Perspectives on Infectious Diseases. 2009;**2009**:372691. DOI: 10.1155/2009/372691

[66] Calisher CH, Goodpasture HC. Human infection with Bhanja virus. The American Journal of Tropical Medicine and Hygiene. 1975;**24**: 1040-1042

[67] Punda V, Beus I, Calisher CH, Vesenjak-Hirjan J. Laboratory infections with Bhanja virus. Zentralblatt fur Bakteriologie. 1980;(Suppl. 9):273-275

[68] Vesenjak-Hirjan J, Calisher CH, Beus I, Marton E. First natural clinical human Bhanja virus infection. Zentralblatt fur Bakteriologie. 1980;(Suppl. 9):297-301

[69] Matsuno K, Weisend C, Travassos da Rosa AP, Anzick SL, Dahlstrom E, Porcella SF, et al. Characterization of the Bhanja serogroup viruses (Bunyaviridae): A novel species of the genus phlebovirus and its relationship with other emerging tick-borne phleboviruses. Journal of Virology. 2013;**87**:3719-3728. DOI: 10.1128/JVI.02845-12

[70] Shahhosseini N, Wong G, Babuadze G, Camp JV, Ergonul O, Kobinger GP, et al. Crimean-Congo hemorrhagic fever virus in Asia, Africa and Europe. Microorganisms. 2021;**9**:1907. DOI: 10.3390/microorganisms9091907

[71] Centers for Disease Control and Prevention. Crimean-Congo Hemorrhagic Fever. Atlanta, Georgia: Centers for Disease Control and Prevention; 2023. Available from: https://www.cdc.gov/vhf/crimean-congo/index.html

[72] Papa A, Papadimitriou E, Christova I. The Bulgarian vaccine Crimean-Congo haemorrhagic fever virus strain. Scandinavian Journal of Infectious Diseases. 2011;**43**:225-229. DOI: 10.3109/00365548.2010.540036

[73] Martinez VP, Bellomo C, San Juan J, Pinna D, Forlenza R, Elder M, et al. Person-to-person transmission of Andes virus. Emerging Infectious Diseases. 2005;**11**:1848-1853. DOI: 10.3201/eid1112.050501

[74] Vial PA, Ferrés M, Vial C, Klingström J, Ahlm C, López R, et al. Hantavirus in humans: A review of clinical aspects and management. The Lancet Infectious Diseases. 2023;**S1473-3099**(23):00128-00127. DOI: 10.1016/S1473-3099(23)00128-7

[75] Kuhn JH, Schmaljohn CS. A brief history of Bunyaviral family *Hantaviridae*. Diseases. 2023;**11**:38. DOI: 10.3390/diseases11010038

[76] Toledo J, Haby MM, Reveiz L, Sosa Leon L, Angerami R, Aldighieri S. Evidence for human-to-human transmission of hantavirus: A systematic review. The Journal of Infectious Diseases. 2022;**226**:1362-1371. DOI: 10.1093/infdis/jiab461

[77] Romero MG, Anjum F. Hemorrhagic Fever Renal Syndrome. [Updated 2022 Jul 19]. Treasure Island (FL): StatPearls Publishing; 2023. Available from: https://www.ncbi.nlm.nih.gov/books/NBK560660/

[78] Sehgal A, Mehta S, Sahay K, Martynova E, Rizvanov A, Baranwal M, et al. Hemorrhagic fever with renal syndrome in Asia: History, pathogenesis, diagnosis, treatment, and prevention. Viruses. 2023;**15**:561. DOI: 10.3390/v15020561

[79] Albariño CG, Palacios G, Khristova ML, Erickson BR, Carroll SA, Comer JA, et al. High diversity and ancient common ancestry of lymphocytic

choriomeningitis virus. Emerging Infectious Diseases. 2010;**16**:1093-1100. DOI: 10.3201/eid1607.091902

[80] Bonthius DJ. The arenaviruses. In: Reiss CS, editor. Neurotropic Viral Infections. Berlin/Heidelberg: Springer; 2016. pp. 149-174. DOI: 10.1007/978-3-319-33133-1_6

[81] Schafer IJ, Miller R, Ströher U, Knust B, Nichol ST, Rollin PE, et al. Notes from the field: A cluster of lymphocytic choriomeningitis virus infections transmitted through organ transplantation - Iowa, 2013. MMWR. Morbidity and Mortality Weekly Report. 2014;**63**:249. DOI: 10.1111/ajt.12802

[82] Ferenc T, Vujica M, Mrzljak A, Vilibic-Cavlek T. Lymphocytic choriomeningitis virus: An under-recognized congenital teratogen. World Journal of Clinical Cases. 2022;**10**:8922-8931. DOI: 10.12998/wjcc.v10.i25.8922

[83] Cordey S, Sahli R, Moraz ML, Estrade C, Morandi L, Cherpillod P, et al. Analytical validation of a lymphocytic choriomeningitis virus real-time RT-PCR assay. Journal of Virological Methods. 2011;**177**:118-122. DOI: 10.1016/j.jviromet.2011.06.018

[84] World Health Organization. Cumulative Number of Confirmed Human Cases of Avian Influenza a(H5N1) Reported to WHO. 2003-2023. Geneva, Switzerland: WHO; 2023. Available from: https://cdn.who.int/media/docs/default-source/global-influenza-programme/2023_march_tableh5n1.pdf?sfvrsn=ec46922b_1&download=true

[85] Li Q, Guan X, Wu P, Wang X, Zhou L, Tong Y, et al. Early transmission dynamics in Wuhan, China, of novel coronavirus-infected pneumonia. The New England Journal of Medicine. 2020;**382**:1199-1207. DOI: 10.1056/NEJMoa2001316

[86] Swayne DE, Suarez DL, Sims LD. Influenza. In: Swayne DE, Boulianne M, Logue C, McDougald LR, Nair V, Suarez DL, editors. Diseases of Poultry. 14th ed. Ames: Wiley Publishing; 2020. pp. 210-256

[87] Suarez DL. Evolution of avian influenza viruses. Veterinary Microbiology. 2000;**74**:5-27. DOI: 10.1016/s0378-1135(00)00161-9

[88] Farahat RA, Khan SH, Rabaan AA, Al-Tawfiq JA. The resurgence of avian influenza and human infection: A brief outlook. New Microbes New Infections. 2023;**53**:101122. DOI: 10.1016/j.nmni.2023.101122

[89] Li YT, Linster M, Mendenhall IH, Su YCF, Smith GJD. Avian influenza viruses in humans: Lessons from past outbreaks. British Medical Bulletin. 2019;**132**:81-95. DOI: 10.1093/bmb/ldz036

[90] Harder TC, Buda S, Hengel H, Beer M, Mettenleiter TC. Poultry food products-a source of avian influenza virus transmission to humans? Clinical Microbiology and Infection. 2016;**22**:141-146. DOI: 10.1016/j.cmi.2015.11.015

[91] Freidl GS, Meijer A, de Bruin E, de Nardi M, Munoz O, Capua I, et al. Influenza at the animal-human interface: A review of the literature for virological evidence of human infection with swine or avian influenza viruses other than a(H5N1). Euro Surveillance. 2014;**19**:20793. DOI: 10.2807/1560-7917.es2014.19.18.20793

[92] Beigel JH, Farrar J, Han AM, Hayden FG, Hyer R, de Jong MD, et al. Writing Committee of the World Health Organization (WHO) consultation on

human influenza a/H5. Avian influenza a (H5N1) infection in humans. The New England Journal of Medicine. 2005;**353**:1374-1385. DOI: 10.1056/NEJMra052211

[93] Gao R, Cao B, Hu Y, Feng Z, Wang D, Hu W, et al. Human infection with a novel avian-origin influenza a (H7N9) virus. The New England Journal of Medicine. 2013;**368**:1888-1897. DOI: 10.1056/NEJMoa1304459

[94] European Centre for Disease Prevention and Control. Testing and Detection of Zoonotic Influenza Virus Infections in Humans in the EU/EEA, and Occupational Safety and Health Measures for those Exposed at Work. Stockholm, Sweden: European Centre for Disease Prevention and Control; 2022. Available from: https://www.ecdc.europa.eu/en/publications-data/zoonotic-influenza-virus-infections-humans-testing-and-detection

[95] Markov PV, Ghafari M, Beer M, Lythgoe K, Simmonds P, Stilianakis NI, et al. The evolution of SARS-CoV-2. Nature Reviews. Microbiology. 2023;**21**:361-379. DOI: 10.1038/s41579-023-00878-2

[96] Valencak TG, Csiszar A, Szalai G, Podlutsky A, Tarantini S, Fazekas-Pongor V, et al. Animal reservoirs of SARS-CoV-2: Calculable COVID-19 risk for older adults from animal to human transmission. Geroscience. 2021;**43**:2305-2320. DOI: 10.1007/s11357-021-00444-9

[97] Stevanovic V, Vilibic-Cavlek T, Tabain I, Benvin I, Kovac S, Hruskar Z, et al. Seroprevalence of SARS-CoV-2 infection among pet animals in Croatia and potential public health impact. Transboundary and Emerging Diseases. 2021;**68**:1767-1773. DOI: 10.1111/tbed.13924

[98] National Institutes of Health. Coronavirus Disease 2019 (COVID-19) Treatment Guidelines. Bethesda, Maryland: National Institutes of Health; 2023. Available from: https://www.covid19treatmentguidelines.nih.gov/

[99] Vilibic-Cavlek T, Bogdanic M, Borko E, Hruskar Z, Zilic D, Ferenc T, et al. Detection of SARS-CoV-2 antibodies: Comparison of enzyme immunoassay, surrogate neutralization and virus neutralization test. Antibodies. 2023;**12**(2):35. DOI: 10.3390/antib1202003

[100] Aslan AT, Balaban HY. Hepatitis E virus: Epidemiology, diagnosis, clinical manifestations, and treatment. World Journal of Gastroenterology. 2020;**26**:5543-5560. DOI: 10.3748/wjg.v26.i37.5543

[101] Samala N, Wang RY, Auh S, Balla AK, Dakhoul L, Alter HJ, et al. Hepatitis E prevalence and infection in solid-organ transplant recipients in the United States. Journal of Viral Hepatitis. 2022;**29**:1134-1142. DOI: 10.1111/jvh.13739

[102] Jha K, Tandukar A, Aryal R, Shrestha P, Bajracharya S, Bista KD. Severe hepatitis E infection in pregnancy: A case report. Annals of Medicine and Surgery (Lond). 2023;**85**:1213-1215. DOI: 10.1097/MS9.0000000000000449

[103] World Health Organization. Hepatitis E. Geneva, Switzerland: World Health Organization; 2023. Available from: https://www.who.int/news-room/fact-sheets/detail/hepatitis-e

[104] Likos AM, Sammons SA, Olson VA, Frace AM, Li Y, Olsen-Rasmussen M, et al. A tale of two clades: Monkeypox viruses. The Journal of General Virology. 2005;**86**:2661-2672. DOI: 10.1099/vir.0.81215-0

[105] European Centre for Disease Prevention and Control. Factsheet for Health Professionals on Mpox (Monkeypox). Stockholm, Sweden: European Centre for Disease Prevention and Control; 2023. Available from: https://www.ecdc.europa.eu/en/all-topics-z/monkeypox/factsheet-health-professionals

[106] Lum FM, Torres-Ruesta A, Tay MZ, Lin RTP, Lye DC, Rénia L, et al. Monkeypox: Disease epidemiology, host immunity and clinical interventions. Nature Reviews. Immunology. 2022;**22**:597-613. DOI: 10.1038/s41577-022-00775-4

[107] Singhal T, Kabra SK, Lodha R. Monkeypox: A review. Indian Journal of Pediatrics. 2022;**89**:955-960. DOI: 10.1007/s12098-022-04348-0

Chapter 13

Oral Health and Zoonotic Diseases

Betsy Joseph, Archana Mootha, Vishnupriya K. Sweety and Sukumaran Anil

Abstract

Zoonotic diseases, transmitted between animals and humans, have significant implications on public health, including oral health. This chapter aims to provide a comprehensive overview of the oral manifestations of zoonotic diseases and their prevention, highlighting the importance of early recognition and management by dental professionals. The chapter will discuss the various oral manifestations associated with common zoonotic diseases, such as periodontal manifestations, mucosal lesions, and salivary gland disorders, emphasizing the need for accurate diagnosis and timely referral to appropriate healthcare providers. Moreover, the chapter will delve into the role of dental professionals in preventing zoonotic disease transmission in clinical settings. It will explore the significance of education and training in recognizing and managing the oral manifestations of zoonotic diseases. Additionally, the chapter will emphasize the implementation of preventive measures, including the appropriate use of personal protective equipment, adherence to stringent infection control protocols, and the development of animal handling policies. By highlighting the intricate relationship between oral health and zoonotic diseases, this chapter aims to underscore the critical role of dental professionals in safeguarding the health and well-being of their patients and communities.

Keywords: zoonotic diseases, oral manifestations, disease prevention, dental professionals, infection control, diagnosis, periodontal disorders, interdisciplinary collaboration

1. Introduction

Zoonotic diseases, also known as zoonoses, are infectious diseases that can be transmitted between animals and humans. These diseases are caused by a variety of pathogens, including viruses, bacteria, parasites, and fungi. Zoonotic diseases can be spread through various mechanisms, such as direct contact with animals, contact with animal products or waste, ingestion of contaminated food or water, and transmission by vectors like insects [1]. Zoonotic diseases have been a part of human history for centuries, with some of the most well-known examples being rabies, Lyme disease, and the H1N1 influenza (swine flu) [2]. The emergence and spread of zoonotic diseases are influenced by several factors, including human encroachment on wildlife habitats, increased interactions between humans and animals, climate change, and global trade and travel [3]. As the human population continues to grow and expand, there is increasing pressure on ecosystems and natural habitats. This encroachment often leads to closer interactions between humans, domestic animals, and wildlife, creating more opportunities for zoonotic diseases to emerge and spread. Urbanization, deforestation, and changes in land use are some of the factors that contribute to this phenomenon [4].

1.1 Oral health and zoonotic disease

Oral health plays a crucial role in the overall well-being of individuals. While it is often overlooked, oral hygiene has significant implications not only for dental health but also for general health, including the prevention and control of zoonotic diseases. Zoonotic diseases are infectious diseases that can be transmitted between animals and humans, with pathogens including viruses, bacteria, parasites, and fungi. Oral health and zoonotic diseases are closely interconnected, with various mechanisms linking the two. Poor oral hygiene can create an environment conducive to the growth and proliferation of harmful microorganisms, including those responsible for zoonotic diseases [5]. Moreover, some zoonotic pathogens can be transmitted through saliva, making oral health an essential factor in preventing disease transmission. For instance, rabies, a viral zoonotic disease, is primarily transmitted through the saliva of infected animals via bites or scratches [6]. A compromised oral health status can weaken the immune system, making individuals more susceptible to infections, including zoonotic diseases [7]. A healthy oral environment is essential for maintaining a strong immune system and reducing the risk of contracting and spreading zoonotic diseases. **Table 1** describes zoonotic diseases and their transmission modes.

Sl No	Condition	Causative organism	Vector	Transmission mode
Viral zoonotic diseases				
1	Monkeypox	Monkeypox virus	Rodents and primates	Human-to-human transmission through respiratory droplets or contact with bodily fluids
2	COVID-19	SARS-CoV-2 virus	Originated in bats, transmitted to humans through an intermediate host, possibly a pangolin	Transmission through respiratory droplets or contact with bodily fluids
3	Hand, foot, and mouth disease	Coxsackie A virus	Not a zoonotic disease itself, but the virus can infect animals and be transmitted to humans	Close personal contact, coughing, contact with infected objects
4	Herpes B Virus infection	Herpes B virus (Macacine herpesvirus 1)	Macaque monkeys	Contact with infected saliva, feces of the macaque monkeys
Fungal zoonotic diseases				
5	Candidiasis	*Candida albicans*	—	Contact with contaminated hands or medical devices.
6	Histoplasmosis	*Histoplasma capsulatum*	Cattle, sheep, horses (target animals)	Infected by inhaling fungal spores from contaminated soil

Sl No	Condition	Causative organism	Vector	Transmission mode
7	Blastomycosis	*Blastomyces dermatitidis*	Direct animal-to-human transmission is rare. Dogs, cats, horses, marine mammals (target animals)	Infected by inhaling fungal spores from moist soil and decaying organic matter
8	Paracoccidiodomycosis	*Paracoccidioides brasiliensis* and *Paracoccidioides lutzii,*	Direct animal-to-human transmission is rare. Dogs and domesticated wild animals, especially armadillos and monkeys (target animals)	Infected by inhaling fungal spores from the environment, injuries of the skin and mucosal membranes
9	Sporotrichosis	*Sporothrix schenckii*	Cats; occasionally dogs, horses, cows, camel, dolphin, goat, mule, bird, pig, rat, armadillo (target animal)	Through contact with infected plant material, soil, or animals, especially cats
10	Aspergillosis	*Aspergillus genus*	All domestic animals and birds	By inhaling fungal spores from the environment
11	Cryptococcosis	*Cryptococcus neoformans* and *Cryptococcus gattii*	Found in the environment, particularly in soil or bird droppings, such as those from pigeons	Mainly by inhalation of fungus, occasionally through breaks in the skin
12	Zygomycosis (mucormycosis)	fungi from the Mucorales order	Not directly transmitted from animals to humans	Inhalation of spores from the environment.
Bacterial zoonotic diseases				
13	Cat-Scratch Disease	*Bartonella henselae*	Infected cats, particularly kittens	Through contact with cat saliva on broken skin or mucous membranes, such as the eyes, nose, or mouth
14	Plague	*Yersinia pestis*	Rodents such as rats, mice, and squirrels	Inhaling respiratory droplets from infected individuals

Table 1.
Zoonotic diseases and their transmission modes.

2. Zoonotic viral diseases with oral manifestations

Viral zoonotic diseases are caused by viruses and can be spread through direct contact with infected animals, consumption of contaminated food, or through vectors like mosquitoes or ticks [8, 9].

2.1 Monkeypox

Monkeypox is a rare viral zoonotic disease primarily found in Central and West Africa. The disease is caused by the Monkeypox virus, a member of the

Orthopoxvirus genus, which also includes the now-eradicated smallpox virus (Variola virus). Monkeypox is similar to smallpox in terms of symptoms and clinical presentation, but it is generally less severe. The virus is transmitted to humans from animals, primarily rodents and primates, and human-to-human transmission can occur through respiratory droplets or contact with bodily fluids. Monkeypox can cause fever, headache, and a rash that progresses to pustules [10].

Monkeypox typically presents with a prodromal phase characterized by fever, headache, muscle aches, and general malaise. This is followed by the development of a characteristic rash, which begins as macules and progresses to papules, vesicles, pustules, and finally crusts. The rash commonly involves the face, palms, and soles but can also spread to other parts of the body, including the oral cavity. Oral lesions in monkeypox may present as painful ulcers or vesicles on the tongue, buccal mucosa, palate, or gingiva (**Figure 1**). These lesions can be accompanied by inflammation and bleeding of the gingiva (gingivitis) or severe inflammation and destruction of the supporting structures of the teeth (periodontitis). In some cases, the oral lesions may precede or coincide with the onset of the characteristic skin rash. The presence of oral lesions can contribute to difficulty eating, drinking, and swallowing, which may result in dehydration and malnutrition, particularly in severe cases [12]. The presence of oral manifestations in monkeypox patients can be a valuable diagnostic clue, particularly in the early stages of the disease when the characteristic rash may not be fully developed. Identifying oral lesions in conjunction with systemic symptoms can help healthcare professionals differentiate monkeypox from other conditions that may present with similar symptoms, such as chickenpox, measles, or other viral infections [13].

2.2 COVID-19

COVID-19 is caused by the SARS-CoV-2 virus; this pandemic began in 2019 and has affected millions worldwide. The virus is believed to have originated in bats and transmitted to humans through an intermediate host, possibly a pangolin [14]. The SARS-CoV-2 virus, responsible for COVID-19, can cause a wide range of symptoms, including oral manifestations [15, 16]. Some patients with COVID-19 have reported symptoms such as dry mouth, loss of taste (ageusia), tongue pain, and oral ulcers [17].

Although respiratory symptoms are the most common manifestations of COVID-19, recent studies have identified various oral symptoms associated with the infection. Some of these oral manifestations include:

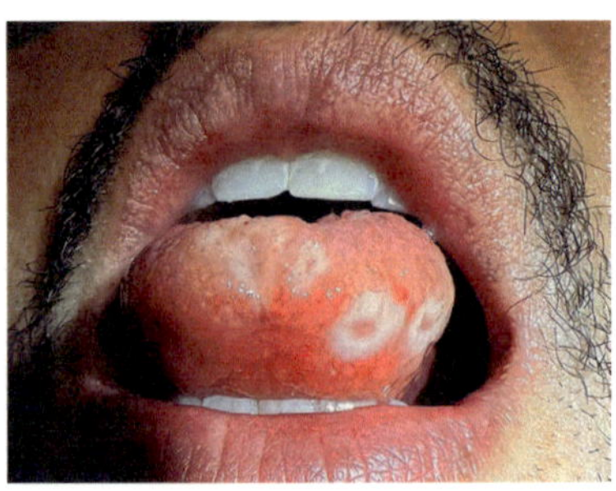

Figure 1.
Ulcerations of the tongue (Adapted from Benslama et al. Monkeypox oral lesions. J Stomatol Oral Maxillofac Surg. 2022; Permission granted for free by Elsevier) [11].

- Xerostomia (dry mouth): COVID-19 patients may experience a reduction in salivary flow due to dehydration, fever, or mouth breathing during the illness. This can lead to dry mouth, which increases the risk of dental caries and periodontal disease.
- Dysgeusia (altered taste): Many COVID-19 patients have reported a loss or alteration of taste sensation, which could be related to the virus's impact on the taste buds or the central nervous system.
- Oral ulcers and lesions: Some COVID-19 patients have presented with oral ulcers, blisters, or other lesions, which may be related to the virus's direct effect on oral tissues or a secondary response to the systemic inflammation caused by the infection (**Figure 2**).
- Gingivitis and periodontitis: The inflammatory response associated with COVID-19 may exacerbate pre-existing periodontal diseases or contribute to the development of new periodontal problems [16].

2.3 Hand, foot, and mouth disease (HFMD)

HFMD is caused by the Coxsackie A virus, which is not a zoonotic disease itself, but the virus can infect animals and be transmitted to humans. HFMD primarily affects infants and young children. The disease is caused by several strains of enteroviruses, most commonly Coxsackievirus A16 and Enterovirus 71 [19]. HFMD is characterized by the presence of a rash and/or blisters on the hands, feet, and mouth, as well as fever, sore throat, and other flu-like symptoms. The disease is characterized by fever, sore throat, and small painful blisters or ulcers in the mouth [20, 21].

Oral manifestations of HFMD can be one of the first and most noticeable symptoms of the disease. Some common oral manifestations include:

- Oral vesicles and ulcers: The primary oral manifestation of HFMD is the appearance of small, painful vesicles and ulcers in the mouth. These lesions typically

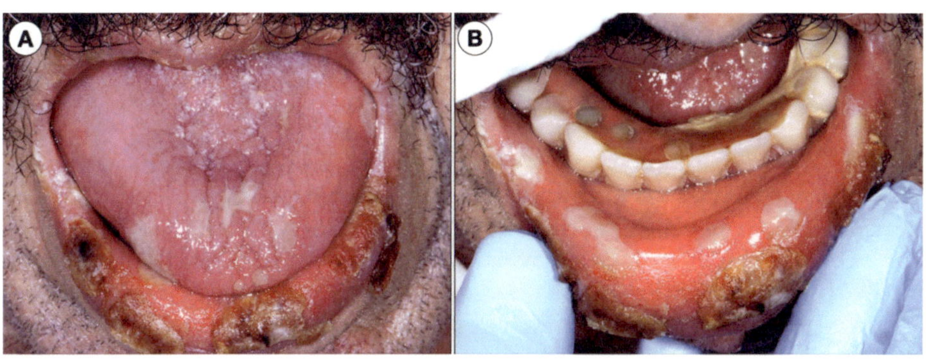

Figure 2.
(A) Clustered ulcers covered with crusts occurring on the lower lip. Ulcerative painful lesions with superficial necrosis affecting the anterior dorsal tongue. (B) Lower lip mucosal ulcers covered with a mucopurulent membrane. (Adapted from: Brandao, et al. Oral lesions in patients with SARS-CoV-2 infection: Could the oral cavity be a target organ? Oral Surg Oral Med Oral Pathol Oral Radiol. 2021; Permission granted for free by Elsevier) [18].

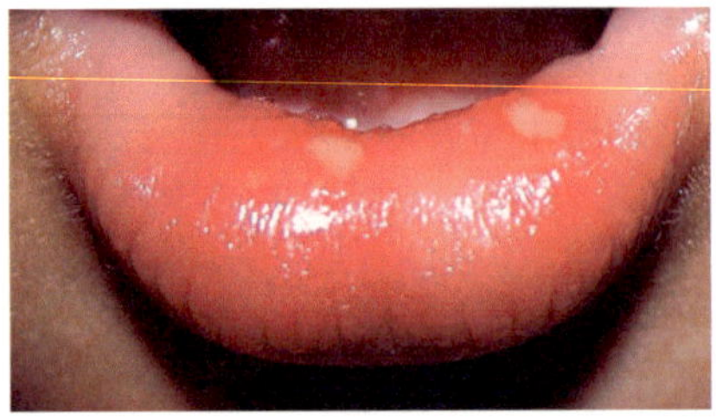

Figure 3.
Oral ulcers on the labial mucosa of lower lip (Rao et al. Hand, foot and mouth disease: Changing Indian scenario. Int J Clin Pediatr Dent. 2012; this work is licensed under a creative commons attribution 3.0 Unported License and is free to share and adapt) [22].

form on the buccal mucosa, tongue, and soft palate. As the vesicles rupture, they leave shallow, red ulcers with a white or yellow base (**Figure 3**).

- Gingivitis: Inflammation of the gingiva (gingivitis) may occur in conjunction with the oral lesions, resulting in red, swollen, and painful gingiva that may bleed easily.

- Difficulty seating and drinking: The oral lesions and gingivitis associated with HFMD can cause significant discomfort, making it challenging for affected individuals to eat, drink, and swallow. This can lead to dehydration, malnutrition, and weight loss, particularly in young children who may be unable or unwilling to communicate their pain.

The oral manifestations of HFMD can significantly impact the quality of life and overall health of affected individuals [23]. The pain and discomfort associated with oral lesions and gingivitis can lead to poor oral hygiene, as the individual may avoid brushing and flossing due to pain. This, in turn, can exacerbate gingival inflammation and increase the risk of secondary bacterial infections. Furthermore, the difficulty in eating and drinking due to oral lesions can have severe consequences for the overall health and well-being of the affected individual, particularly in young children [24]. Proper nutrition and hydration are crucial for maintaining a healthy immune system and supporting the body's ability to fight off the viral infection.

2.4 Herpes B virus infection

Herpes B virus, also known as Macacine herpesvirus 1, is a virus that primarily infects macaque monkeys but can also infect humans. In humans, Herpes B virus infections are rare but can be serious, even fatal [25]. In humans, the virus can cause vesicular lesions in the oral cavity, similar to those caused by herpes simplex virus [26].

Oral manifestations of Herpes B virus infection in humans can include:

- Oral ulcers: Herpes B virus infection can cause painful ulcers to develop on the gingiva, tongue, or inside the cheeks.

- Gingivitis: The virus can cause inflammation of the gingiva, leading to redness, swelling, and bleeding.

- Pharyngitis: Herpes B virus can cause sore throat, difficulty swallowing, and inflammation of the pharynx.
- Oral herpes: In some cases, Herpes B virus infection can lead to oral herpes, characterized by cold sores or blisters on the lips, inside the mouth, or on the tongue.

Herpes B virus infection can also cause the lymph nodes in the neck to become swollen and tender. A high fever is a common symptom of Herpes B virus infection, along with headache, muscle aches, and fatigue. It's important to note that Herpes B virus infection can be extremely serious and potentially life-threatening, especially if left untreated [27].

3. Fungal zoonotic diseases with oral manifestations

Fungal zoonotic diseases are infections caused by fungi that can be transmitted between animals and humans. Although oral manifestations are relatively rare, some fungal zoonotic diseases can present with symptoms in the oral cavity [28]. The oral manifestations of fungal zoonotic diseases can often be mistaken for other conditions, making accurate diagnosis and appropriate treatment crucial. Treatment for these conditions typically involves antifungal medications, and in some cases, surgical intervention may be necessary [29].

3.1 Candidiasis

Candidiasis, commonly known as thrush, is caused by the Candida species, particularly *Candida albicans*. While Candida is a commensal organism and is commonly found in the human body, it can cause infections in individuals with weakened immune systems or predisposing factors. Oral candidiasis presents as white patches on the tongue, inner cheeks, and other oral mucosal surfaces [30]. These patches may be painful and can bleed when scraped. In severe cases, the infection can spread to the esophagus and cause difficulty swallowing [29].

3.2 Histoplasmosis

Caused by the fungus *Histoplasma capsulatum*, histoplasmosis primarily affects the lungs. The fungus is found in soil, especially in areas with bird or bat droppings [31]. Although not directly transmitted from animals to humans, people can become infected by inhaling fungal spores from contaminated soil. Histoplasmosis can occasionally present with oral manifestations, especially in immunocompromised individuals [32]. Oral histoplasmosis may present as ulcers, nodules, or granulomatous lesions on the oral mucosa, tongue, or palate. These lesions can be painful and may mimic other oral conditions, such as squamous cell carcinoma or tuberculosis [33].

3.3 Blastomycosis

Caused by the fungus *Blastomyces dermatitidis*, blastomycosis primarily affects the lungs and can also involve the skin, bones, and other organs. The fungus is found in moist soil and decaying organic matter. Humans can become infected by inhaling fungal spores from the environment; direct animal-to-human transmission is rare [34]. Blastomycosis can occasionally involve the oral cavity, particularly in disseminated cases. Oral manifestations of blastomycosis may include ulcers, nodules, or verrucous lesions on the oral mucosa, tongue, or palate [35]. These lesions can be painful and may be mistaken for other oral conditions, such as oral cancer or fungal infections like histoplasmosis.

3.4 Paracoccidioidomycosis (South American blastomycosis)

Paracoccidioidomycosis, caused by the fungi *Paracoccidioides brasiliensis* and *Paracoccidioides lutzii,* primarily affects the lungs and can also involve the skin, lymph nodes, and other organs [36]. The fungi are found in soil, and humans can become infected by inhaling fungal spores from the environment. Direct animal-to-human transmission is rare. Paracoccidioidomycosis can present with oral manifestations, especially in the chronic form of the disease. The classic oral presentation, known as "mulberry-like stomatitis," consists of granulomatous lesions with a mulberry-like appearance on the oral mucosa, lips, and gingiva [37, 38]. These lesions can be painful and may cause difficulty eating or speaking.

3.5 Sporotrichosis

Caused by the fungus *Sporothrix schenckii*, this disease is commonly transmitted to humans through contact with infected plant material, soil, or animals, especially cats [39]. Infection occurs when fungal spores enter the skin through cuts or scratches, resulting in skin lesions, nodules, and sometimes more severe systemic infections [40]. Although oral involvement in sporotrichosis is uncommon, there have been reported cases where the fungus *Sporothrix schenckii* has caused oral manifestations. These can include ulcers, nodules, or granulomatous lesions on the oral mucosa, tongue, or palate. The lesions may be painful and can mimic other oral conditions, making diagnosis challenging [41].

3.6 Aspergillosis

Aspergillosis is caused by fungi from the *Aspergillus genus*, which are found in soil, decaying vegetation, and other organic matter. While Aspergillus is not directly transmitted from animals to humans, people can become infected by inhaling fungal spores from the environment. Aspergillosis primarily affects the lungs and can cause a range of symptoms, from mild allergic reactions to severe, invasive infections [42]. Although primarily a respiratory infection, it can sometimes involve the oral cavity, particularly in immunocompromised individuals. Oral manifestations of aspergillosis may include necrotizing ulcers, palatal perforations, or fungal masses (aspergillomas) within the oral cavity [43]. These lesions can be painful and may cause difficulty eating or speaking. Accurate diagnosis is essential, as oral aspergillosis can resemble other oral conditions, such as malignancies or other fungal infections [44].

3.7 Cryptococcosis

Cryptococcosis, caused by the fungi *Cryptococcus neoformans* and *Cryptococcus gattii,* is primarily a pulmonary and central nervous system infection. While these fungi are not directly transmitted from animals to humans, they are found in the environment, particularly in soil or bird droppings, such as those from pigeons [45]. Humans can become infected by inhaling fungal spores from the environment. However, in rare cases, it can involve the oral cavity, especially in individuals with weakened immune systems. Oral manifestations of cryptococcosis may include ulcers, nodules, or granulomatous lesions on the oral mucosa, tongue, or palate [40, 46]. These lesions may be painful and can mimic other oral conditions, making accurate diagnosis crucial.

3.8 Zygomycosis (Mucormycosis)

Zygomycosis, also known as mucormycosis, is caused by fungi from the Mucorales order, which are found in soil, decaying organic matter, and certain foods. Although not directly transmitted from animals to humans, people can become infected through inhalation of fungal spores or direct contact with contaminated materials, particularly if they have a weakened immune system or existing health conditions [47]. It is a rare but potentially life-threatening infection that can affect various organs and tissues, including the oral cavity. Oral manifestations of zygomycosis may include necrotizing ulcers, black eschars, or destruction of oral tissues, such as the palate or gingiva [48]. These lesions can be extremely painful and may cause significant morbidity and mortality if not treated promptly (**Figure 4**).

To minimize the risk of contracting fungal zoonotic diseases, individuals should take precautions such as wearing gloves and protective clothing when handling soil or animals, avoiding areas with heavy accumulations of bird or bat droppings, maintaining good hygiene practices, and ensuring proper ventilation in indoor environments [50]. For individuals with weakened immune systems or underlying health conditions, additional preventive measures may be necessary, such as wearing masks in high-risk environments or taking antifungal medications as prophylaxis.

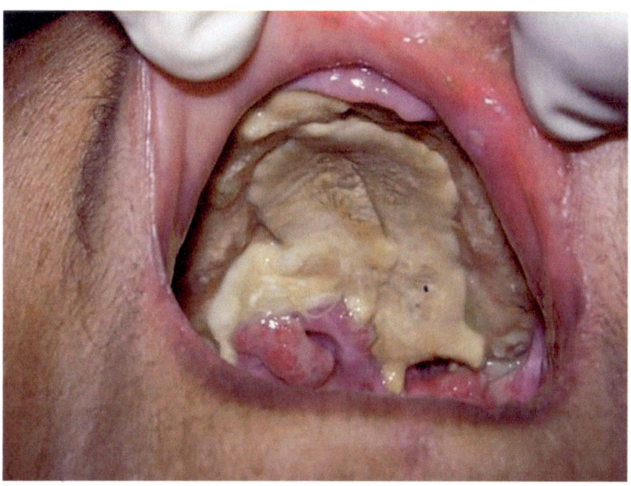

Figure 4.
Intra-oral photograph showing total denudation of the entire palate with extensive necrosis of overlying mucosa (Verma et al. Necrosis of maxilla, nasal, and frontal bone secondary to extensive rhino-cerebral mucormycosis. Natl J Maxillofac Surg. 2013; this is an open-access article distributed under the terms of the creative commons attribution-noncommercial-share alike 3.0 Unported, which permits unrestricted use, distribution, and reproduction) [49].

4. Bacterial zoonotic diseases with oral manifestations

4.1 Cat-scratch disease

Cat-scratch disease (CSD), also known as cat-scratch fever, is a bacterial zoonotic infection caused by *Bartonella henselae*. The disease is primarily transmitted to humans through scratches or bites from infected cats, particularly kittens [51]. While CSD typically presents with symptoms such as fever, fatigue, and swollen lymph nodes, it can also manifest with oral health issues. *Bartonella henselae*, the bacterium responsible for the cat-scratch disease, is commonly found in the saliva of infected cats. Transmission to humans usually occurs when an infected cat scratches or bites a person, introducing the bacteria into the skin. In some cases, the bacteria may also be transmitted through contact with cat saliva on broken skin or mucous membranes, such as the eyes, nose, or mouth. The primary symptoms of cat-scratch disease include swollen and painful lymph nodes near the site of the scratch or bite, fever, headache, and fatigue. These symptoms generally appear within one to three weeks after exposure to the bacteria and can last for several weeks or months [52].

While the most common manifestations of cat-scratch disease involve lymph nodes and flu-like symptoms, the infection can also affect oral health in several ways. CSD may cause oral ulcers or sores in the oral cavity [53]. These ulcers can be painful and make eating or drinking difficult. Infected individuals may experience periodontitis or gingivitis, which can cause redness, swelling, and bleeding of the gingiva. In rare instances, CSD may cause erythema or redness of the oral mucosa, leading to discomfort and potential complications if left untreated [54]. Once these bacteria are introduced into the oral cavity, they can potentially cause secondary infections that may lead to more severe oral health issues, such as periodontitis or dental abscesses.

4.2 Plague

Plague, a severe and potentially fatal zoonotic infection, is caused by the bacterium *Yersinia pestis*. The primary mode of transmission to humans is through the bite of infected fleas, which commonly infest rodents such as rats, mice, and squirrels. Additional transmission routes include direct contact with infected animals or their tissues and inhaling respiratory droplets from infected individuals. Plague presents in three main forms: bubonic, septicemic, and pneumonic, each with distinct symptoms and health consequences [55]. Although the primary symptoms of plague involve swollen lymph nodes (buboes), fever, chills, and weakness, the disease may also manifest with oral complications in some instances.

Infections caused by *Yersinia pestis* can result in acute gingival bleeding, characterized by swollen, tender gingiva that bleed easily. This symptom is particularly worrisome in the context of septicemic plague, where the bacteria have disseminated through the bloodstream, causing intravascular coagulation and potential bleeding in various body parts, including the oral cavity. Plague may also cause the formation of oral ulcers or sores in the mouth, which can be painful and interfere with eating or drinking. In severe cases of septicemic or pneumonic plague, the infection might lead to necrosis or tissue death in different parts of the body, including the oral cavity [56]. Necrotic lesions in the mouth can be extremely painful and result in significant damage to the oral tissues.

5. Zoonotic disease prevention in dental practice settings

In dental care setups, practitioners may come into contact with zoonotic pathogens through direct contact with infected animals or indirectly through contaminated instruments, surfaces, or airborne transmission [57]. Therefore, it is crucial for dental care professionals to adopt preventive measures to minimize the risk of zoonotic diseases in their practice.

5.1 Education and training

Continuous education and training of dental professionals on zoonotic diseases are vital for effective prevention. Dental care professionals should be knowledgeable about the different types of zoonoses, their transmission modes, and the necessary precautions to take. This knowledge can be acquired through formal education, professional development courses, and regular workshops. Dental professionals should also be trained in identifying potential zoonotic disease symptoms and handling suspected cases.

5.2 Personal protective equipment (PPE)

The use of appropriate PPE, including gloves, masks, eye protection, and gowns, is essential in preventing the transmission of zoonotic pathogens. Dental professionals should adhere to strict protocols regarding the use, disposal, and replacement of PPE to minimize the risk of cross-contamination and infection [58].

The following PPE components should be considered:

a. Gloves: Disposable gloves should be worn during all procedures involving potential exposure to blood, body fluids, or contaminated surfaces. Gloves should be changed between patients and disposed of properly.

b. Masks: Dental professionals should wear surgical masks or respirators to protect against the inhalation of aerosols or droplets containing pathogens. Masks should be replaced regularly and disposed of properly.

c. Eye protection: Safety goggles or face shields should be worn to protect the eyes from splashes, sprays, or airborne particles.

d. Gowns: Disposable gowns should be used to protect clothing from contamination. Gowns should be changed between patients and disposed of properly.

5.3 Infection control and sterilization procedures

Dental care professionals should follow strict infection control protocols, including regular cleaning and sterilization of dental instruments, surfaces, and equipment. The use of disposable items, such as single-use dental needles and saliva ejectors, can help minimize the risk of cross-contamination. Proper disposal of contaminated waste, such as used gloves, masks, and sharps, should be practiced to prevent environmental contamination.

a. Instrument sterilization: All reusable dental instruments should be thoroughly cleaned and sterilized between patients using appropriate methods such as autoclaving or chemical sterilization.

b. Surface disinfection: Surfaces in the dental operatory, including countertops, dental chairs, and light handles, should be regularly cleaned and disinfected using EPA-registered disinfectants.

c. Equipment maintenance: Dental equipment, such as handpieces and ultrasonic scalers, should be maintained, cleaned, and sterilized according to the manufacturer's recommendations.

d. Use of disposable items: Whenever possible, single-use items such as dental needles and saliva ejectors should be utilized to minimize the risk of cross-contamination.

e. Proper waste disposal: Contaminated waste, including used gloves, masks, and sharps, should be disposed of in designated biohazard containers.

5.4 Animal handling policies

In cases where dental care professionals encounter animals in their practice, such as service animals or therapy pets, strict animal handling policies should be in place. These policies should include guidelines on hand hygiene, avoiding direct contact with animals when possible, and immediately reporting any incidents of bites or scratches. Additionally, dental care setups should ensure that animals present in the clinic have been properly vaccinated and are free of any known zoonotic diseases.

a. Hand hygiene: Dental professionals should practice proper hand hygiene before and after handling animals, including washing hands with soap and water or using alcohol-based hand sanitizers.

b. Avoiding direct contact: Whenever possible, dental professionals should avoid direct contact with animals, especially if they have open wounds or broken skin.

c. Reporting incidents: Any incidents of bites or scratches should be immediately reported, and appropriate medical attention should be sought.

d. Animal vaccination and health checks: Dental care setups should ensure that animals present in the clinic have been properly vaccinated and are free of any known zoonotic diseases. Regular health check-ups should be conducted by a veterinarian to ensure the animals' well-being and to minimize the risk of disease transmission.

5.5 Airborne transmission prevention

To minimize the risk of airborne transmission of zoonotic pathogens, dental care setups should invest in proper ventilation systems, air purifiers, and high-efficiency particulate air (HEPA) filters. Regular maintenance and cleaning of these systems are essential to ensure their efficiency in preventing the spread of airborne pathogens [59]. The following measures can be taken to prevent airborne transmission:

a. Ventilation systems: Dental care setups should have adequate ventilation systems in place to ensure proper air circulation and reduce the concentration of airborne pathogens.

b. Air purifiers: The use of air purifiers with HEPA filters can help remove airborne particles, including pathogens, from the air, reducing the risk of transmission.

c. Regular maintenance and cleaning: Ventilation systems and air purifiers should be regularly maintained and cleaned according to the manufacturer's recommendations to ensure their efficiency in preventing the spread of airborne pathogens.

5.6 Surveillance and reporting

Dental care professionals should be vigilant in monitoring for signs and symptoms of zoonotic diseases in both patients and staff. Any suspected cases should be promptly reported to relevant public health authorities, and appropriate measures, such as isolation and contact tracing, should be implemented to prevent further transmission [60]. The following steps can be taken to enhance surveillance and reporting:

a. Monitoring for symptoms: Dental professionals should be trained to identify potential signs and symptoms of zoonotic diseases and to report any suspected cases to the appropriate public health authorities.

b. Reporting incidents: Any incidents of potential zoonotic disease transmission, such as animal bites or scratches, should be promptly reported to the relevant public health authorities.

c. Implementing control measures: In the event of a suspected case, dental care setups should implement appropriate measures, such as isolation, contact tracing, and enhanced infection control procedures, to prevent further transmission.

As zoonotic diseases continue to pose a significant threat to global health, it is crucial for dental care setups to prioritize preventive measures to minimize the risk of transmission. By adopting comprehensive policies and protocols, including education, the use of PPE, infection control, animal handling, airborne transmission prevention, and surveillance, dental care professionals can contribute to the global effort to combat zoonotic diseases and protect the health of their patients and auxiliary staff.

6. Conclusion

The connection between oral health and zoonotic diseases highlights the importance of maintaining good oral hygiene to reduce the risk of disease transmission. By adopting a comprehensive approach that includes oral health practices, public awareness, vaccination and disease control, and interdisciplinary collaboration, we can effectively address the challenges posed by zoonotic diseases and promote better health outcomes for both humans and animals. By implementing a One Health approach and addressing the root causes of zoonotic disease emergence and spread, we can work toward reducing the impact of these diseases on human, animal, and environmental health. Preventing and controlling zoonotic diseases require a collaborative, interdisciplinary approach known as One Health, which recognizes the interconnectedness of human, animal, and environmental health. This approach involves cooperation among various sectors, including public health, veterinary medicine, agriculture, and wildlife management, to monitor and respond to zoonotic disease threats effectively.

Conflict of interest

The authors declare no conflict of interest.

Author details

Betsy Joseph[1,2]*, Archana Mootha[3], Vishnupriya K. Sweety[2] and Sukumaran Anil[4]

1 Saveetha Dental College and Hospital, Saveetha Institute of Medical and Technical Sciences, Chennai, India

2 Pushpagiri Institute of Medical Sciences and Research Centre, Medicity, Tiruvalla, Kerala, India

3 Department of Biomaterials Science, Graduate School of Biomedical and Health Sciences, Hiroshima University, Hiroshima, Japan

4 Department of Dentistry, Oral Health Institute, Hamad Medical Corporation, Qatar University, Doha, Qatar

*Address all correspondence to: jobets121@gmail.com

References

[1] Cross AR, Baldwin VM, Roy S, Essex-Lopresti AE, Prior JL, Harmer NJ. Zoonoses under our noses. Microbes and Infection. 2019;**21**(1):10-19

[2] Weiss RA, Sankaran N. Emergence of epidemic diseases: Zoonoses and other origins. Faculty Review. 2022;**11**:2

[3] Hassell JM, Begon M, Ward MJ, Fevre EM. Urbanization and disease emergence: Dynamics at the wildlife-livestock-human Interface. Trends in Ecology & Evolution. 2017;**32**(1):55-67

[4] Wilke ABB, Beier JC, Benelli G. Complexity of the relationship between global warming and urbanization - an obscure future for predicting increases in vector-borne infectious diseases. Current Opinion Insect Science. 2019;**35**:1-9

[5] Rahman MT, Sobur MA, Islam MS, Ievy S, Hossain MJ, El Zowalaty ME, et al. Zoonotic diseases: Etiology, impact, and control. Microorganisms. 2020;**8**(9):1-34

[6] Varela K, Brown JA, Lipton B, Dunn J, Stanek D, Behravesh CB, et al. A review of zoonotic disease threats to pet owners: A compendium of measures to prevent zoonotic diseases associated with non-traditional pets: Rodents and other small mammals, reptiles, amphibians, backyard poultry, and other selected animals. Vector Borne and Zoonotic Diseases. 2022;**22**(6):303-360

[7] Sampson V, Kamona N, Sampson A. Could there be a link between oral hygiene and the severity of SARS-CoV-2 infections? British Dental Journal. 2020;**228**(12):971-975

[8] Scully C, Samaranayake LP. Emerging and changing viral diseases in the new millennium. Oral Diseases. 2016;**22**(3):171-179

[9] Rajeev R, Prathiviraj R, Kiran GS, Selvin J. Zoonotic evolution and implications of microbiome in viral transmission and infection. Virus Research. 2020;**290**:198175

[10] Titanji BK, Tegomoh B, Nematollahi S, Konomos M, Kulkarni PA. Monkeypox: A contemporary review for healthcare professionals. Open Forum Infectious Diseases. 2022;**9**(7):ofac310

[11] Benslama L, Foy JP, Bertolus C. Monkeypox oral lesions. Journal of Stomatol Oral Maxillofacultory Surgery. 2022;**123**(6):596

[12] Joseph B, Anil S. Oral lesions in human monkeypox disease and their management-a scoping review. Oral Surgery, Oral Medicine, Oral Pathology, Oral Radiology. 2023;**135**(4):510-517

[13] Waltzek TB, Cortes-Hinojosa G, Wellehan JF Jr, Gray GC. Marine mammal zoonoses: A review of disease manifestations. Zoonoses and Public Health. 2012;**59**(8):521-535

[14] Adil MT, Rahman R, Whitelaw D, Jain V, Al-Taan O, Rashid F, et al. SARS-CoV-2 and the pandemic of COVID-19. Postgraduate Medical Journal. 2021;**97**(1144):110-116

[15] Ghosh A, Joseph B, Anil S. Does periodontitis influence the risk of COVID-19? A scoping review. Clinical Experience in Dental Research. 2022;**8**(5):1011-1020

[16] Anand PS, Jadhav P, Kamath KP, Kumar SR, Vijayalaxmi S, Anil S. A case-control study on the association between

periodontitis and coronavirus disease (COVID-19). Journal of Periodontology. 2022;**93**(4):584-590

[17] Soares CD, Souza LL, de Carvalho MGF, Pontes HAR, Mosqueda-Taylor A, Hernandez-Guerrero JC, et al. Oral manifestations of coronavirus disease 2019 (COVID-19): A comprehensive Clinicopathologic and Immunohistochemical study. The American Journal of Surgical Pathology. 2022;**46**(4):528-536

[18] Brandao TB, Gueiros LA, Melo TS, Prado-Ribeiro AC, Nesrallah A, Prado GVB, et al. Oral lesions in patients with SARS-CoV-2 infection: Could the oral cavity be a target organ? Oral Surgery, Oral Medicine, Oral Pathology, Oral Radiology. 2021;**131**(2):e45-e51

[19] Saguil A, Kane SF, Lauters R, Mercado MG. Hand-foot-and-mouth disease: Rapid evidence review. American Family Physician. 2019;**100**(7):408-414

[20] Muzumdar S, Rothe MJ, Grant-Kels JM. The rash with maculopapules and fever in children. Clinics in Dermatology. 2019;**37**(2): 119-128

[21] Zhu P, Ji W, Li D, Li Z, Chen Y, Dai B, et al. Current status of hand-foot-and-mouth disease. Journal of Biomedical Science. 2023;**30**(1):15

[22] Rao PK, Veena K, Jagadishchandra H, Bhat SS, Shetty SR. Hand, foot and mouth disease: Changing Indian scenario. International Journal of Clinical Pediatric Dentistry. 2012;**5**(3):220-222

[23] Han Y, Ji H, Shen W, Duan C, Cui T, Chen L, et al. Disease burden in patients with severe hand, foot, and mouth disease in Jiangsu Province: A cross-sectional study. Human Vaccines & Immunotherapeutics. 2022;**18**(5):2049168

[24] Toida M, Watanabe F, Goto K, Shibata T. Usefulness of low-level laser for control of painful stomatitis in patients with hand-foot-and-mouth disease. Journal of Clinical Laser Medicine & Surgery. 2003;**21**(6):363-367

[25] Katz D, Shi W, Gowda MS, Vasireddi M, Patrusheva I, Seoh HK, et al. Identification of unique B virus (Macacine herpesvirus 1) epitopes of zoonotic and macaque isolates using monoclonal antibodies. PLoS One. 2017;**12**(8):e0182355

[26] Birek C. Herpesvirus-induced diseases: Oral manifestations and current treatment options. Journal of the California Dental Association. 2000;**28**(12):911-921

[27] Hu G, Du H, Liu Y, Wu G, Han J. Herpes B virus: History, zoonotic potential, and public health implications. Biosafety and Health. 2022;**4**(4):213-219

[28] Farah CS, Lynch N, McCullough MJ. Oral fungal infections: An update for the general practitioner. Australian Dental Journal. 2010;**55**(s1):48-54

[29] Telles DR, Karki N, Marshall MW. Oral fungal infections: Diagnosis and management. Dental Clinics of North America. 2017;**61**(2):319-349

[30] Hellstein JW, Marek CL. Candidiasis: Red and white manifestations in the Oral cavity. Head and Neck Pathology. 2019;**13**(1):25-32

[31] Arauz AB, Papineni P. Histoplasmosis. Infectious Disease Clinics of North America. 2021;**35**(2):471-491

[32] Seyedmousavi S, Guillot J, Tolooe A, Verweij PE, de Hoog GS. Neglected fungal zoonoses: Hidden threats to man and animals. Clinical Microbiology and Infection. 2015;**21**(5):416-425

[33] Ng KH, Siar CH. Review of oral histoplasmosis in Malaysians. Oral Surgery, Oral Medicine, Oral Pathology, Oral Radiology, and Endodontics. 1996;**81**(3):303-307

[34] Saccente M, Woods GL. Clinical and laboratory update on blastomycosis. Clinical Microbiology Reviews. 2010;**23**(2):367-381

[35] Mutalik VS, Bissonnette C, Kalmar JR, McNamara KK. Unique oral presentations of deep fungal infections: A report of four cases. Head and Neck Pathology. 2021;**15**(2):682-690

[36] Hahn RC, Hagen F, Mendes RP, Burger E, Nery AF, Siqueira NP, et al. Paracoccidioidomycosis: Current status and future trends. Clinical Microbiology Reviews. 2022;**35**(4):e0023321

[37] Costa MC, de Carvalho MM, Sperandio FF, Ribeiro Junior NV, Hanemann JAC, Pigossi SC, et al. Oral Paracoccidioidomycosis affecting women: A systematic review. Mycoses. 2021;**64**(2):108-122

[38] Webber LP, Martins MD, de Oliveira MG, Munhoz EA, Carrard VC. Disseminated paracoccidioidomycosis diagnosis based on oral lesions. Contemporary Clinical Dental. 2014;**5**(2):213-216

[39] Valeriano CAT, Ferraz CE, Oliveira MME, Inacio CP, de Oliveira EP, Lacerda AM, et al. Cat-transmitted disseminated cutaneous sporotrichosis caused by Sporothrix brasiliensis in a new endemic area: Case series in the northeast of Brazil. JAAD Case Report. 2020;**6**(10):988-992

[40] DiNardo AR, Schmidt D, Mitchell A, Kaufman Y, Tweardy DJ. First description of oral Cryptococcus neoformans causing osteomyelitis of the mandible, manubrium and third rib with associated soft tissue abscesses in an immunocompetent host. Clinical Microbiological Case Report. 2015;**1**(3):1-12

[41] Abrahao AC, Agostini M, de Oliveira TR, Noce CW, Junior AS, Cabral MG, et al. Oral manifestations of sporotrichosis: A neglected disease. Journal of Clinical and Experimental Dentistry. 2023;**15**(1):e82-e87

[42] Mousavi B, Hedayati MT, Hedayati N, Ilkit M, Syedmousavi S. Aspergillus species in indoor environments and their possible occupational and public health hazards. Current Medical Mycology. 2016;**2**(1):36-42

[43] Chermetz M, Gobbo M, Rupel K, Ottaviani G, Tirelli G, Bussani R, et al. Combined orofacial Aspergillosis and Mucormycosis: Fatal complication of a recurrent paediatric glioma-case report and review of literature. Mycopathologia. 2016;**181**(9-10):723-733

[44] Faustino ISP, Ramos JC, Mariz B, Papadopoulou E, Georgaki M, Nikitakis NG, et al. A rare case of mandibular aspergillus osteomyelitis in an immunocompetent patient. Dental Journal (Basel). 2022;**10**(11):2-8

[45] Kwon-Chung KJ, Fraser JA, Doering TL, Wang Z, Janbon G, Idnurm A, et al. Cryptococcus neoformans and Cryptococcus gattii, the etiologic agents of cryptococcosis. Cold Spring Harbor Perspectives in Medicine. 2014;**4**(7):a019760

[46] Santiso GM, Messina F, Gallo A, Marin E, Depardo R, Arechavala A, et al. Tongue lesion due to Cryptococcus

neoformans as the first finding in an HIV-positive patient. Revista Iberoamericana de Micología. 2021;**38**(1):19-22

[47] Vasudevan B, Hazra N, Shijith KP, Neema S, Vendhan S. Mucormycosis: The scathing invader. Indian Journal of Dermatology. 2021;**66**(4):393-400

[48] Janjua OS, Shaikh MS, Fareed MA, Qureshi SM, Khan MI, Hashem D, et al. Dental and Oral manifestations of COVID-19 related Mucormycosis: Diagnoses, management strategies and outcomes. Journal of Fungi. 2022;**8**(1):44

[49] Verma A, Singh V, Jindal N, Yadav S. Necrosis of maxilla, nasal, and frontal bone secondary to extensive rhino-cerebral mucormycosis. Natural Journal of Maxillofacatory Surgery. 2013;**4**(2):249-251

[50] Soare AY, Watkins TN, Bruno VM. Understanding Mucormycoses in the age of "omics". Frontiers in Genetics. 2020;**11**:699

[51] Goldstein EJC, Abrahamian FM. Diseases transmitted by cats. Microbiological Spectroscopy. 2015;**3**:5

[52] Klotz SA, Ianas V, Elliott SP. Cat-scratch disease. American Family Physician. 2011;**83**(2):152-155

[53] Mandel L, Surattanont F, Miremadi R. Cat-scratch disease: Considerations for dentistry. Journal of the American Dental Association (1939). 2001;**132**(7):911-914

[54] Da Silva K, Chussid S. Cat scratch disease: Clinical considerations for the pediatric dentist. Pediatric Dentistry. 2009;**31**(1):58-62

[55] Yang R. Plague: Recognition, treatment, and prevention. Journal of Clinical Microbiology. 2018;**56**(1):1-6

[56] Giuffra V, Milanese M, Minozzi S. Dental health in adults and subadults from the 16th-century plague cemetery of Alghero (Sardinia, Italy). Archives of Oral Biology. 2020;**120**:104928

[57] Khanagar SB, Al-Ehaideb A, Vishwanathaiah S, Maganur PC, Naik S, Siddeeqh S. Exposure risks and preventive strategies considered in dental care settings to combat coronavirus disease (COVID-19). HERD. 2021;**14**(1):278-289

[58] Patil S, Moafa IH, Bhandi S, Jafer MA, Khan SS, Khan S, et al. Dental care and personal protective measures for dentists and non-dental health care workers. Disease-a-Month. 2020;**66**(9):101056

[59] Yue L. Ventilation in the dental clinic: An effective measure to control droplets and aerosols during the coronavirus pandemic and beyond. The Chinese Journal of Dental Research. 2020;**23**(2):105-107

[60] Sacoor S, Chana S, Fortune F. The dental team as part of the medical workforce during national and global crises. British Dental Journal. 2020;**229**(2):89-92

Chapter 14

SARS-CoV-2 Secondary Spillover: From Doubt to Evidence

AbdulRahman A. Saied, Faten F. Mohammed and Asmaa A. Metwally

Abstract

The severe acute respiratory syndrome coronavirus 2 (SARS-CoV-2) is the culprit behind the coronavirus disease 2019 (COVID-19) and it is believed that bats may have been the source. SARS-CoV-2 can naturally infect humans and various animal species, including pets, farm animals, zoo animals, and wild animals that might serve as potential reservoirs for the viral transmission to humans. Most infected animals with SARS-CoV-2 are associated with exposure to infected humans; therefore, SARS-CoV-2 is characterized by zoonosis and reverse zoonosis. It is critical to quickly detect and classify variants of concern of SARS-CoV-2 in both domestic and wild animals. In addition, it's possible that novel variants emerging due to viral mutation, making the infection of incidental animal hosts worrying. Here, we discuss the most recent information on the spreading of SARS-CoV-2 among animals and humans, the importance of genomic research, and active surveillance of these animals that may help us to understand the spread of viruses and the emergence of variants.

Keywords: SARS-CoV-2, animal-to-human transmission, evidence, coronaviruses, vaccines

1. Introduction

In 1937, coronavirus (CoV) was discovered to be the cause of the first respiratory infection; the virus had a terrible impact on poultry. In 1965, it was established that CoV was to blame for 15–30% of human common colds [1]. Three novel, highly pathogenic human respiratory coronaviruses (HCoVs) that have caused global infections in the last twenty years, are the severe acute respiratory syndrome coronavirus (SARS-CoV) in 2003, Middle-East respiratory syndrome coronavirus (MERS-CoV) in 2012, and severe acute respiratory syndrome coronavirus 2 (SARS-CoV-2) in 2019 [2]. They are all assumed to have evolved from an animal reservoir through viral spillover into humans via an intermediate host [3], highlighting the role of animals as reservoirs. (CoVs) have the propensity for rapid adaptation to various geographic settings and to transmit consistently to new species [4]. SARS-CoV-2 has been detected in Wuhan's Huanan food market, China following its jumping from animals into humans (spill-over).

 IntechOpen

CoVs cause respiratory, gastrointestinal, neurological, and other widespread disorders in various hosts, such as birds, companion animals, livestock, zoo animals, and wild animals. CoVs are the most extensive diverse group of positive-sense, single-stranded RNA-enveloped viruses. CoV has "crown"-shaped spikes that project from its envelope, giving the appearance of a stellar corona and that's why is termed "coronavirus." The spikes, the large type 1 transmembrane spike (S) glycoprotein, enable viral adherence, host entrance, and subsequent infections. The *Coronaviridae* family of the *Nidovirales* order includes the *Orthocoronavirinae* subfamily. According to the International Committee on the Taxonomy of Viruses (ICTV), the *Orthocoronavirinae* subfamily is further divided into four genera: *Alphacoronavirus*, *Betacoronavirus*, *Gammacoronavirus*, and *Deltacoronavirus*. Gamma and delta CoVs predominantly infect birds and some mammals, while alpha and beta CoVs most commonly infect mammals such as bats, rats, domestic animals, and humans.

SARS-CoV-2, the etiological agent of the COVID-19 pandemic, is a member of the *Coronaviridae* family, *Betacoronavirus* genus, and *Sarbecovirus* subgenus [5]. As of 16 July 2023, 6.9 million deaths have been reported out of over 768 million confirmed cases worldwide by the WHO [6].

This virus is very infectious and spreads very quickly with a high rate of genome mutation. Since the outbreak started in late 2019, the virus has continued to affect many populations in wide geographic areas to reach everywhere mostly [7, 8]. Since then, there have been claims about the contribution of animals to the viral transmission from animals to humans. Even though this disease is zoonotic, both the public and many researchers pay less attention to this point in the pandemic. The fact that SARS-CoV-2 causes primarily human-to-human transmission, causing a devastating pandemic; however, it also results in severe respiratory infections of animals (spillback), which cause illness in animals [9]. Many different exotic animal species have the potential to transmit the CoVs to people, especially in locations where these animals are kept for food [10–12].

The COVID-19 outbreak shows that specific risk factors, such as sufficient contact between infected individuals and recipient animals, the availability of animal hosts for multiplying viral infection, and the capacity of animal host populations to ensure viral survival, maybe the primary factors in the emergence of newly emerging contagious zoonotic diseases [13, 14]. The main problem is that the virus spreads to animal species that are vulnerable to it, as SARS-CoV-2 has shown remarkable host adaptability.

At least 31 different animal species, such as domestic cats (*Felis catus domesticus*), mink (*Neovison vison*), white-tailed deer (*Odocoileus virginianus*), domestic dogs (*Canis lupus familiaris*), non-domestic felid species, gorillas (*Gorilla gorilla*), black-tailed marmoset (*Mico melanurus*), mule deer (*Odocoileus hemionus*), hyena (*crocuta crocuta*), Asian small-clawed otter (*Aonyx cinereus*), manatee (*Trichechus manatus*), giant anteater (*Myrmecophaga tridactyla*), and golden hamsters (*Mesocricetus auratus*), are recognized to be vulnerable to SARS-CoV-2. SARS-CoV-2 has been observed to spread rapidly among animal groups, including mink and white-tailed deer, raising worry that viral variants may accumulate among these animals.

The group habitation and interaction network structure in these sensitive animal species may contain another virus library that can be reintroduced into humans [15]. Now, after three years, studies have revealed SARS-CoV-2's spreading from animal to human. More interestingly, different kinds of animals can do this kind of viral transmission (White-tailed deer [16–18], Cat [19], Pet hamsters [20, 21], African lion [22], and Contaminated hair of Dog [23]), and one of them helped in the SARS-CoV-2 variant's transmission that is highly transmissible among humans (Mink [24, 25]) (**Figure 1**).

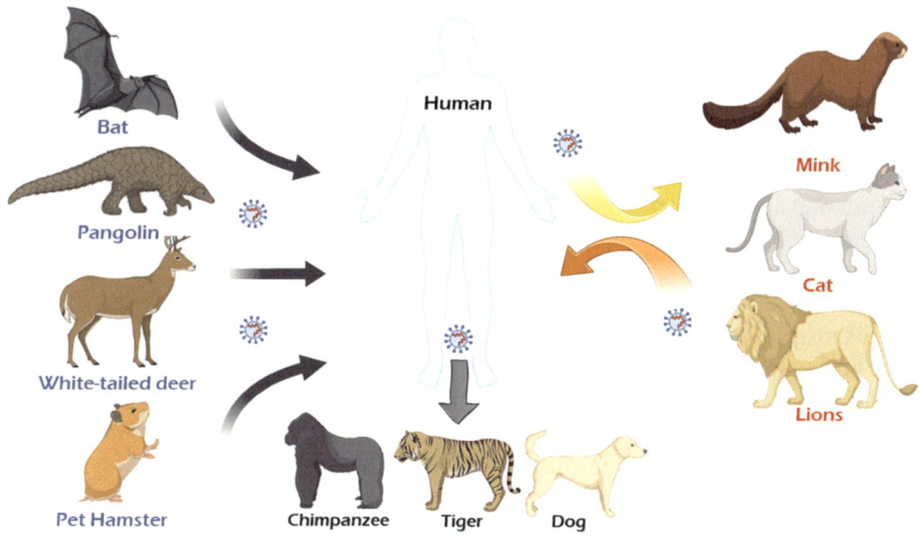

Figure 1.
SARS-CoV-2 transmission among humans and animals.

Wild animals that can adapt effectively to an environment where humans predominate, such as rats, bats, and primates, will spread more viruses to humans as the human population rises [26]. Because of population growth, humans now occupy most of the living area traditionally allotted for animals, resulting in frequent interactions between people and animals. These animals are at significant risk of transferring the virus to humans since they reside near human homes, farms, and crops. Restricting human contact with wild animals is essential to reduce the possibility of SARS-CoV-2 transmitting from wild animals to humans and to protect wild animals [27].

The initial victims of the COVID-19 outbreak in Wuhan, Hubei Province, China, were workers or consumers who had previously had a lot of contact with animals, raising the possibility that SARS-CoV-2 can be spread from animals to people [28–30]. Also, it was recorded that numerous coronaviruses have been found in Cameroon, some of which are closely related to human coronavirus 229E [31].

SARS-CoV-2 may have evolved further in new hosts due to interspecies transmission, which would have led to new spread, such as the SARS-CoV-2 mutation in minks and human exposure to minks [32, 33], which enforced the Netherlands and Denmark to substantial mink culling late 2020. In a previous similar scenario, several months after SARS-CoV was under control within the impacted nations, similar outbreaks occurred in animals at the end of 2003. A restaurant serving civet cats reared on a farm was related to fresh human infections with SARS-CoV [34], which prompted China's mass culling of civet cats.

Human-to-animal spreading of SARS-CoV-2 may occur when wildlife is handled or eaten [35]. Additionally, despite being a respiratory virus, SARS-CoV-2 is excreted in the feces and connected with certain cases of diarrhea in people [36]. Additionally, some animal food sources have a reputation for raising concerns that diseases could spread through direct contact with or consumption of wild animals and/or animals used for farming [37]. It is crucial to keep monitoring the animal-source of SARS-CoV-2 and adapt control and preventative methods to prevent a large-scale communal transmission brought on by the virus moving from animals to humans in the future.

Relying solely on the development of vaccines while neglecting this approach could result in the loss of many lives [38].

1.1 Bats

Since the first identification and early outbreak at the end of 2019 of the COVID-19 pandemic, epidemiological investigations have revealed that the infectious agent is of animal origin, likely from bats [39], through an unidentified intermediary animal host [40]. SARS-CoV-2 was first found in bats and later transmitted to pangolins or other wild species, where it interacted with viruses that were already present in these animals to become able to infect people [7]. SARS-CoV and MERS-CoV are just two of the coronaviruses that have spread from bats to other animals. There have been discovered a large number of bat-originating coronaviruses (Bat-CoV), including Bat-CoV-RaTG13 (RaTG13), RpYN06, PrC31, RmYN02, Bat-SL-CoVZC45, and Bat-SL-CoVZXC 21 [7, 41, 42].

The RTG13 identified in the Chinese chrysanthemum-headed bat (*Rhinolophus sinicus*) shared 96.2%, 97.5%, and 89.2% nucleotide and amino acid sequence similarities with SARS-CoV-2 for the spike (S) protein and the receptor-binding domain (RBD), respectively [41]. Because SARS-CoV-2's mutation spectrum resembles that of coronavirus RaTG13, it is likely that the SARS-CoV-2 emerged from RaTG13 in a bat-like host cell environment before being transmitted to humans. This research confirms SARS-CoV-2's natural origins and suggests that it started in bats [43].

1.2 Hamsters

In Hong Kong, China, the earliest documented instance of naturally occurring SARS-CoV-2 infection in hamsters [44]. An epidemiological investigation determined that the SARS-CoV-2 variant AY.127 was transmitted from pet hamsters to customers and workers at pet shops, which was connected to the origin of this case in Hong Kong [20, 21, 45]. The human patient in this case had a SARS-CoV-2 strain that shared substantial sequence similarity with the positive Syrian hamster (*Mesocricetus auratus*) sample, both of which belonged to the AY.127 lineage [20], whereas the possibility that a dog serving as a passive mechanical carrier of the SARS-CoV-2 transmitted the Omicron BA.2 subvariant to Chinese people [23].

1.3 Minks

COVID-19 has been found in farmed mink, and transmission from among mink and human (mink to mink, human to mink, and mink to human) has been established [46]. Over one million minks have been exterminated due to reports like these in countries like Spain and the Netherlands [47]. Other than the Netherlands and Denmark, reports of SARS-CoV-2-infected minks have also been recorded in Spain and the US. Denmark's discovery of mink-associated variant and its human transmission, even those who do not interact with mink [25], where the spike protein in this strain underwent mutations. Additionally, the variant associated with minks had enhanced binding to the mink angiotensin-converting enzyme 2 (ACE2) receptor, potentially indicating host adaptability [48]. SARS-CoV-2 has been detected in 11 wild minks in Utah, USA, which are thought to have escaped from a farm nearby where they were captured [49]. The SARS-CoV-2 infection in two wild minks in Spain has been confirmed to be phylogenetically identical to the Wuhan variant [50], thus demonstrating the power of SARS-CoV-2 to spread to wild populations of species that have a high vulnerability to the virus, such as mink.

It's possible that the evolution of a variant that has enhanced adherence to the cat ACE2 receptor might have an impact on transmission from cat to cat and raise the possibility that cats could act as virus reservoirs [51]. Interestingly, feline coronaviruses showed a mutation of feline enteric coronavirus into feline infectious peritonitis virus [52].

In 474 farms across 12 different countries as of August 2022, SARS-CoV-2 was being studied in farm-raised mink [53]. Farmed minks have drawn attention from all around the world because of their extremely high SARS-CoV-2 vulnerability, an infection that is both symptomatic and subclinical, high mortality, and capability to spread the virus to other mink and animal species [54–57]. Denmark discovered SARS-CoV-2-positive mink between June 2020 and November 2020 on 290 farms and 4000 human sequences with suspected mink-related mutations [53, 58].

There have been reports of SARS-CoV-2-infected minks (*Neovison vision*) in the Netherlands, Denmark, the USA, Canada, Spain, France, Italy, and other countries. [59]. In the Netherlands, it was recorded that SARS-CoV-2 may have been transmitted from animal-to-human among mink farms. Whole-genome sequencing revealed that 68% of people who lived in mink farms, worked there, or had contact with them had SARS-CoV-2 infection [46]. It was reported that, SARS-CoV-2 animal-to-human transmission in the Netherlands from infected farm minks to farmworkers [46].

Naturally, the caretaker's infection spread to the minks. Infections of SARS-CoV-2 were identified in two-thirds of the mink farm inhabitants and employees who were screened [46]. Munnink et al. sequenced the whole genomes of the SARS-CoV-2 strains from 16 mink farms in the Netherlands that were of mink and human origin. They also disclosed the first evidence of human-to-animal transmission, raising the possibility that minks could serve as the SARS-CoV-2 virus' possible intermediate host . The most likely way for minks to infect humans with SARS-CoV-2 is through the dust or aerosols of infected bedding from mink farms [60].

Closeness of people to animals, including dogs, cats, minks, and captive wild animals, is often a contributing element in COVID-19 natural events. One cat that tested positive for RNA and seven stray cats that were seropositive for SARS-CoV-2 indicate that there is a possibility of mink-to-cat transmission [61]. Human-to-mink transmission of SARS-COV-2 then mink-to-human transmission poses the greatest public health risk besides mink-to-feline transmission and among minks [46].

The earliest known minks' infection with SARS-CoV-2 was found to have occurred spontaneously on a mink farm in the Dutch proven of North Brabant. After that, numerous mink farms in the Netherlands had an outbreak of the SARS-CoV-2 virus [54, 62, 63]. The disease was shown to have been introduced by humans and subsequently spread among mink, according to a detailed outbreak analysis at Dutch mink farms. After that, the virus changed within the minks, creating a mink SARS-CoV-2 strain. According to whole-genome sequencing, several mink farm workers were infected with the mink strain, proving that minks can also spread SARS-CoV-2 to people [46, 62].

Given the high sensitivity of minks to SARS-CoV-2 and the viral development in minks, it is plausible to expect that variants might regularly be transmitted from minks to people or other species, potentially enhancing viral transmission [56, 62]. Additionally, mink and 12 human specimens from affected Danish farms and nearby settlements have the Cluster 5 variant, which has been shown to be less susceptible to neutralizing antibodies [64, 65]. The spike protein alone contained 35 changes and four deletions in the Cluster 5 version [58].

The Danish government authorized roughly 17 million minks depopulation in November 2020; Cluster 5 has yet to be discovered in humans since September 2020 [58, 64, 65]. These findings have emphasized the significance of comprehensive epidemiologic studies to assess the effects of SARS-CoV-2 epidemics in farmed mink on human and animal health [66], as well as indications of anthropogenic and zoonotic transmission [25, 46] and the possibility for species-wide spillover transmission [54, 56, 67], including susceptible free-roaming wildlife [53, 68].

1.4 Pets

With the early discovery of SARS-CoV-2 in pets, worries about zoonotic transmission from animals in close contact with people have grown [69]. There are 370 million pet cats and 470 million pet dogs who reside with their human owners, according to some estimates. The SARS-CoV-2 virus has been found in a few pets and wild animals, including cats [70, 71], which are more susceptible than dogs to this virus [72, 73], and susceptibility studies have revealed that the virus can replicate in cats as well [74]. Neutralizing antibodies in pets against SARS-CoV-2 were reported and correlated to COVID-19 incidence in humans [75]. The same scenario was reported in SARS-CoV, which can replicate with disease signs in cats [76]. Domestic cats in Hong Kong's Amoy Gardens apartment block with SARS-infected residents were infected with the virus [76]. Since late March 2020, natural infections in domestic cats contracted from COVID-19-positive owners have been documented in the United States [77], Italy [78, 79], Spain [80–82], Netherlands [83], France [84], Brazil [72], Belgium, and Hong Kong. Also, large non-domestic cats were reported to have naturally contracted SARS-CoV-2, probably by reverse zoonosis [85]. According to some scientists, the severity of the COVID outbreak in northern Italy was exacerbated by the high rates of dog ownership in this area [86]. Others stated that serious consideration is needed in light of the minimal evidence of SARS-CoV-2 infection in domestic animals like dogs and cats and the recognized similarities in ACE2 receptor binding sites between humans and some domesticated species [87].

Viral transmissibility has been attenuated via serial passages with SARS-CoV-2 strain in cats, which may be due to weaker interactions of SARS-CoV-2 with feline ACE2 compared to human receptors [51]. The infection rate within the domestic cat population is low, and reports are describing the relatively short duration of shedding and resistance to reinfection in cats [88, 89], speculating that SARS-CoV-2 occurs in domestic cats with a narrow transmission bottleneck [90, 91]. Lu et al. [92] suggested there are 5 variations that exist at feline ACE2 receptor than human ACE2. Additionally, Wu et al. [93] recognized that the feline ACE2 receptor's binding affinity to the SARS-CoV-2 RBD was 3 to 4 times weaker due to mutated amino acids at sites 24 and 34. This finding explains why the SARS-CoV-2 transmission from cat-to-cat is less persistent over time than the sustained transmission from human-to-human. However, it is unknown if domestic and wild cat populations could act as SARS-CoV-2 reservoirs for human exposure [51]. Previous research was constrained by the tiny sample size and laboratory tests of young, healthy, and adult cats. We need a larger population, more elderly cats, cats with comorbid conditions, and cats with coinfections to better understand the typical course of infection and immunity in community populations of cats [51, 94, 95]. During the outbreak in Thailand, a domestic cat was infected with another critical respiratory virus, H5N1 virus, after eating a pigeon carcass infected with H5N1 virus [96, 97]. Pigeons can contract SARS-CoV-2 as well [98] due to the existence of angiotensin-converting enzyme 2 (ACE2) receptor in their body that is utilized by SARS-CoV-2, suggesting that feral cats can catch the infection from infected pigeons [99]; however, this hypothesis needs to be investigated. Household cats (*Felis domesticus*) can catch SARS-CoV and SARS-CoV-2 infections from infected owners, and they can easily spread the virus to previously uninfected animals that share their room [76]. Because cats are frequent indoor pets, there is worry about disease transfer to humans [97].

SARS-CoV was discovered in domestic cats in 2003 [100], and recombinant events of *Betacoronavirus* were recorded in cats [101]. Domestic dogs, cats, and mustelids in China, Hong Kong, Europe, and the United States were all found to have natural SARS-CoV-2 infections [102, 103] as a result of a reverse zoonotic transmission route [46, 104]. Additionally, it was noted that ACE2 is highly homologous in both humans and cats [105].

However, owners who tested positive for COVID-19 were responsible for the majority of SARS-CoV-2 infections in animals [106, 107], and there was some indication of human-to-animal transfer, although it was minimal. As a result, several researchers hypothesized that even if dogs were carriers of the SARS-CoV-2 virus, they would not have a major epidemiological role in human SARS-CoV-2 transmission [69]. Songkhla Province in southern Thailand announced the first confirmed incidence of cat-to-human transmission [19, 108]. A recent study suggested that a cat may have transmitted the zoonotic SARS-CoV-2 virus to a human in Thailand [19]. Because of this, petting or kissing infected pets can cause owners to contract the virus through intimate contact with their hair, paws, or pads; therefore, there is a possibility that domestic pets could spread SARS-CoV-2 [83].

Following contact with an infected cat belonging to an infected patient, a Thai veterinarian was discovered to have COVID-19. Genetic studies supported the idea that SARS-CoV-2 was transmitted from the owner to the cat, and then from the cat to the veterinarian. It is assumed that this brief, but extremely close, interaction led to transmission from the cat's sneeze. Bangkok was most likely the origin of the SARS-CoV-2 infection chain in this cluster. It is generally known that cats can contract the SARS-CoV-2 virus from people, especially when they are in close proximity to those who are already showing symptoms of the infection. This cat likely only had a week before becoming infected with SARS-CoV-2 and perhaps passing the infection on to patient A, the veterinarian who examined the infected cat and caught the infection from it, because infected cats have relatively short incubation and infectious periods.

Investigation revealed that the purported dog-to-human transmission of variant was passive and mechanical because the dog's nasopharyngeal swab samples for SARS-CoV-2 were negative despite the dog's hair and kennel being positive [23]. By having intimate contact with the pet dog, the owners could mechanically contract SARS-CoV-2 [23]. These results may confirm the critical hypothesis for outbreak investigations that SARS-CoV-2 transmitters can spread the virus through intimate contact with infected dogs. Furthermore, Chan et al. assert that human-to-human transmission of the SARS-CoV-2 Delta variant AY.127 caused a COVID-19 outbreak at a pet store in Hong Kong [45]. Therefore, veterinarians and owners should be cautious when dealing with cat environments and flea-infested cats. Canine Coronavirus-Human Pneumonia-2018

(CCoV-HuPn-2018), a unique canine-feline recombinant *alphacoronavirus*, was recently discovered. It was initially found in a case of human pneumonia in Sarawak, Malaysia [109]. CCoV-HuPn-2018 might be the eighth coronavirus to infect humans, following SARS-CoV-2 [109, 110]. Despite the fact that the influenza A (H7N2) virus of avian origin only sporadically passes from human to human [111], it's notable that Lee et al. [112] confirmed the first instance of H7N2 cat-to-human transmission occurred following an outbreak among cats in New York City animal shelters. Even though this danger is minimal, the fact that it exists and the possibility of it returning pose a health concern [113]. We urgently want a One Health surveillance effort since there is no clear evidence for this scenario with SARS-CoV-2 in cats.

1.5 Deer

Since just one study has identified the white-tailed deer (WTD; *Odocoileus virginianus*) variant version of SARS-CoV-2 that has been isolated from humans in Canada, it raises the prospect that the virus could spread from deer to humans [114]. The results are significant because they demonstrate that handling and processing WTD corpses may expose workers to infected SARS-CoV-2, which could cause the virus to spread from deer to humans. This is accurate even if few samples contained the live virus [115].

SARS-CoV-2 samples from WTD have substantially higher mutations than those found in samples from humans, which shows that SARS-CoV-2 has been circulating and evolving in the deer population. Some of the changes that have been noticed could be the result of host adaptation. For instance, the ORF1a: L4111F mutation has been identified in WTD-derived samples from various geographical locations and is present throughout all human sequences in the GISAID database at a low frequency (0.5%). This shows that this mutation originated independently in deer following human spills. The lack of or extremely low frequency of fixed mutations in the S gene, which shows that host-specific adaptation was not required for spillover from humans to deer, supports SARS-CoV-2's designation as a "generalist" virus [116].

2. Conclusions

All pathogenic human coronaviruses originate in animals; therefore, concerns about the possibility of interspecies transmission between people and animals have arisen as a result of SARS-CoV-2 emerging after cross-species jumping in animals; as a result, a vaccine strategy for companion animals is conceivable and plausible (**Table 1**) [118].

The SARS-CoV-2 virus has been naturally acquired by domestic animals (dogs, cats, and ferrets), captive species (tiger, lion, snow leopard, puma, otter, and gorilla), and wild and farmed minks, according to the OIE database. It is possible that the transmission of SARS-CoV-2 in populations of wild animals is periodically to blame for the reappearance of COVID-19 in people at the human-animal interface (**Figure 2**) [119].

FAO, OIE, and WHO released a joint statement on March 7, 2022, encouraging all nations to cooperate to lessen the danger of SARS-CoV-2 transmission between humans and animals to decrease the risk of variant emergence and safeguard both people and wildlife [120]. It is crucial to carry out viral surveillance and sequencing in animals, especially those who have frequent interaction with people.

Animal vaccine	Description	Target animals
Carnivac-Cov (inactivated vaccine)	The first COVID-19 vaccine for animals developed by Russia have been shown to elicit robust responses in animals vulnerable to SARS-CoV-2 infection such as dogs, cats, foxes, and minks. It contains an inactivated SARS-CoV-2 virus strain. Vaccination with Carnivac-Cov induced immunity that lasted for at least six months after the vaccination	Dogs, cats, foxes, and minks
LinearDNA™ COVID-19 vaccine	LinearDNA™ ("linDNA") vaccine encoding the RBD domain of SARS-CoV-2. linDNA developed through a joint effort between Applied DNA Sciences (United States) and EvviVax (Italy). Clinical trials showed that the vaccine is safe and immunogenic and support the development of vaccines for preventing viral spread in susceptible species, especially those in close contact with humans. Recently, a linearDNA vaccine was successfully elicited neutralizing antibodies and cellular immunity against SARS-CoV-2. LineaRx announced the successful expression *in vitro* of its linDNA SARS-CoV-2 vaccine candidate encapsulated within lipid nanoparticles (LNP). The linDNA-LNP vaccine will be used in upcoming *in vivo* animal studies to assess the performance of linDNA-LNP vaccines and will inform the final design of the Company's lead veterinary asset, a linDNA-LNP canine lymphoma vaccine candidate.	Domestic cats (Now is reported to be focused on inoculating mink instead)
Zoetis vaccine	The captive orangutans and bonobos at the San Diego Zoo in the United States of America became the first non-human primates to receive an experimental COVID-19 vaccine developed specifically for animals by the veterinary pharmaceutical company Zoetis. It has been authorized for experimental use on a case-by-case basis by the United States Department of Agriculture (USDA).	Dogs, cats, and minks
Ancovax	India's first COVID-19 vaccine for animals. It contains an inactivated SARS-CoV-2 (Delta) antigen capable of neutralizing both Delta and Omicron variants	Dogs, lions, leopards, mice, and rabbits

Table 1.
Examples of animal COVID-19 vaccines used in domestic and wild animals [117].

Finally, the One Health strategy must be used urgently to adequately track the virus in animal populations by observation of livestock, pets, and trading networks. Although the idea of One Health is not new, effective public health initiatives necessitate cooperation between the human, veterinary, and environmental health sectors since humans interact with both wild and domestic animals regularly. Despite the minimal number of reported cases of animal-to-human SARS-CoV-2 transmission [121], it is critical to recognize the significant risks associated with zoonotic transmissions or spillover of the SARS-CoV-2 virus from animals to humans and motivate us to conduct genomic research on these animals as they are under active observation to learn more about viral circulation and how variants emerge.

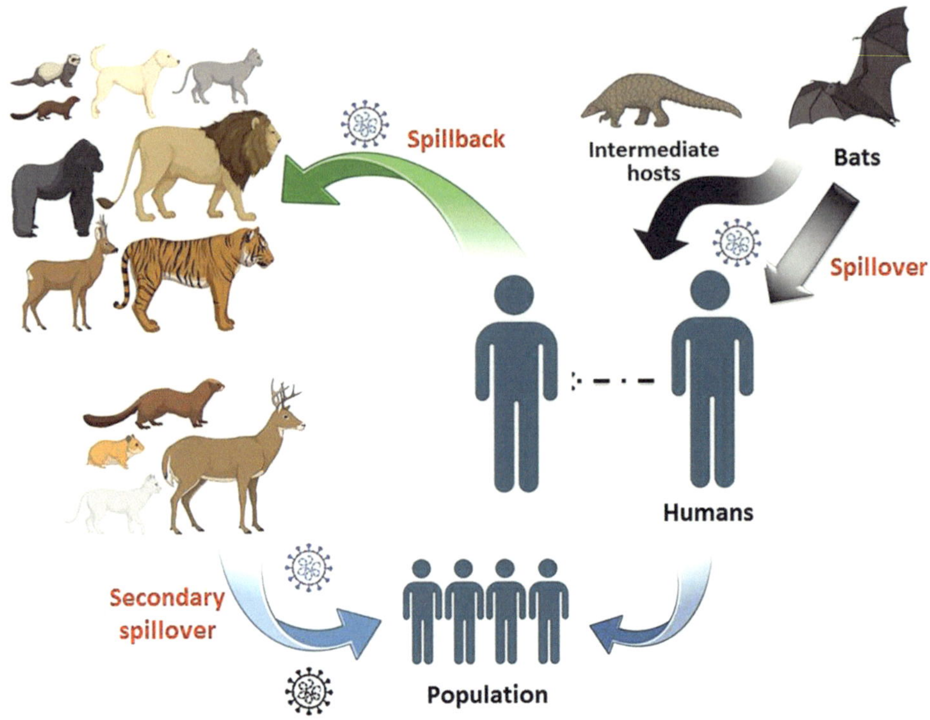

Figure 2.
Spillover and spillback of SARS-CoV-2 among domestic and wild animals, and humans.

Author details

AbdulRahman A. Saied[1*], Faten F. Mohammed[2,3] and Asmaa A. Metwally[4]

1 Ministry of Tourism and Antiquities, Aswan Office, Aswan, Egypt

2 Department of Pathology, College of Veterinary Medicine, King Faisal University, Al Ahsa, Saudi Arabia

3 Faculty of Veterinary Medicine, Department of Pathology, Cairo University, Giza, Egypt

4 Faculty of Veterinary Medicine, Department of Surgery, Anesthesiology, and Radiology, Aswan University, Aswan, Egypt

*Address all correspondence to: saied_abdelrahman@yahoo.com

References

[1] Saied AA, Metwally AA, Mohamed HM, Haridy MA. The contribution of bovines to human health against viral infections. Environmental Science and Pollution Research. 2021;**28**(34):46999-47023

[2] Zhu Z, Lian X, Su X, Wu W, Marraro GA, Zeng Y. From SARS and MERS to COVID-19: A brief summary and comparison of severe acute respiratory infections caused by three highly pathogenic human coronaviruses. Respiratory Research. 2020;**21**:1-14

[3] Kuhlmeier E, Chan T, Agüí CV, Willi B, Wolfensberger A, Beisel C, et al. Detection and molecular characterization of the SARS-CoV-2 Delta variant and the specific immune response in companion animals in Switzerland. Viruses. 2023;**15**:245

[4] Graham RL, Donaldson EF, Baric RS. A decade after SARS: Strategies for controlling emerging coronaviruses. Nature Reviews Microbiology. 2013;**11**:836-848

[5] Gorbalenya AE, Baker SC, Baric RS, de Groot RJ, Drosten C, Gulyaeva AA, et al. The species severe acute respiratory syndrome-related coronavirus: Classifying 2019-nCoV and naming it SARS-CoV-2. Nature Microbiology. 2020;**5**:536-544

[6] WHO. Weekly Epidemiological Update on COVID-19 - 20 July 2023. 2023. Available from: https://www.who.int/publications/m/item/weekly-epidemiological-update-on-covid-19---20-july-2023

[7] Qiu X, Liu Y, Sha A. SARS-CoV-2 and natural infection in animals. Journal of Medical Virology. 2023;**95**:e28147

[8] Pappas G, Vokou D, Sainis I, Halley JM. SARS-CoV-2 as a Zooanthroponotic infection: Spillbacks. Secondary Spillovers, and Their Importance, Microorganisms. 2022;**10**:2166

[9] Sooksawasdi Na Ayudhya S, Kuiken T. Reverse zoonosis of COVID-19: Lessons from the 2009 influenza pandemic. Veterinary Pathology. 2021;**58**:234-242

[10] Ribeiro J, Araújo MB, Santana J, Strubbe D, Vaz AS, Reino L. Impacts of the SARS-CoV-2 pandemic on the global demand for exotic pets: An expert elicitation approach. Global Ecology and Conservation. 2022;**35**:e02067

[11] Rotstein DS, Peloquin S, Proia K, Hart E, Lee J, Vyhnal KK, et al. Investigation of SARS-CoV-2 infection and associated lesions in exotic and companion animals. Veterinary Pathology. 2022;**59**:707-711

[12] Shankar EM, Che KF, Yong YK, Girija AS, Velu V, Ansari AW, et al. Asymptomatic SARS-CoV-2 infection: Is it all about being refractile to innate immune sensing of viral spare-parts, clues from exotic animal reservoirs. Pathogens and Disease. 2021;**79**(1):ftaa076

[13] Córdoba-Aguilar A, Ibarra-Cerdeña CN, Castro-Arellano I, Suzan G. Tackling zoonoses in a crowded world: Lessons to be learned from the COVID-19 pandemic. Acta Tropica. 2021;**214**:105780

[14] Zhai S, Li C, Sun M, Zhang J, Zheng C, Liao M. Natural infections of SARS-CoV-2 increased in animals: How should humans interact with animals? Journal of Medical Virology. 2022;**94**:3503

[15] Aleta A, Martin-Corral D, Pastore y Piontti A, Ajelli M, Litvinova M,

Chinazzi M, et al. Modelling the impact of testing, contact tracing and household quarantine on second waves of COVID-19. Nature Human Behaviour. 2020;**4**:964-971

[16] Kuchipudi SV, Surendran-Nair M, Ruden RM, Yon M, Nissly RH, Vandegrift KJ, et al. Multiple spillovers from humans and onward transmission of SARS-CoV-2 in white-tailed deer. Proceedings of the National Academy of Sciences. 2022;**119**(6):e2121644119

[17] Pickering B, Lung O, Maguire F, Kruczkiewicz P, Kotwa JD, Buchanan T, et al. Divergent SARS-CoV-2 variant emerges in white-tailed deer with deer-to-human transmission. Nature Microbiology. 2022;**7**(12):2011-2024

[18] Hale VL, Dennis PM, McBride DS, Nolting JM, Madden C, Huey D, et al. SARS-CoV-2 infection in free-ranging white-tailed deer. Nature. 2022;**602**(7897):481-486

[19] Sila T, Sunghan J, Laochareonsuk W, Surasombatpattana S, Kongkamol C, Ingviya T, et al. Suspected cat-to-human transmission of SARS-CoV-2, Thailand, July–September 2021. Emerging Infectious Diseases. 2022;**28**:1485

[20] Yen H-L, Sit THC, Brackman CJ, Chuk SSY, Gu H, Tam KWS, et al. Transmission of SARS-CoV-2 delta variant (AY. 127) from pet hamsters to humans, leading to onward human-to-human transmission: A case study. Lancet. 2022;**399**:1070-1078

[21] Kok K-H, Wong S-C, Chan W-M, Wen L, Chu AW-H, Ip JD, et al. Co-circulation of two SARS-CoV-2 variant strains within imported pet hamsters in Hong Kong, Emerg. Microbes and Infection. 2022;**11**:689-698

[22] Siegrist AA, Richardson KL, Ghai RR, Pope B, Yeadon J, Culp B, et al. Probable transmission of SARS-CoV-2 from african lion to zoo employees, Indiana, USA, 2021. Emerging Infectious Diseases. 2023;**29**(6):1102

[23] Zhou C, Wu A, Ye S, Zhou Z, Zhang H, Zhao X, et al. Possible transmission of COVID-19 epidemic by a dog as a passive mechanical carrier of SARS-CoV-2, Chongqing, China, 2022. Journal of Medical Virology. 2023;**95**:e28408

[24] Rabalski L, Kosinski M, Mazur-Panasiuk N, Szewczyk B, Bienkowska-Szewczyk K, Kant R, et al. Zoonotic spill-over of SARS-CoV-2: Mink-adapted virus in humans. Clinical Microbiology and Infection. 2022;**28**(3):451-e1

[25] Hammer AS, Quaade ML, Rasmussen TB, Fonager J, Rasmussen M, Mundbjerg K, et al. SARS-CoV-2 transmission between mink (Neovison vison) and humans, Denmark. Emerging Infectious Diseases. 2021;**27**:547

[26] Decaro N, Lorusso A. Novel human coronavirus (SARS-CoV-2): A lesson from animal coronaviruses. Veterinary Microbiology. 2020;**244**:108693

[27] Decaro N, Martella V, Saif LJ, Buonavoglia C. COVID-19 from veterinary medicine and one health perspectives: What animal coronaviruses have taught us. Research in Veterinary Science. 2020;**131**:21-23

[28] Lin Q, Zhao S, Gao D, Lou Y, Yang S, Musa SS, Wang MH, Cai Y, Wang W, Yang A. Wang, L. Yang, A conceptual model for the coronavirus disease 2019 (COVID-19) outbreak in Wuhan, China with individual reaction and governmental action. International Journal of Infectious Diseases. 2020;93:211-216

[29] Huang C, Wang Y, Li X, Ren L, Zhao J, Hu Y, et al. Clinical features

of patients infected with 2019 novel coronavirus in Wuhan, China. Lancet. 2020;**395**:497-506

[30] Zhu N, Zhang D, Wang W, Li X, Yang B, Song J, et al. A novel coronavirus from patients with pneumonia in China, 2019. New England Journal of Medicine. 2020;**382**(8):727-733

[31] Ntumvi NF, Ndze VN, Gillis A, Le Doux Diffo J, Tamoufe U, Takuo J-M, et al. Wildlife in Cameroon harbor diverse coronaviruses, including many closely related to human coronavirus 229E. Virus Evolution. 2022;**8**:veab110

[32] Devaux CA, Pinault L, Delerce J, Raoult D, Levasseur A, Frutos R. Spread of mink SARS-CoV-2 variants in humans: A model of sarbecovirus interspecies evolution. Frontiers in Microbiology. 2021;**12**:2842

[33] Zhang L, Cui Z, Li Q, Wang B, Yu Y, Wu J, et al. Ten emerging SARS-CoV-2 spike variants exhibit variable infectivity, animal tropism, and antibody neutralization. Communications Biology. 2021;**4**:1196

[34] Wang M, Yan M, Xu H, Liang W, Kan B, Zheng B, et al. SARS-CoV infection in a restaurant from palm civet. Emerging infectious diseases. 2005;**11**(12):1860

[35] Banerjee A, Doxey AC, Mossman K, Irving AT. Unraveling the zoonotic origin and transmission of SARS-CoV-2. Trends in Ecology & Evolution. 2021;**36**:180-184

[36] D'amico F, Baumgart DC, Danese S, Peyrin-Biroulet L. Diarrhea during COVID-19 infection: Pathogenesis, epidemiology, prevention, and management. Clinical Gastroenterology and Hepatology. 2020;**18**:1663-1672

[37] Espinosa R, Tago D, Treich N. Infectious diseases and meat production. Environmental and Resource Economics. 2020;**76**:1019-1044

[38] Saied AA, Metwally AA. SARS-CoV-2 variants of concerns in animals: An unmonitored rising health threat. Virus Disease. 2022;**33**(4):466-476

[39] Zhou P, Yang X-L, Wang X-G, Hu B, Zhang L, Zhang W, et al. A pneumonia outbreak associated with a new coronavirus of probable bat origin. Nature. 2020;**579**:270-273

[40] Conforti A, Sanchez E, Salvatori E, Lione L, Compagnone M, Pinto E, et al. A linear DNA encoding the SARS-CoV-2 receptor binding domain elicits potent immune response and neutralizing antibodies in domestic cats. Molecular Therapy Methods & Clinical Development. 2023;**28**:238-248. DOI: 10.1016/j.omtm.2022.12.015

[41] Zhang S, Qiao S, Yu J, Zeng J, Shan S, Tian L, et al. Bat and pangolin coronavirus spike glycoprotein structures provide insights into SARS-CoV-2 evolution. Nature Communications. 2021;**12**:1607. DOI: 10.1038/s41467-021-21767-3

[42] Caserta LC, Martins M, Butt SL, Hollingshead NA, Covaleda LM, Ahmed S, et al. White-tailed deer (Odocoileus virginianus) may serve as a wildlife reservoir for nearly extinct SARS-CoV-2 variants of concern. Proceedings of the National Academy of Sciences. 2023;**120**:e2215067120

[43] Zhao J, Cui W, Tian B. The potential intermediate hosts for SARS-CoV-2. Frontiers in Microbiology. 2020;**11**:580137

[44] World Organisation for Animal Health. SARS-CoV-2 in Animal-Situation Report 9(oie.int). Available from: https://www.woah.org/app/uploads/2022/02/sars-cov-2-situation-report-9.pdf

[45] Chan JF-W, Siu GK-H, Yuan S, Ip JD, Cai J-P, Chu AW-H, et al. Probable animal-to-human transmission of SARS-CoV-2 Delta variant AY. 127 causing a pet shop-related COVID-19 outbreak in Hong Kong. Clinical Infectious Diseases. 2022;**75**(1):e76-e81

[46] Oude Munnink BB, Sikkema RS, Nieuwenhuijse DF, Molenaar RJ, Munger E, Molenkamp R, et al. Transmission of SARS-CoV-2 on mink farms between humans and mink and back to humans. Science . 2021;**371**(6525):172-177

[47] Ekstrand K, Flanagan AJ, Lin IE, Vejseli B, Cole A, Lally AP, et al. Animal transmission of SARS-CoV-2 and the welfare of animals during the COVID-19 pandemic. Animals. 2021;**11**:2044

[48] Welkers MRA, Han AX, Reusken CBEM, Eggink D. Possible host-adaptation of SARS-CoV-2 due to improved ACE2 receptor binding in mink. Virus Evolution. 2021;7:veaa094

[49] Shriner SA, Ellis JW, Root JJ, Roug A, Stopak SR, Wiscomb GW, et al. SARS-CoV-2 exposure in escaped mink, Utah, USA. Emerging Infectious Diseases. 2021;**27**:988-990. DOI: 10.3201/eid2703.204444

[50] Aguiló-Gisbert J, Padilla-Blanco M, Lizana V, Maiques E, Muñoz-Baquero M, Chillida-Martínez E, et al. First description of SARS-CoV-2 infection in two feral American mink (Neovison vison) caught in the wild Animals. 2021;**11**(5):1422

[51] Davis MF, Innes GK. The Cat's in the bag: Despite limited cat-to-cat severe acute respiratory syndrome coronavirus 2 transmission, one health surveillance efforts are needed. The Journal of infectious diseases. 2021;**223**:1309-1312

[52] Olsen M, Cook SE, Huang V, Pedersen N, Murphy BG. Perspectives: Potential therapeutic options for SARS-CoV-2 patients based on feline infectious peritonitis strategies: Central nervous system invasion and drug coverage. International Journal of Antimicrobial Agents. 2020;**55**:105964

[53] World Organization for Animal Health. WOAH World Organization for Animal Health (WOAH). Available from: https://wahis.woah.org/#/home

[54] Oreshkova N, Molenaar RJ, Vreman S, Harders F, Munnink BBO, Hakze-van Der Honing RW, et al. SARS-CoV-2 infection in farmed minks, the Netherlands, April and may 2020. Eurosurveillance. 2020;**25**:2001005

[55] Wolters WJ, de Rooij MMT, Molenaar RJ, de Rond J, Vernooij JCM, Meijer PA, et al. Manifestation of SARS-CoV-2 infections in mink related to host-, virus-and farm-associated factors, the Netherlands 2020. Viruses. 2022;**14**:1754

[56] van Aart AE, Velkers FC, Fischer EAJ, Broens EM, Egberink H, Zhao S, et al. SARS-CoV-2 infection in cats and dogs in infected mink farms. Transboundary and Emerging Diseases. 2022;**69**:3001-3007

[57] Chaintoutis SC, Thomou Z, Mouchtaropoulou E, Tsiolas G, Chassalevris T, Stylianaki I, et al. Outbreaks of SARS-CoV-2 in naturally infected mink farms: Impact, transmission dynamics, genetic patterns, and environmental contamination. PLoS Pathogens. 2021;**17**:e1009883

[58] Larsen HD, Fonager J, Lomholt FK, Dalby T, Benedetti G, Kristensen B, et al. Preliminary report of an outbreak of SARS-CoV-2 in mink and mink farmers associated with community spread, Denmark, June to November 2020. Eurosurveillance. 2021;**26**:2100009

[59] World Organization for Animal Health, Events in Animal.

COVID-19-WOAH-World Organization for Animal Health. Available from: https://www.woah.org/en/what-we-offer/emergency-and-resilience/covid-19/#ui-id-3

[60] Sharun K, Tiwari R, Natesan S, Dhama K. SARS-CoV-2 infection in farmed minks, associated zoonotic concerns, and importance of the one health approach during the ongoing COVID-19 pandemic. Veterinary Quarterly. 2020;**41**(1):50-60

[61] Edwards SJL, Santini JM. Anthroponotic risk of SARS-CoV-2, precautionary mitigation, and outbreak management. The Lancet Microbe. 2020;**1**:e187-e188. DOI: 10.1016/S2666-5247(20)30086-0

[62] Lu L, Sikkema RS, Velkers FC, Nieuwenhuijse DF, Fischer EAJ, Meijer PA, et al. Adaptation, spread and transmission of SARS-CoV-2 in farmed minks and associated humans in the Netherlands. Nature Communications. 2021;**12**:6802

[63] Molenaar RJ, Vreman S, Hakze-van der Honing RW, Zwart R, de Rond J, Weesendorp E, et al. Clinical and pathological findings in SARS-CoV-2 disease outbreaks in farmed mink (Neovison vison). Veterinary Pathology. 2020;**57**:653-657

[64] Lassaunière R, Fonager J, Rasmussen M, Frische A, Strandh CP, Rasmussen TB, et al. Working paper on SARS-CoV-2 spike mutations arising in Danish mink, their spread to humans and neutralization data. Copenhagen Statens Serum Institut. 2020. Available from: https://files.ssi.dk/mink-cluster-5-short-report_afo2

[65] WHO. SARS-CoV-2 Mink-Associated Variant Strain—Denmark. Available from: https://www.who.int/emergencies/disease-outbreak-news/item/2020-don301

[66] Cossaboom CM, Wendling NM, Lewis NM, Rettler H, Harvey RR, Amman BR, et al. One health investigation of SARS-CoV-2 in people and animals on multiple mink farms in Utah. Viruses. 2023;**15**:96

[67] Boklund A, Hammer AS, Quaade ML, Rasmussen TB, Lohse L, Strandbygaard B, et al. SARS-CoV-2 in Danish mink farms: Course of the epidemic and a descriptive analysis of the outbreaks in 2020. Animals. 2021;**11**:164

[68] USDA. SARS-CoV-2 in Animals in the United States. Available from: https://www.aphis.usda.gov/aphis/dashboards/tableau/sars-dashboard

[69] Lauzi S, Stranieri A, Giordano A, Lelli D, Elia G, Desario C, et al. Do dogs and cats passively carry SARS-CoV-2 on hair and pads? Viruses. 2021;**13**:1357

[70] Tiwari R, Dhama K, Sharun K, Iqbal Yatoo M, Malik YS, Singh R, et al. COVID-19: Animals, veterinary and zoonotic links. The Veterinary Quarterly. 2020;**40**:169-182

[71] Sharun K, Tiwari R, Patel SK, Karthik K, Iqbal Yatoo M, Malik YS, et al. Coronavirus disease 2019 (COVID-19) in domestic animals and wildlife: Advances and prospects in the development of animal models for vaccine and therapeutic research. Human Vaccines & Immunotherapeutics. 2020;**16**(12):3043-3054

[72] Calvet GA, Pereira SA, Ogrzewalska M, Pauvolid-Corrêa A, Resende PC, de Tassinari WS, et al. Investigation of SARS-CoV-2 infection in dogs and cats of humans diagnosed with COVID-19 in Rio de Janeiro, Brazil. PLoS One. 2021;**16**:e0250853

[73] Decaro N, Balboni A, Bertolotti L, Martino PA, Mazzei M, Mira F, et al.

SARS-CoV-2 infection in dogs and cats: Facts and speculations. Frontiers in Veterinary Science. 2021;**8**:80

[74] Shi J, Wen Z, Zhong G, Yang H, Wang C, Huang B, et al. Susceptibility of ferrets, cats, dogs, and other domesticated animals to SARS–coronavirus 2. Science (80-.). 2020;**368**:1016-1020

[75] Barroso-Arévalo S, Sánchez-Morales L, Barasona JA, Domínguez L, Sánchez-Vizcaíno JM. SARS-CoV-2 Seroprevalence studies in pets, Spain. Emerging Infectious Diseases. 2023;**29**:1136

[76] Martina BEE, Haagmans BL, Kuiken T, Fouchier RAM, Rimmelzwaan GF, Van Amerongen G, et al. SARS virus infection of cats and ferrets. Nature. 2003;**425**:915

[77] Newman A, Smith D, Ghai RR, Wallace RM, Torchetti MK, Loiacono C, et al. First reported cases of SARS-CoV-2 infection in companion animals - New York, march-April 2020. MMWR. Morbidity and Mortality Weekly Report. 2020;**69**:710-713. DOI: 10.15585/mmwr.mm6923e3

[78] Patterson EI, Elia G, Grassi A, Giordano A, Desario C, Medardo M, et al. Evidence of exposure to SARS-CoV-2 in cats and dogs from households in Italy. Nature Communications. 2020;**11**:1-5

[79] Musso N, Costantino A, La Spina S, Finocchiaro A, Andronico F, Stracquadanio S, et al. New SARS-CoV-2 infection detected in an Italian pet cat by RT-qPCR from deep pharyngeal swab. Pathogens. 2020;**9**:746

[80] Ruiz-Arrondo I, Portillo A, Palomar AM, Santibáñez S, Santibáñez P, Cervera C, et al. Detection of SARS-CoV-2 in pets living with COVID-19 owners diagnosed during the COVID-19 lockdown in Spain: A case of an asymptomatic cat with SARS-CoV-2 in Europe. Transboundary and Emerging Diseases. 2020;**68**(2):973-976

[81] Ruiz-Arrondo I, Portillo A, Palomar AM, Santibáñez S, Santibáñez P, Cervera C, et al. Detection of SARS-CoV-2 in pets living with COVID-19 owners diagnosed during the COVID-19 lockdown in Spain: A case of an asymptomatic cat with SARS-CoV-2 in Europe. Transboundary and Emerging Diseases. 2021;**68**:973-976. DOI: 10.1111/tbed.13803

[82] Segalés J, Puig M, Rodon J, Avila-Nieto C, Carrillo J, Cantero G, et al. Detection of SARS-CoV-2 in a cat owned by a COVID-19– affected patient in Spain. Proceedings of the National Academy of Sciences. 2020;**117**:24790-24793

[83] Hossain MG, Javed A, Akter S, Saha S. SARS-CoV-2 host diversity: An update of natural infections and experimental evidence. Journal of Microbiology, Immunology, and Infection. 2021;**54**:175-181

[84] Sailleau C, Dumarest M, Vanhomwegen J, Delaplace M, Caro V, Kwasiborski A, et al. First detection and genome sequencing of SARS-CoV-2 in an infected cat in France. Transboundary and Emerging Diseases. 2020;**67**(6):2324-2328

[85] Bartlett SL, Diel DG, Wang L, Zec S, Laverack M, Martins M, et al. SARS-CoV-2 infection and longitudinal fecal screening in Malayan tigers (Panthera tigris jacksoni), Amur tigers (Panthera tigris altaica), and African lions (Panthera leo krugeri) at the Bronx zoo, New York, USA. Journal of Zoo and Wildlife Medicine. 2021;**51**:733-744

[86] Goumenou M, Spandidos DA, Tsatsakis A. Possibility of transmission through dogs being a contributing factor to the extreme Covid-19 outbreak in North Italy. Molecular Medicine Reports. 2020;**21**:2293-2295

[87] Leroy EM, Gouilh MA, Brugère-Picoux J. The risk of SARS-CoV-2 transmission to pets and other wild and domestic animals strongly mandates a one-health strategy to control the COVID-19 pandemic. One Health (Amsterdam, Netherlands). 2020;**10**:100133. DOI: 10.1016/j.onehlt.2020.100133

[88] Bao L, Song Z, Xue J, Gao H, Liu J, Wang J, et al. Susceptibility and attenuated transmissibility of SARS-CoV-2 in domestic cats. The Journal of Infectious Diseases. 2021;**223**(8):1313-1321

[89] Gaudreault NN, Carossino M, Morozov I, Trujillo JD, Meekins DA, Madden DW, et al. Experimental re-infected cats do not transmit SARS-CoV-2. Emerging Microbes & Infections. 2021;**10**(1):638-650

[90] Braun KM, Moreno GK, Halfmann PJ, Hodcroft EB, Baker DA, Boehm EC, et al. Transmission of SARS-CoV-2 in domestic cats imposes a narrow bottleneck. PLoS Pathogens. 2021;**17**:e1009373

[91] Sharun K, Saied AA, Tiwari R, Dhama K. SARS-CoV-2 infection in domestic and feral cats: Current evidence and implications. The Veterinary Quarterly. 2021;**41**:228-231

[92] Lu R, Zhao X, Li J, Niu P, Yang B, Wu H, et al. Genomic characterisation and epidemiology of 2019 novel coronavirus: Implications for virus origins and receptor binding. Lancet. 2020;**395**:565-574

[93] Wu L, Chen Q, Liu K, Wang J, Han P, Zhang Y, et al. Broad host range of SARS-CoV-2 and the molecular basis for SARS-CoV-2 binding to cat ACE2. Cell Discovery. 2020;**6**:1-12

[94] Villanueva-Saz S, Giner J, Tobajas AP, Pérez MD, González-Ramírez AM, Macías-León J, et al. Serological evidence of SARS-CoV-2 and co-infections in stray cats in Spain. Transboundary and Emerging Diseases. 2022;**69**(3):1056-1064

[95] Klaus J, Palizzotto C, Zini E, Meli ML, Leo C, Egberink H, et al. SARS-CoV-2 infection and antibody response in a symptomatic cat from Italy with intestinal B-cell lymphoma. Viruses. 2021;**13**:527

[96] Enserink M, Kaiser J. Avian flu finds new mammal hosts. Science. 2004;**305**:1385-1385. DOI: 10.1126/science.305.5689.1385a

[97] Songserm T, Amonsin A, Jam-on R, Sae-Heng N, Meemak N, Pariyothorn N, et al. Avian influenza H5N1 in naturally infected domestic cat. Emerging Infectious Diseases. 2006;**12**:681

[98] Devaux CA, Pinault L, Osman IO, Raoult D. Can ACE2 receptor polymorphism predict species susceptibility to SARS-CoV-2? Frontiers in Public Health. 2021;**8**:608765

[99] Qiu Y, Zhao Y-B, Wang Q, Li J-Y, Zhou Z-J, Liao C-H, et al. Predicting the angiotensin converting enzyme 2 (ACE2) utilizing capability as the receptor of SARS-CoV-2. Microbes and Infection. 2020;**22**:221-225

[100] Sit THC, Brackman CJ, Ip SM, Tam KWS, Law PYT, To EMW, et al. Infection of dogs with SARS-CoV-2. Nature. 2020;**586**:776-778. DOI: 10.1038/s41586-020-2334-5

[101] Hedman HD, Krawczyk E, Helmy YA, Zhang L, Varga C. Host

diversity and potential transmission pathways of SARS-CoV-2 at the human-animal Interface. Pathogens. 2021;**10**:180

[102] Kiros M, Andualem H, Kiros T, Hailemichael W, Getu S, Geteneh A, et al. COVID-19 pandemic: Current knowledge about the role of pets and other animals in disease transmission. Virology Journal. 2020;**17**:1-8

[103] Bonilla-Aldana DK, Dhama K, Rodriguez-Morales AJ. Revisiting the one health approach in the context of COVID-19: A look into the ecology of this emerging disease. Advances in Animal and Veterinary Sciences. 2020;**8**:234-237

[104] Enserink M. Coronavirus Rips through Dutch Mink Farms. Triggering Culls. Science. 2020;**368**:1169-1169

[105] Sreenivasan CC, Thomas M, Wang D, Li F. Susceptibility of livestock and companion animals to COVID-19. Journal of Medical Virology. 2021;**93**:1351-1360

[106] Leroy EM, Gouilh MA, Brugère-Picoux J. The risk of SARS-CoV-2 transmission to pets and other wild and domestic animals strongly mandates a one-health strategy to control the COVID-19 pandemic. One Health. 2020;**10**:100133

[107] Pagani G, Lai A, Bergna A, Rizzo A, Stranieri A, Giordano A, et al. Human-to-cat SARS-CoV-2 transmission: Case report and full-genome sequencing from an infected pet and its owner in northern Italy. Pathogens. 2021;**10**:252

[108] Mallapaty S. First reported case of a person getting COVID from a cat. Nature. 29 Jun 2022. DOI: 10.1038/d41586-022-01792-y

[109] Vlasova AN, Diaz A, Damtie D, Xiu L, Toh T-H, Lee JS-Y, et al. Novel canine coronavirus isolated from a hospitalized patient with pneumonia in East Malaysia. Clinical Infectious Diseases. 2022;**74**(3):446-454

[110] Abdelgadir A, Vlasova AN, Gray GC. Susceptibility of different cell lines to the novel canine coronavirus CCoV-HuPn-2018. Influenza and Other Respiratory Viruses. 2021;**15**(6):824

[111] Belser JA, Lash RR, Garg S, Tumpey TM, Maines TR. The eyes have it: Influenza virus infection beyond the respiratory tract. The Lancet Infectious Diseases. 2018;**18**:e220-e227

[112] Lee CT, Slavinski S, Schiff C, Merlino M, Daskalakis D, Liu D, et al. Outbreak of influenza a (H7N2) among cats in an animal shelter with cat-to-human transmission—New York City. Clinical Infectious Diseases. 2017;**65**(11):1927-1929

[113] Jain S, Murray EL. The cat's meow: using novel serological approaches to identify cat-to-human influenza a (H7N2) transmission. The Journal of Infectious Diseases. 2019;**219**:1685-1687

[114] Porter SM, Hartwig AE, Bielefeldt-Ohmann H, Bosco-Lauth AM, Root JJ. Susceptibility of wild canids to SARS-CoV-2. Emerging Infectious Diseases. 2022;**28**(9):1852-1855

[115] Martins M, Boggiatto PM, Buckley A, Cassmann ED, Falkenberg S, Caserta LC, et al. From deer-to-deer: SARS-CoV-2 is efficiently transmitted and presents broad tissue tropism and replication sites in white-tailed deer. PLoS Pathogens. 2022;**18**:e1010197

[116] MacLean OA, Lytras S, Weaver S, Singer JB, Boni MF, Lemey P, et al. Natural selection in the evolution of SARS-CoV-2 in bats created a generalist virus and highly capable

human pathogen. PLoS Biology. 2021;**19**:e3001115

[117] Choudhary OP, Saied AA. COVID-19 vaccination in animals: A strategy for combating the global outbreak–correspondence. International Journal of Surgery. 2022;**105**:106848

[118] Saied AA. Besides human booster doses: Could vaccinating highly susceptible animals to SARS-CoV-2 be the needed urgent strategic step? International Journal of Surgery. 2022;**104**:106761

[119] Sharun K, Tiwari R, Saied AA, Dhama K. SARS-CoV-2 vaccine for domestic and captive animals: An effort to counter COVID-19 pandemic at the human-animal interface. Vaccine. 2021;**39**:7119-7122

[120] WHO. Joint Statement on the Prioritization of Monitoring SARS-CoV-2 Infection in Wildlife and Preventing the formation of Animal Reservoirs. 2022. Available from: https://www.who.int/news/item/07-03-2022-joint-statement-on-the-prioritization-of-monitoring-sars-cov-2-infection-in-wildlife-and-preventing-the-formation-of-animal-reservoirs

[121] CDC. Animals and COVID-19. 2023. Available from: https://www.cdc.gov/coronavirus/2019-ncov/daily-life-coping/animals.html